Acupuncture in Physiotherapy

For Butterworth Heinemann:

Senior Commissioning Editor: *Heidi Allen*
Associate Editor: *Robert Edwards*
Project Manager: *Jane Dingwall*
Illustration Manager: *Bruce Hogarth*
Design Direction: *George Ajayi*
Illustrations: *Amanda Williams*

Acupuncture in Physiotherapy

Val Hopwood PhD, FCSP, SRP, Dip Ac Nanjing

Course Leader
MSc Acupuncture
Coventry University
United Kingdom

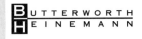

OXFORD AUCKLAND BOSTON JOHANNESBURG MELBOURNE NEW DELHI

BUTTERWORTH-HEINEMANN
An imprint of Elsevier Limited

First published 2004

ISBN 0 7506 5328 0

British Library Cataloguing in Publication Data
A catalogue record for this book is available from the British Library

Library of Congress Cataloging in Publication Data
A catalog record for this book is available from the Library of Congress

Notice
Medical knowledge is constantly changing. Standard safety precautions must be followed, but as new research and clinical experience broaden our knowledge, changes in treatment and drug therapy may become necessary or appropriate. Readers are advised to check the most current product information provided by the manufacturer of each drug to be administered to verify the recommended dose, the method and duration of administration, and contraindications. It is the responsibility of the practitioner, relying on experience and knowledge of the patient, to determine dosages and the best treatment for each individual patient. Neither the Publisher nor the author assumes any liability for any injury and/or damage to persons or property arising from this publication.

The Publisher

The
Publisher's
policy is to use
**paper manufactured
from sustainable fores**

Printed in China

Contents

Preface

This book is written primarily for physiotherapists who use acupuncture. It moves beyond the basic theories taught by the Acupuncture Association of Chartered Physiotherapists (AACP)-approved tutors in the introductory courses now studied by thousands of UK physiotherapists. It is intended as both an intermediate text and an encouragement to look further than simplistic musculoskeletal pain applications for this ancient technique.

Several assumptions are made: first, that all readers will be familiar with the anatomy of the human body; second, that they will be familiar with both normal and abnormal manifestations of physiology as taught to medical professionals in the UK; and third, that they will be practising within the physiotherapy discipline although not necessarily within the National Health Service of the UK.

Much of the material in this book will serve as an introduction to the study of acupuncture at a postgraduate level where students are expected to evolve their own practice, based on a combination of the available scientific evidence, the rich clinical history of Traditional Chinese Medicine and the basic skills of their profession.

Val Hopwood
Southampton 2004.

Overview of the main TCM theories and their place in modern practice

Introduction

This book is the sum of many hours of reading and researching, mostly of modern acupuncture texts, looking for a handle or key to the mysteries of acupuncture. Have I found one? I'm not certain, but I know that I answer questions with more intelligence than I once might have done because the information I have gleaned has informed my thoughts. I still feel that there is a great deal I don't know, but I also begin to feel that some of what I have learnt is unnecessary baggage. I am not yet ready to abandon all the original ideas of Traditional Chinese Medicine (TCM), even though my professional background is in so-called scientific medicine; consequently my practice is, at best, an uneasy balance between the two.

Historically, the acupuncture training available to physiotherapists has been provided by both TCM and medical trainers, leading to wide variety in the philosophical underpinnings to practice. As a response, physiotherapists are using their own form of acupuncture in the conditions that they understand and in ways that the Chinese probably did not envisage. This does not make us better, just different.

The teachers and colleagues with whom I work have slowly been moving to this new form of acupuncture, intuitively filtering the ancient philosophies when applied to clinical practice and incorporating the newest research when it seems to offer an explanation.

Most of the work done by physiotherapists can be identified as the relief of pain and the search for a neurological cure. This is, of course, a sweeping generalization and does not take into account a great deal of work focused on other fields such as basic movement, the cardiovascular system, respiration and child development. However, the majority of physiotherapists in the UK are still employed in National Health Service (NHS) outpatient departments dealing with various forms of pain on a daily basis.

This professional interest in alleviating painful problems offers a direct application for acupuncture, a truly holistic approach. An understanding of the physiological mechanisms underlying both acupuncture and pain itself is important. New research information about these mechanisms could, and indeed should, change the application of acupuncture if it is shown that the effects can be improved. Equally, if no effects can be demonstrated, we may need to think again. To quote White and Ernst: 'If acupuncture turns out in the end to only be a superior form of placebo then we should still use it, for we have few active treatments with as few side effects...' (Ernst & White 1999). It is perhaps as well that these authors have not

spent much time systematically reviewing the evidence for some physiotherapy modalities. I would venture to suggest that physiotherapists are
very familiar with the placebo effect.

It may be that this book will inform the debate. It will sometimes be
advisable to think of the symptoms and pattern in TCM terms before the
Western diagnostic method. When the signs and symptoms are divorced
from their rigid medical background it is possible actually to see new patterns and logic. A good example is the field of neurology. Essentially, the
problems experienced by the patient include a wide range of changes and
deficits, most of which are common to all the identified conditions although
of differing severity. All of these can be related directly to malfunction of
part of the nervous system, as we currently understand it. Taken in the
broadest possible sense, and in no particular order, the following are symptoms that might be expected in a patient with severe multiple sclerosis:

- decreased mobility
- autonomic changes
- fatigue
- muscle spasm
- contractures
- cognitive damage
- communication problems
- emotional lability
- breathing and coughing problems
- bladder symptoms
- visual symptoms.

Few patients are unlucky enough to suffer from all these problems, but the
nature of nerve damage implicit in the diagnosis of the condition means
that they are all possible. Neurological conditions are often difficult to distinguish (with the possible exception of a straightforward stroke), because
they have a great deal in common with one another. Table 1.1 shows the

Table 1.1   Neuro-
symptoms

Symptom	Multiple sclerosis	Stroke	Parkinson's disease	Motor neuron disease
Decreased mobility	✓	✓	✓	✓
Fatigue	✓ ✓		✓	✓
Respiratory problems	✓	✓		✓ ✓
Muscle spasm	✓	✓	✓	✓
Contractures	✓	✓	✓	✓
Autonomic changes	✓	✓	✓ ✓	✓
Cognition or mood	✓	✓	✓	
Communication	✓	✓	✓ ✓	✓
Bladder problems	✓	✓		✓
Visual problems	✓	✓		

symptoms described above and how they relate to some of the diseases commonly treated by neurophysiotherapists.

Obviously the full selection is rarely found in each specified disease, although the potential remains. The actual perceived physiological reason may also differ but the end result for the patient is the same. The double ticks indicate some of the defining diagnostic symptoms. When these symptoms are considered from the vantage point of TCM theory they fall into patterns or syndromes suggesting their treatment. It becomes evident that the treatment of stroke will not be dissimilar to that of multiple sclerosis, apart from the obvious problem of laterality, because the basic physiological function within the body will need to be stimulated in similar ways. This is heresy to a neurology physiotherapist – and quite possibly to a traditional acupuncturist too. However, the staging proposed by Blackwell (see Ch. 8) will apply across the range of neurological problems, with minor adjustments, because it is firmly rooted in Zang Fu theory, which in itself regards organ physiology as function (Blackwell & MacPherson 1993).

When the body is considered purely in terms of function, diagnosis becomes much easier and follows the TCM logic patterns. The ancient Chinese did not get everything right; in fact they got some aspects of body function spectacularly wrong. From the lofty height of Western scientific knowledge, we can make allowance for that and still perceive and use the patterns.

In this book I hope to highlight the parts of Chinese medical theory that have illuminated my approach to acupuncture within physiotherapy. I will only nod towards those parts that are too rooted in ancient philosophy to have much relevance, and adapt the modern research ideas that seem to justify some of what we do. I am happy to be accused of 'cherry-picking' as long as my patients benefit from this broad-minded approach to the subtle energies of the body. This makes for an uneasy mixture but it is beginning to resolve itself into a new animal 'acuphysio' 'physiopuncture' or simply 'directed sensory stimulation' – call it what you will.

This book is arranged like the layers of an onion (Fig. 1.1) because this is the best way to tempt the sceptical physiotherapist deeper into the mysteries. The deepest layers are the first that will be explored, progressing

Figure 1.1   Acupuncture 'onion'

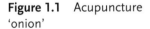

Subdermal
Musculotendinous
Meridian
Extra meridians
Chiaos
Qi at the centre

to the more superficial ideas and finishing with the surface applications. Hopefully this will be a form of revision for therapists who are hoping to use this book to extend their basic skills. However, I will start with an overview of the basic building blocks, the ancient ideas of development, reproduction, Qi, Blood and Body fluids, and examine why these might have some meaning for therapists working in a busy modern hospital.

Discussion of Zang Fu organ activities will illustrate the TCM physiology of function, and the use of these ideas links well to the known symptomatology of disease. This aspect of acupuncture is the one most difficult to sell to NHS managers when requesting funding for advanced training. I hope to provide sufficient evidence of this approach in action to reassure them that this type of training is never wasted. To quote Jane Lyttelton (1992, p 242):

> Chinese medicine provides a particularly attractive model for wholistic health care. It sees health and well-being as a state of balance between a person and every aspect of that person's context. This indicates primarily a respectful and caring relationship with the natural environment and a lifestyle appropriate to the exigencies of natural forces and climates. It can also be extrapolated to include relationships between the body's constitution and the way we work and play, where we live, what we eat, how we modulate our relationships with others etc, etc. The interdependence of mind and body goes without saying in such a comprehensive view of health. Illness is not usually an arbitrary and unlucky event but an expression of a lack of balance, and as such it is up to the individual to take care of their lifestyle to keep their health.

Acupuncture: history and concepts

A considerable amount of the original Chinese philosophy underpinning TCM was the attempt to explain the phenomena of the perceptible world as natural occurrences, without referring to mysterious forces such as gods, demons or ancestors. Medicine and religion were closely linked in the early history of the area now known as China.

When considering acupuncture treatment it is important to be clear what is meant by the term acupuncture. It is necessary to place acupuncture in context; it has a long recorded history – the first written records, the Huang Di Nei Jing, are dated at about 200 BC – and has evolved as part of the TCM paradigm together with Chinese herbal medicine. It is also necessary to examine the basic concepts within TCM, as a common failing among acupuncture researchers is to test what they believe acupuncture ought to be, rather than what it is.

The history of acupuncture cannot be divorced from the history of Chinese culture itself. The Middle and Late Zhou dynasties were particularly important and much of the theory accepted today was first recorded then. Various theories were widely discussed and some gained temporary dominance. The origins of Chinese Medicine are fairly obscure; the great heroes, Fu Xi, Shen Nong and Huang Di, were said to have lived in the Shang dynasty, but were not actually written about until much later. Table 1.2 gives a brief summary of the history of acupuncture starting from

Table 1.2 Brief summary of Chinese history in relation to acupuncture

Period	Dates	Summary
Shang	1523 to 1027 BC	The classical Chinese bronze age *Demonological beliefs and propitiation of ancestors indicate that a medicine distinct from religion has yet to develop* *Fu Xi, Shen Nong and Huang Di influential*
Early Zhou	1027 to 772 BC	Classical feudalism *Advances in agriculture allow greater armies and workforces led by hereditary and absolute rulers* *Medicine still within shamanistic ritual-based religion*
Middle Zhou	772 to 480 BC	Declining feudalism *Recorded history begins. Confucianism arises, medicine begins to develop as an institution*
Late Zhou	480 to 221 BC	Warring states *Chaos of warring principalities* *Daoism arises and five-phase theory begins to develop*
Qin	221 to 206 BC	Period of book burning *Autocratic rule, with governmental bureaucracy*
Han	206 BC to AD 220	Period of systematization *Medicine of systematic correspondence dominates acupuncture. Nei Jing and Nan Jing written* *Sanitation developed*
Six Dynasties	AD 220 to 589	Period of disunity *Buddhist influences active in China. Medicine becomes more formal with the development of a technical literature*
Sui	AD 590 to 617	Period of reunification *Chinese culture, including acupuncture, spreads throughout Asia*
Tang	AD 618 to 906	Period of culmination *Developments dominated by the search for alchemical mortality*
Five Dynasties	AD 907 to 960	Period of disunity *Weak government in China* *Medical colleges established in Korea and Japan*

Continues

Table 1.2   cont'd

Period	Dates	Summary
Song	AD 960 to 1264	Neo-Confucianism *Medicine of systematic correspondences dominates and drug therapy is incorporated into the Qi paradigm*
Yuan	AD 1264 to 1368	Period of Mongol control *European influences felt* *First independent medical college established*
Ming	AD 1368 to 1643	Period of restoration *Democratization of the Confucian bureaucracy leads to an explosion of information and more individualism*
Qing	AD 1644 to 1911	The end of the Empire *Severe decline in traditional medicine. Acupuncture largely lost*

1523 BC and coming nearly to an end in 1911. It is useful to remind ourselves of this long history and the vast wealth of empirical evidence.

The concepts were applied to both individuals and society at large. In individual terms, the ancient Chinese physicians preached moderation in all things, such as alcoholic intake and gastronomic excess. There have been many schools of thought over the centuries, emphasizing different aspects but all broadly agreeing on the underlying theories, the most important of which is that concerning 'Qi'.

Qi

In the beginning, the concept of Qi had nothing to do with medicine. It was at the core of Chinese philosophical thinking, attempting to define the relations between matter and change, substance and activity. Later, 'Qi became a popular concept and was even used in many vernacular expressions. For instance Sheng Qi, 'to produce Qi', means to be angry; Qi Ying, 'overflowing with Qi', means to be pleased with oneself; Yun Qi, the 'moving Qi', means chance; Qi Xing, the 'nature of Qi', means the character of a person.' (Ernst & White 1999).

Qi is a speculation about the nature of being. It is, at once, both a very simple and a complex concept. It is frequently described as the life force or vital energy of a living thing. Without Qi there is no life. Qi represents the vital energy of the body but it also has a material form. It is both substance and function. This means that one can talk of the Qi of the Lungs, referring to their functional ability, and also the clean Qi or inspired air. Chinese Medicine embraces both ideas, using further subdivisions of Qi according to where it is found in the body and the function ascribed to it.

As Qi is vital to life, it follows that if it is in poor condition, deficient in some way or not able to circulate freely throughout the body, then pain or ill-health may result. This, in fact, is the basic idea informing most acupuncture treatment and TCM. Slowing or blockage of the Qi is reversed or prevented, and the body functions normally again. Qi is disseminated through the body in meridians or channels and can be influenced via the acupuncture points found on the channels.

General health or constitution depends on the quality of the Inherited Qi. This forms half the total; the quality of the rest depends on the air breathed and the food and drink ingested, hence a sensible diet and good living conditions will aid good general health. Another form of Qi, the Wei Qi, is a defensive form of Qi, protecting the body from invasion by disease, circulating just below the skin and fending off invasion by Pathogens. Although said to be found together in the meridians, Qi and Blood are seen as two separate entities. Qi is a very wide concept, described fully in Chapter 2. Its existence is difficult to prove or disprove, but Qi is essential to an understanding of Chinese Medicine.

Yin and Yang

One of the major assumptions in TCM is that disease is also due to an internal imbalance of Yin, translated literally as 'the shady side of the mountain' and Yang, translated as 'the sunny side of the mountain'. The living body exists as a delicate balance between the two. Put very simply, Yang represents fire, noise, function and day, whereas Yin represents water, quiet, substance and night. Yin is essentially internal, while Yang defines the outer boundaries of the body. Although Yin and Yang are extreme opposites, one cannot exist without the other: we cannot understand hot without cold. The balance of Yin and Yang within it determines the state of the body.

The two aspects are interdependent, Yin being regarded as the interior, material foundation of Yang, whereas Yang is an exterior manifestation of the function of Yin. The Yin–Yang aspects within a body are in a continual state of flux; the lessening of one leads to an increase in the other because they are contained within a closed system. The functional activities in the healthy body can be considered in terms of Yin and Yang.

Each of the organs is predominantly Yin or Yang but has nonetheless an element of the opposite within it. Thus the Liver is said to be a Yin organ because Yin energy predominates, but it also has Yang within it. If this balance is altered and the Yang assumes greater prominence, the Liver is said to be out of balance and will begin to show signs of 'dis-ease', with the appearance of symptoms associated with TCM Liver pathology. Treatment would be directed at supplementing the Liver Yin, but if the imbalance was too great or caused possibly by the interaction of imbalances in other organs then the Liver Yang could be drained or decreased in order to restore balance and the controlling organs or meridians supplemented. Specific acupuncture points on the appropriate meridians, either Yin or Yang in nature, are used. This type of treatment could be undertaken to prevent the occurrence of stroke, an extreme state of imbalance in a vulnerable patient.

If there is an excess of Yin Qi the Yang Qi is diminished and cold will be the predominant symptom of disease. Excess Yang consumes Yin and disease where the predominant symptom is heat occurs (Figs 1.2 & 1.3). The Yin–Yang design expresses this theory very well. There is no absolute Yin or Yang: each always contains the germ of the other (Fig. 1.4).

Figure 1.2 Yin–Yang
hyperactivity

Figure 1.3 Yin–Yang
hypoactivity

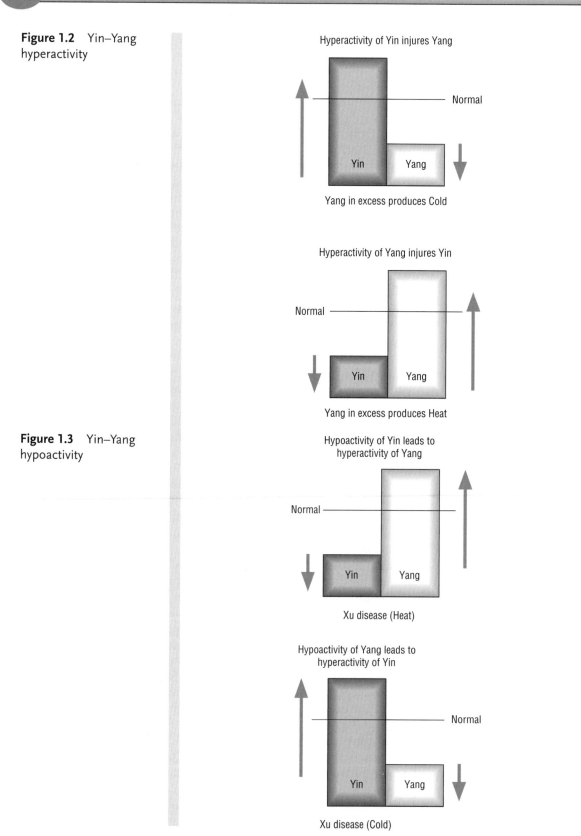

Hyperactivity of Yin injures Yang

Normal

Yin   Yang

Yang in excess produces Cold

Hyperactivity of Yang injures Yin

Normal

Yin   Yang

Yang in excess produces Heat

Hypoactivity of Yin leads to
hyperactivity of Yang

Normal

Yin   Yang

Xu disease (Heat)

Hypoactivity of Yang leads to
hyperactivity of Yin

Normal

Yin   Yang

Xu disease (Cold)

Figure 1.4 The Yin–Yang symbol

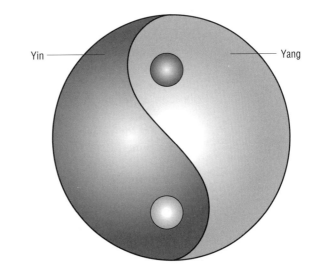

Yin ————   ———— Yang

Table 1.3 Yin–Yang psychological types

Yang	Yin
Active	Passive
Dynamic	Static
Rage, fury	Resentful, grudging
Light-hearted	Melancholy, depressed
Joy, delight	Grief, sadness
Courage	Timidity
Uncontrolled desires	Discretion, prudence
Extroverted	Introverted

The theory is inextricably bound up with the corresponding ideas of Excess (Shi) and Deficiency (Xu) in the Eight Principles of diagnosis, described later in this chapter. Yin–Yang theory can also be applied to the psychological state of the patient, as shown in Table 1.3.

In simple terms, this means that the patient sitting quietly in the corner of the waiting room, who, it is suspected, has been there for some time without making a fuss, may have a current Yin–Yang balance demonstrating predominantly Yin characteristics. On the other hand, the patient who is currently complaining bitterly and loudly about their lengthy wait, who you are having difficulty in responding to politely because they appear to be resolutely invading your space, may prove to be predominantly Yang. It is, of course, never as simple, as that.

Yin–Yang research

The basic idea underpinning most TCM diagnostics should be amenable to scientific proof one way or the other. However, even if the theory of this imbalance is accepted, the customary illustration (as in Figs 1.2 & 1.3) is a bar graph representing the relative amount of Yin versus Yang, as well as an absolute amount of each relative to an undefined zero point representing a balanced or healthy state.

A recent study set out to test the hypothesis that a numerical score can reliably be assigned to the concepts of Yin and Yang (Langevin et al 2003). Six acupuncturists interviewed 12 healthy human volunteers successively on the same day. Each acupuncturist gave each patient a score for Yin and a score for Yang on a scale of −10 to +10, zero representing a balance. The acupuncturists were blind to one another's scores. The evidence from this study suggests that Yin and Yang could be quantified in a reliable manner. The inter-rater correlation was relatively high and significant differences in mean scores across patients were detected at $P < 0.001$ for Yin, Yang and Yin–Yang. Further work needs to be done on groups of patients with active pathology (i.e. an assumed imbalance of Yin and Yang), but the possibility of meaningful numerical measurement exists.

Pathogens

Diagnosis in TCM takes many factors into consideration, not least of which are the Pathogens. These are classified as either External or Internal. The External Pathogens are really based on climatic influences: Wind, Cold, Damp and Heat. These are considered to be capable of entering the body to cause disease. When present in excess, a body with deficient defences, or Wei Qi, will be susceptible to invasion by them. Thus, External Pathogens can become internalized, moving deeper from the meridians into the organ systems where they can cause considerable damage to the delicate energy balances. Each type of pathogenic invasion produces distinctive symptoms, allowing the Pathogen to be recognized. Cold tends to produce a deep pain, generally static in nature with loss of joint movement – 'freezing' in effect. Damp is associated with excess fluid, oedema, heaviness, swelling of the lower limbs and a dull pain, often a headache. Wind is characterized by a volatile or mobile symptomatology. Joint pain caused by Wind will not have a constant focus but is likely to move from joint to joint. Heat is relatively straightforward, causing an increase in internal heat, shown by a rise in body temperature or drying of body fluids and a burning type of pain.

More than one Pathogen can invade at the same time; if a patient is suffering from influenza, there will be a fever and also muscular aches that wander all over the body. This is defined as an invasion of the Pathogens Wind and Heat.

Internal Pathogens are those arising from within the body itself and are thought to be excess emotions. These emotions are a normal part of life, and normal emotional activity does not lead to illness. Illness results from emotions only when the emotional pressure is too strong, or the patient is highly sensitive for some other health reason. Anger, fear or worry taken to excess can lead to pathogenic damage to the energy systems within the body. Particular emotions are said to affect specific body organs (Table 1.4); for example, the Liver is particularly susceptible to damage by anger and the Lungs by grief.

Table 1.4   Emotions and their effects

Organ	Normal TCM activity	Damaging emotion
Heart Contains the Shen or spirit–mind	Consciousness Logical thinking Insight	Overjoy
Liver Contains the Hun or Ethereal Soul	Command of self Mental balance	Anger or depression
Lung Contains the Po or Animal Spirit	Sensations Emotions	Grief
Kidney Controls Zhi or the will	Motivation	Fear
Spleen Connected to Yi or idea	Centrality, grounding, cognition, memory	Obsession

Research

The effect of the External Pathogens on body functions has always been known in preindustrial societies. It was thought quite logical that external conditions could affect the body and might be instrumental in causing disease; however, finding scientific proof of this is more problematic. Strangely, Western medicine is more comfortable with the idea of the Internal Pathogens, the emotions, being a possible cause of ill-health.

There has been some work that links joint pain to weather conditions. The pressure within a joint space, within the capsule, is believed to be slightly less than that of the atmosphere surrounding it. This has the effect of making the capsule pull in slightly, tending to maintain the integrity of the joint – holding it together, as it were. If the external atmospheric pressure should drop, the relative pressure within the joint will be higher, causing some outward movement and tending to put structures on a slight stretch. If these structures are tender or sensitive, there is the very real possibility that a painful arthritic joint could be perceived as more painful on a rainy day. Work on this effect in patients with rheumatic joint disease has been carried out in Israel (Guedj & Weinberger 1990) and has shown clear links with meteorology.

Zang Fu

Chinese physiology is a little different to that understood in Western medicine. As mentioned above, the driving force behind all body functions is Qi. Varying forms of Qi are found in the major organs of the body, with variations in function according to location. The organs are defined by their function, some being perceived much as in modern medicine, others having additional functions. The internal organs are collectively termed Zang Fu, and the first details of this functional physiology are found in the Nei Ching Su Wen dating from the first century BC (Veith 1972).

The Heart was thought to house the mind, ancient Chinese Medicine having no concept of the brain. However, the circulation of blood was understood in much the same way as in the West. The Lungs were seen as being importantly linked with the Kidneys in the control of water circulation throughout the body, whereas the Kidneys themselves were thought to house the original Qi from the parents and to be vital to the reproductive cycle. The characteristics of each organ are very important to the TCM paradigm and will be considered separately in Chapter 3. The concept of wholism, of organs working together to maintain body harmony, runs through all Chinese Medicine.

Pulses and tongue

Pulse diagnosis is an important aspect of TCM and requires considerable expertise. Since the late Han dynasty, radial pulse palpation has been believed to indicate the general health of the patient. The 12 channels are thought to be reflected, one each at two depths in each of six finger positions along the surface of the radial artery just proximal to the wrist.

Pulse-takers look for a variation of strength in one position relative to the others. This indicates a problem with the channel or organ that corresponds to that position. It is a skill that takes a long time to learn and, although I am certain that some information can be obtained from the chief characteristic of the pulse (i.e. whether it is strong or weak), I have never devoted sufficient time to learning the finer points of this diagnostic technique to write about it with any confidence. I am not aware of any good controlled research into the relation of the Zang Fu pulses to Western pathology, or into inter-rater reliability between diagnosticians. Just because there is no proof that pulse-taking is useful does not, of course, mean that it is not useful in the hands of a skilled practitioner.

The tongue is also thought to indicate the state of health by demonstrating the deficiencies and excesses within the Zang Fu system. A normal tongue has a pink body and a light white coating. It is normal in size: it does not look too big for the space it lies in, nor does it deviate to one side or the other. The patient can also put it out and hold it steady for a reasonable length of time.

The invasion of pathogenic factors can also be seen in the variations of colour, texture and quality of the tongue body and coating. The different areas of the tongue are sometimes seen as indicating the organs zoned by their place in the Sanjiao, although there are several ways to interpret the information offered by the tongue. Assessment of the tongue is generally more helpful when attempting to identify a long-term or chronic change. It is often used to detect an underlying Heat problem. It rarely indicates an acute situation.

A full account of this useful diagnostic tool can be found in the definitive text written by Maciocia (1987).

Chinese diagnosis

With the preceding concepts in mind, it is possible to understand the process of diagnosis, particularly that of Eight Principle diagnosis. This considers the following pairings:

Yin–Yang	Cold–Hot
Internal–External	Deficiency–Excess

A series of questions is asked and all body functions are observed. This process includes a detailed reading of the pulses and observation of the tongue. First, an assessment is made of the relative strengths of Yin and Yang within the patient. This may well localize the symptoms into one of the Zang Fu organs, but will lead to further judgement on whether the disease process remains relatively superficial or whether it has penetrated the body. The symptoms, including those that are either Hot or Cold in nature, will begin to form into recognizable patterns or syndromes leading to the identification of a Deficient or Excess condition according to whether the Qi, or energy, appears to be insufficient or in overabundance. Thus, the exact nature of the imbalance can be defined, leading to the possibility of treatment of both the symptoms and the cause.

Box 1.1 allows the therapist to consider the Eight Principles and to select the most important characteristics as they apply to the patient. It is clear that no patient will fit neatly into one category, but the art of Chinese Medicine is to decide where the main problem lies before assessing the possible contributing factors.

This type of diagnostic process is undertaken before the administration of acupuncture or Chinese herbal medicine, the two modalities often being used together. It will also determine the acupuncture points to be chosen and any ancillary techniques, such as cupping (a stimulus to the superficial circulation), moxibustion (a form of localized intensive heat) or, in more modern treatments, electroacupuncture.

Acupuncture points and meridians

Acupuncture meridians or channels are conduits that carry and distribute Qi, or vital energy, throughout the body. Each of the organs is represented by a channel, and diseases of a particular organ can be treated by using acupuncture points on the channel representing that organ. In Chinese medical thinking, the meridians have a functional rather than an anatomical base; their existence was deduced from the many sensations – painful or abnormal, spontaneous or provoked – that occur even when in good health. These sensations tend to have a linear location. However, atlases have evolved that give precise anatomical locations for each acupuncture point (Deng et al 1990).

The concept of channels exists exclusively in TCM, but what evidence do we have for them within our conventional paradigm? A considerable amount of work has been carried out, particularly in China, on the possible anatomical basis of meridians and acupuncture points.

Propagated channel sensation (PCS) has been investigated extensively by many Chinese authors. PCS refers to the sensations experienced by a small proportion of individuals when acupuncture points are needled; as mentioned above, these sensations tend to run along the acupuncture meridians, although it is not clear whether the subjects, who are presumably

Box 1.1 Differentiation according to the Eight Principles

Yin	Yang
(Ideas suggested in text: water, quiet, substance, etc.)	(Ideas suggested in text: fire, noise, function, etc.)
Interior	**Exterior**
Called Li in Chinese	Called Biao in Chinese
Disharmonious states of the Zang Fu organs	Disturbances of channels and collaterals
May involve increase in temperature and gastrointestinal problems	Mostly peripheral symptoms
	Acute pain in the extremities
Usually chronic in nature	Affected by climatic factors
Often caused by an excess of emotional factors or inadequate or contaminated foods	Typically peripheral neuralgia or painful joint disease
Deficiency	**Excess**
Xu conditions	Shi conditions
Characterized by deficient Qi or Blood	Excessive Qi or Blood in organs or channels
Usually chronic	Acute pain, cramps, increased muscle tone
Excessive tiredness, exhaustion, dizziness, pallor	Loud voice
Faint voice	Upright posture
Stooping posture	Increased secretion of Body fluids
Depression, passivity, subdued mood	Redness of the face
Slow movements	Excitement, mania
Long sleeping period but disturbed sleep	Difficulty falling asleep
Weak pulse	Strong pulse
Cold	**Heat**
Han	Re
External Pathogens invade a body with weakened Qi	Increased Yang activity in the body, leads to exhaustion of Yin, particularly fluids
Pale face, pale mucous membranes	Red face, flushed mucous membranes
Cold extremities	Warm extremities
Hypothermia	Fever
Cold makes the symptoms worse	Symptoms made worse by heat
Need for warm drinks	Thirst for cold drinks
Dilute urine	Dark scanty urine
Watery stools	Constipated
Slow pulse, pale tongue	Fast pulse, red tongue

all Chinese, know in advance where the meridian pathways are supposed to be (Bensoussan 1991).

Changes in skin resistance and temperature have also been suggested as providing evidence for the existence of meridians (Zhaowei et al 1985). Reviewing this work Macdonald (1989) acknowledged that sensations may follow meridian lines, but suggested that such phenomena can be explained without postulating the existence of a meridian system. Other Western physicians, notably Felix Mann (1992), have suggested that the acupoints do not exist, as such, offering large acupuncture areas with variable positions instead.

The most interesting modern work has been done by Zang-He Cho, who looked for evidence of acupuncture point stimulation in the cortex on functional magnetic resonance imaging (fMRI) scans (Cho et al 1998). In a controlled experiment, Cho stimulated UB 67 Zhiyin (situated on the little toe), a point said to have an effect on the eye, and measured the effects on fMRI. He observed activation in the visual cortex area. He also used GB 37 Guangming, a point said to have similar effects, and observed the same response. These two points produced a similar effect in the cortex to the stimulus of a flashing light. This evidence is supported by the stimulation of a point believed to affect the ear, GB 43 Xiaxi, which appeared to activate the auditory cortex. The transmission route for these stimuli to the brain remains unclear, but gives some credence to the idea of meridians. The acupuncture stimulation appears to be projected to the higher brain centres such as the visual and auditory cortices. It is postulated that information is relayed from these sites to other key processing areas, including the prefrontal cortex and limbic systems. It is likely that acupuncture signals projected to these higher cortical areas will induce pain modulation and may also affect other survival-related functions. This group of researchers proposed a project to map all the other acupuncture points systematically, but have, so far, not published this ambitious work.

Other researchers have taken up the challenge. Wu et al (1999) have made some interesting findings that add to the current confusion but may open the way to a more logical appraisal of the effects of acupuncture. They used 15 healthy volunteers and attempted to define the action of both electroacupuncture on accepted acupoints and sham acupuncture on non-meridian points by neuroimaging. They found that both interventions activated the pain-related neuromatrix but the response to electroacupuncture was significantly higher, particularly in the hypothalamic–limbic system.

Darras et al (1993) concluded that meridian pathways could be marked by injecting radioactively labelled technetium into acupuncture points, and that these pathways were separate from lymph vessels and other identifiable structures. Lazorthes et al (1990), who thought that the pathways were, in fact, probably part of the lymphatic system, successfully contested this theory later.

In China, research on the meridian phenomena continues, but most Western researchers appear to dismiss the idea of a meridian system. At the very least, it must be concluded that on current evidence the existence of the meridians exactly as described by the TCM doctors remains unproven. The evidence of Cho et al and of Wu et al cannot be discounted, however; although the meridians may not look exactly like those in the atlases, there is clearly a form of communication from the periphery to the brain that needs to be investigated fully.

References

Bensoussan A 1991 The vital meridian, a modern exploration of acupuncture. 1st edn. Melbourne: Churchill Livingstone.

Blackwell R, MacPherson H 1993 Multiple sclerosis. Staging and patient management. Journal of Chinese Medicine 42: 5–12.

Cho ZH, Chung SC, Jones JP et al 1998 New findings of the correlation between acupoints and corresponding brain cortices using functional MRI. Proceedings of the National Academy of Sciences USA 95: 2670–2673.

Darras JC, Albarede P, de Vernejoul P 1993 Nuclear medicine investigation of transmission of acupuncture information. Acupuncture in Medicine 11: 22–28.

Deng L, Li D, Chen K et al 1990 The location of acupoints: state standard of the People's Republic of China, 1st edn. Beijing: Foreign Languages Press.

Ernst E, White A 1999 Acupuncture: a scientific appraisal, 1st edn. Oxford: Butterworth Heinemann.

Guedj D, Weinberger A 1990 Effects of weather conditions on rheumatic patients. Annals of the Rheumatic Diseases 49: 158–159.

Langevin HM, Badger GJ, Povolny BK et al 2003 Yin/Yang score: an inter-rater reliability pilot study. Clinical Acupuncture and Oriental Medicine 4: 41–50.

Lazorthes Y, Esquerre JP, Simon J et al 1990 Acupuncture meridians and radio tracers. Pain 40: 109–112.

Lyttelton, J 1992 Of molecules, meridians and medicine: the feminist influence – putting the Yin back into health care. American Journal of Acupuncture 20: 237–243.

Macdonald A 1989 Acupuncture analgesia and therapy. In: Wall PD, Melzack R, eds. The textbook of pain, 2nd edn, pp 906–919. Edinburgh: Churchill Livingstone.

Maciocia G 1987 Tongue diagnosis in Chinese Medicine. Seattle: Eastland Press.

Mann F 1992 Re-inventing acupuncture: a new concept of Ancient Medicine, 1st edn. Oxford: Butterworth Heinemann.

Veith I 1972 The Yellow Emperor's classic of internal medicine, translated with an introductory study by Ilza Veith. Berkley: University of California Press.

Wu MT, Hsieh JC, Xiong J et al 1999 Central nervous pathway for acupuncture stimulation: localisation of processing with functional MR imaging of the brain – preliminary experience. Radiology 212: 133–141.

Zhaowei M, Zongxiang Z, Xianglong H 1985 Progress in the research of meridian phenomena in China during the last five years. Journal of Traditional Chinese Medicine 5: 145–152.

Qi, Blood and Body fluids – the core of the onion

KEY CONCEPTS

☯ Qi is the basis of and essential to life.

☯ Qi has many manifestations, classified according to function.

☯ Blood is closely associated with Qi, and this circulation is influential in the diseases of old age.

☯ The effective circulation of Body fluids is an important factor in health.

☯ Bi syndrome, the most commonly seen condition in physiotherapy departments, has its origin in the effect of external Pathogens on the circulation of Qi and fluids.

☯ Heart disease and stroke can be explained in these terms.

☯ There has been little research into Qi but considerable investigation of Bi syndrome or arthritic pain.

Introduction

Working from the inside out, it becomes imperative to decide on the essence of the human being. What is at the core of our very being? What in fact produces our being? Ancient Chinese theories are quite explicit. There is heaven above and earth below, and between the two the human is to be found as a sort of link or conduit for cosmic energy.

As a fully paid-up member of my own quasi-scientific culture, some of the ideas of Qi are difficult to understand. It seems from the outside to be as much a matter of faith as anything else. It also seems dangerously like intellectual suicide even to explore it, far less start a textbook for physiotherapists with as full an explanation as I can manage. Through many years of acupuncture study and practice I have decided that the roots of acupuncture and Traditional Chinese Medicine (TCM) theory are important – not necessarily to be believed in, as with a religion, but to be understood and evolved gently, as indeed has been happening for thousands of years, into something that can accompany the spirit of scientific enquiry and the evidence base as it now exists.

The consistent theme of TCM in the ancient writings is a holistic approach toward the prevention and treatment of human illness that involves helping the patient to harmonize with the universe at many different levels: body, mind, spirit, lifestyle and diet. The spiritual reality of both the patient and the practitioner was an inseparable part of the treatment. Classical Chinese doctors saw their mission as assisting the person to achieve balance and harmony with the universe, not just clearing up symptoms of low back pain and Kidney deficiency.

Students of acupuncture are taught that Qi is the basis of all life and that the smooth circulation of healthy Qi is essential for a healthy body. At the same time, one of the most influential modern Chinese texts, *Essentials of Chinese Acupuncture*, used by large numbers of foreign students while studying acupuncture in China, does not actually mention Qi, preferring to describe the dichotomy of Yin and Yang instead. It prefaces this description with the comment that the theories of Yin–Yang 'involved a naive concept of materialism and dialectics' and neatly avoids the issue. It is said that modern TCM has systematically eliminated the spiritual element under the communists, referring to it as 'spiritual pollution'.

Perhaps this reluctance to tackle the most important concept (from a Western point of view) arises from the fact that Qi really is integral to Chinese culture. The following quote from Zhang & Rose (2001, p 171) sums it up well:

> *Qi is such an integral part of the experience of life and language in China that it can seem almost impossible to pull this one thread out of the embroidery of Chinese culture without entirely unravelling it. What we've experienced far too often in the past is that those who start to tug on it will pull too quickly and the thread will break. Or they will give up and never find how far it winds through the fabric of Chinese thought. Perhaps, worst of all they succeed at freeing a small fragment of the thread of Qi from the complex brocade of its multi-dimensional meanings and we are left with a paltry impression of how Qi functions to connect so much that is vital and thriving in the Chinese imagination.*

While accepting the inherent truth of this statement, it is worthwhile examining some of the many threads, if only to get some idea of the range and variety involved. A working knowledge of this basic concept will help to make the difference between an acupuncture 'technician' and a true acupuncture practitioner.

Qi is variously described as 'life force', 'vital energy', 'basic energy', 'moving power'. One of the reasons Qi is so difficult to define is that it is most often defined by function. The Chinese character for Qi (Fig. 2.1) implies that it is both something of substance and at the same time insubstantial, with part being translated as 'vapour' or 'steam' and part being translated as 'rice'. Maciocia (1989) makes the point that the subtle aspect of Qi, the steam, is produced from the very much less subtle substance when rice is cooked. This juxtaposition of opposites informs a great deal of Chinese theory and achieves great subtlety in the Yin–Yang theory.

The Chinese creation story is found in the *Tao Teh Ching*; the basic idea is that creation is the coming into being of bipolar energy. In his translation, Arthur Waley (1934, ch XLII) describes it as follows:

> *Tao gave birth to the One: the One gave birth successively to two things, three things, up to ten thousand. These ten thousand things cannot turn their backs to the shade without having the sun on their bellies and it is upon this blending of the breaths that their harmony depends.*

Figure 2.1 Chinese character for Qi.

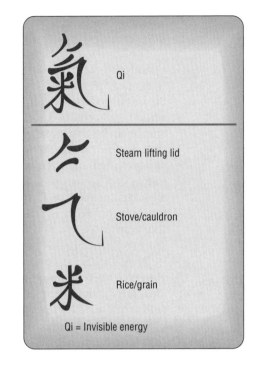

Qi

Steam lifting lid

Stove/cauldron

Rice/grain

Qi = Invisible energy

This idea of sun and shade leads to the idea of Yin and Yang, and makes the aspect of interdependence quite clear. One cannot exist without the other. Birth requires death.

The One Law of Fu Hsi (a legendary emperor who, according to various authorities, lived about 4000 years ago) states: 'The universe represents the interplay of the two activities Yin and Yang and their vicissitudes'. This is followed by the 12 axioms or propositions, which attempted to explain the dichotomy of Yin and Yang (Lawson-Wood & Lawson-Wood 1973, p 13):

1. *That which produces and composes the Universe is Tao, Inner Nature.*
2. *Inner Nature polarises itself, one pole becomes charged with Yang activity and the other with Yin activity.*
3. *Yang and Yin are opposites.*
4. *Beings and phenomena in the Universe are multiple and complex aggregates of Universe aether charged with Yang and Yin in all proportions.*
5. *Beings and phenomena are diverse dynamic equilibria: nothing in the Universe is stable or finished; all is in unceasing motion, because polarisation is without beginning or end.*
6. *Yin and Yang are attracted to one another.*
7. *Nothing is wholly Yin or wholly Yang. Yin and Yang are characterised only relatively: all is Yin and Yang aggregate.*
8. *Nothing is neutral. Polarisation is ceaseless and universal.*
9. *The force of attraction between two beings is a function of the difference between their charges of opposite activities (expressed $A = f(x - y)$).*
10. *Like activities repel one another. The repulsion between two beings of the same polarity is the greater the closer their similarity.*
11. *Yin produces Yang. Yang produces Yin.*
12. *All beings are charged: Yang interiorly and Yin exteriorly.*

Lawson-Wood & Lawson-Wood (1973) claim that the above propositions do not merely deal with creation but can also be seen as a 'Story of Continuum'.

The Chinese envisaged human beings as microcosms of the universe that surrounded them, the link between heaven and earth, part of one unbroken, integrated, interrelated whole, the Tao. This type of holistic thinking predates the mind–body separation that has prevailed in Western medicine since the seventeenth century. This universal system exists in a continuous process of change and transformation, and human beings are seen as only a part of that. All theories are therefore applied to the macrocosm of the universe as well as to humanity. Thus the concept of Qi is far more than just the vital energy of a human person: it is linked to the cosmic energy also. Matter is Qi taking shape; the formation of mountains, the growth of forests, the movement of the seas and the life present in all environments are all manifestations of Qi in action. That said, it is human beings with whom we are most concerned in this book, and human Qi that will be examined.

Qi is a difficult concept for Western medical practitioners to adopt. However, the term 'energy medicine' used by the US National Institutes of Health for acupuncture is helpful. Even so, the total concept of Qi remains stubbornly outside current scientific understanding. It is more than just an energy to be understood by the application of physical laws. There is also a psychical component: Chinese theory unites mind and body. The same character, Xin, is used for 'Heart' and 'Mind', and the internal organs are all associated with specific emotions that may damage them if occurring in excess. This means that the Qi, or energy within the system, can be affected by these emotions too. The further application of this idea can be seen when the Zang Fu organ system is examined.

There are four components of a human being, taken from the early literature of China and Japan. *Shen* is translated as 'spirit' or 'mind', *Jing* as 'Essence', *Hun* as 'aetheric soul' and *Po* as 'corporeal soul'. These four concepts are widely discussed and their interpretation owes more to the society in which they were used, perhaps, than to their true origin.

Po is an easy concept in that it is inherently visual; it is sometimes translated as 'the white part' and signifies the skeleton, left behind after death. The Po, Yin in nature, controls the development of the fetus. The Hun is said to be Yang in nature, and is sometimes translated as 'unresting flight'. The vital energy of Jing is seen as a driving force for development, a product of both the nutritional substances and the reproductive processes. Finally, the composite, Shen Ming – spirit and intelligence – is regarded as the sum of all these. Yi, representing 'idea', and Zhi, representing 'will', are further mental or emotional subdivisions found in Five Element theory, and are shown along with the psychospiritual affinities of the Zang organs and the Five Elements in Table 2.1.

We are the product of the Qi belonging to our parents; indeed, one of the translations of sexual intercourse in the Chinese language is 'combining Qi'. This basic energy is combined in the individual to become the pre-Heaven, Yuan, source or Congenital Qi stored in the Kidneys. There are many names for this substance, but it is best understood as the blueprint for our constitution or basic health. In Chinese thinking, the congenitally disabled child has been dealt a poor hand and, although acupuncture may be used to relieve distressing symptoms, the basic flaw in development

Table 2.1 Mental faculties and the Five Elements

	Translation	Governs	Element	Zang organ
Shen	Spirit–mind	Consciousness Logical thinking Insight	Fire	Heart
Yi	Idea	Cognition Memory Imagination	Earth	Spleen
Po	Animal spirit	Sensations Emotions Body awareness	Metal	Lung
Zhi	Will	Motivation Determination Decision	Water	Kidney
Hun	Ethereal soul	Emotions Mental balance Spiritual 'soul'	Wood	Liver

cannot be changed. This ties in neatly with modern thinking about DNA and hereditary disease. Together, the Yin and Yang of the Kidney construct the substance and stimulate the soma and the psyche.

Qi itself can be described in many ways but is only truly defined by function. Reading Chinese texts can be very confusing, with many names being given to the Qi according to where in the body it is to be commonly found and what it is thought to be doing. The concept of Qi circulation is integral to an understanding of the many functions of Qi. It is present within the blood circulation and is thought to support and energize that activity. It can be imagined as entering the body for the first time when the infant draws its first breath. This, by convention, is thought to be at 2 o'clock in the morning, when babies are prone to being born naturally. (Air is a form of Qi that is combined with food and drink within the body to form Qing Qi.) The first breath vitalizes the process, and the circulation of Qi through the main body organs begins at that point. Qi is to be found in all parts of the body at all times but, owing to the activity of circulation, a concentration can be found in certain parts at certain times (Fig. 2.2).

Moving on from the Lungs, like the leading edge of a small tidal wave, the Qi concentration progresses to the next organ around the circle, in this case the Large Intestine. It remains in a more concentrated form within this organ and the associated meridian for 2 hours, until 6 am, then moves again to the Stomach. This concept has a clear clinical application in that the organ or meridian may be expected to respond better to the stimulus of acupuncture if treated at the appropriate time. On examination of the 24-hour circulation diagram, it does become apparent that some of these times would be anything but clinically convenient, so other ways must also be used to stimulate the organs or meridians in question. One can question this process and ask what happens when crossing time zones, as the modern traveller frequently does. Does the hour of Qi concentration

Figure 2.2 Diagram of body clock. Lu, Lung; LI, Large Intestine; St, Stomach; Sp, Spleen; Ht, Heart; SI, Small Intestine; UB, Urinary Bladder; Kid, Kidney; Pe, Pericardium; SJ, Sanjiao; GB, Gall Bladder; Liv, Liver.

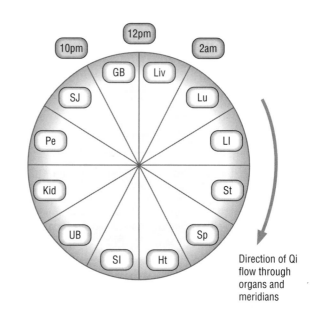

Direction of Qi flow through organs and meridians

alter? The purists would respond that this is the reason for jet-lag: the body needs time to adjust.

The circulation of Qi enables visualization of the geography of the meridians (Fig. 2.3). The Qi commences in the Yin Lung meridian, runs from the thorax down the inner surface of the arm and forearm to the tip of the thumb, where it transfers into the Yang Large Intestine meridian to

Figure 2.3 Schematic representation of Yin–Yang channels and the flow of Qi. (Redrawn with kind permission from Hopwood et al 1997.)

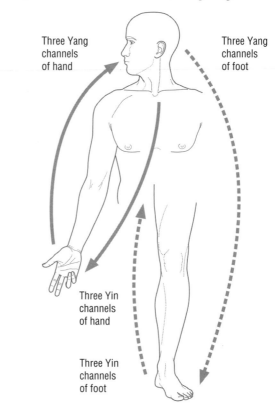

Three Yang channels of hand

Three Yang channels of foot

Three Yin channels of hand

Three Yin channels of foot

Figure 2.4 Circulation of Qi in the 12 channels.

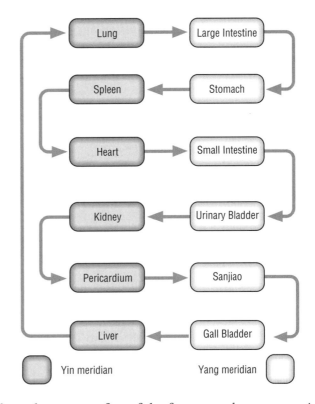

run back up the outer surface of the forearm and arm to terminate just below the nostril on the opposite side. (The Large Intestine meridian is in fact the only one to cross the midline.) The Qi runs from here into the Yang Stomach meridian, down the anterolateral aspect of the body and leg to the toes, where it joins the Yin Spleen meridian to run back up into the trunk. Thus, one-third of the 24-hour circulation is completed with the energy transferring from Yin to Yang meridians and covering the whole of the body. It then begins the process again, this time starting in the Yin Heart channel (Fig. 2.4).

Defining types of Qi

The list in Table 2.2 is for reference only, in order to clarify the exact nature of the Qi under discussion within any described syndrome. It will be clear that the nomenclature is variable, partly depending on translation but sometimes depending on variety in TCM theories.

Table 2.2 Classification of Qi

Category	Alternative names	Function
Central Qi	Zhong Qi, Zhong Jiao Qi	Qi found in the middle Jiao
Channel Qi	Jing Qi, Essence (Jing Luo Qi, also found in Luo vessels)	Vital energy found in the 12 principal channels
Clean Qi	Qing Qi	Pure fraction of that acquired through air and food

Continues

Table 2.2 cont'd

Category	Alternative names	Function
Collateral Qi	Luo Qi	Found in collaterals
Congenital Qi	Yuan Qi, Source Qi, Pre-Heaven Qi	Qi inherited from parents; one's constitution
Da Qi	Big Qi, Kong Qi	Vital energy acquired through breathing
Defensive Qi	Wei Qi	The Yang aspect of channel Qi; protects Blood, organs and tissues, and circulates outside the channels in the muscles, tendons and superficial tissues; defends the body from exogenous Pathogens
Grain Qi	Gu Qi, Nutritive Qi	Qi from food and drink (grain and water) Part of acquired Qi (Hou Tian Zhi Qi)
Internal Qi	Nei Qi	Found in more internal body regions; tends to be Yin in character
Jing Qi		Stored in Kidney; differs from Jing Luo Qi; essential energy derived from both Pre-Heaven and Post-Heaven Qi
Organ Qi	Zang Fu Zhi Qi	Qi present in the Zang Fu organs, maintaining their healthy functions
Qing Qi (see Clean Qi)	Post-Heaven Qi	Result of transformation of food by Spleen and of air by Lung
Ying Qi	Constructive Qi, Rong Qi, Xian Tian Zhi Qi	The Yin aspect of Channel Qi; nourishes Blood, organs and tissues
Zong Qi	Ancestral or Initial Qi	Differs from Congenital Qi: it is one's own original Qi and starts all Qi activity within the body
Zheng Qi	Zheng means 'correct'	Part of Zhen Qi protecting the body from pathogenic (or Xie) Qi
Zhen Qi	True Qi; Zhen means 'true'	All the Qi that nourishes the body, whatever the source

There are two basic categories to be borne in mind: that which is effectively inherited and unalterable and can loosely be compared with the genetic material, DNA, and that which can be altered and controlled, either in quality or distribution. A further subdivision can be into Yin and Yang types of energy.

The most important inference to be drawn from this discussion of the nature of Qi is that somehow, by stimulating the acupuncture points on the meridians, it seems to be possible to influence these complex and sophisticated physiological functions. The complicated aspect of this is that Qi and Blood are considered to circulate together in the meridians; often the two concepts are so closely linked that they cannot be separated.

Slowing or stagnation of the flow of Blood

Any obstacle to the free flow of blood will have implications for both the Qi and other Body fluids. The duration of the natural progression from youthful vigour to slow and cautious old age is dependent on the constitution. In TCM terms this is taken to mean the relative efficiency of the Qi and Blood activities and the basic physiology. This implies that the diagnosis of Blood stagnation becomes a very important one. Blood will be discussed as a single entity in the following pages, although it must be borne in mind that Qi and the other Body fluids are often flowing with it.

A severe pain in the tissues is often caused by either a deficiency of Qi or the stagnation of Qi and Blood. This pain is often quite superficial and associated with many musculoskeletal problems. It is characteristically a stabbing pain that does not move. There is a TCM saying that describes this well: 'Tong Zhi Bu Tong, Bu Tong Zhi Tong'. This translates very roughly as 'free flow, no pain'. The ideas of pain and the free flow of Blood and Qi are linked; the play on words depends on the pronunciation. The meaning is, literally, obstruction causes pain, removing the obstruction relieves the pain. This is a basic tenet of all acupuncture used for pain relief.

Stiffness in the joints is often the first sign of stagnation, although it may be relatively painless. If it progresses to serious pain, there may be echoes in lower layers and 'sickness' or physiological symptoms involving the Zang Fu organs.

Stagnation is relatively easy to palpate; light massage will indicate skin anomalies. These changes are largely functional and will not show up in any tests, radiographs, etc. When palpating the skin, a light brush with the fingertips will indicate skin that is trophically compromised: a roughness to the texture, a slight stickiness or greasiness to the fingertip, or the evidence of deep open pores will alert the therapist. The latter sign is sometimes called 'orange peel' skin and is quite distinctive (see cellulite, Ch. 11).

Degeneration of underlying joints may be present but is not necessarily a sign of stagnation; the two signs may exist independently. (This is similar to the radiographic evidence of osteoarthritic changes – these do not necessarily mean that the joint is painful.)

Two types of stagnation may be manifest in the superficial layers of the body – that of Qi and that of Blood – and both will respond to acupuncture. There is a TCM saying: 'The Blood nourishes the Qi and the Qi leads the Blood'. Qi is more Yang than Blood, which tends to be Yin. It is relatively easy to distinguish between them; the main points are given in Box 2.1.

Box 2.1   Qi or Blood stagnation?

Qi stagnation	Blood stagnation
Dull pain	Sharp, strong pain
Less severe pain	Severe pain
Mobile	Fixed
Palpable changes less likely	Clearly palpable by therapist; dry, scaly skin. Possible varicosities
Patient vague about location	Patient indicates clearly
Affected by stress or emotion	Unaffected
Improves with gentle massage	No immediate improvement with light massage, but deep, invigorating massage may help in treatment
Responds to acupuncture	Responds to acupuncture
Distal acupuncture points are most important	Fixed local points are more effective; these may include Ah Shi and Extra points
Overall regulation of body energy required	Does not affect internal functions

The acupuncture points generally recommended for moving stagnation of the Blood are listed in Table 2.3. All stagnation is considered as a Shi (Full or Excess) condition, but as it may occur only locally this could be within a context of overall Xu (or Deficiency). Stagnation may, of course, be due simply to local trauma; a visible haematoma is a good example of this. Another helpful TCM phrase is: 'An island of Shi in a sea of Xu'.

The excess may vary in type. It may be full or empty in nature. When *full*, the pain is worse on waking in the morning or after a period of inactivity. When *empty*, the pain is worse after activity and in the evening; the patient has little energy, which is soon used up.

There is a need to identify the type of stagnation in order to treat it successfully. However, stagnation is a problem associated with most diseases of the elderly and is consequently difficult to treat: owing to a general decrease in the abundance and energy of Qi, there will be a tendency to relapse (see Ch. 12).

From a physiotherapeutic point of view, the use of light massage to stimulate the superficial circulation makes good sense. Use of the TCM adjunctive technique of cupping is also relevant. Improving the oxygen exchange in the tissues by increasing subcutaneous perfusion will clearly improve the health of the tissues and increase their resistance to minor injury or infection.

Table 2.3   Blood stagnation points

	Acupuncture points
Upper body	LI 11, LI 4, Lu 7, Lu 5
Lower body	St 36, St 41, Sp 10, Sp 6

Fluids or Jin Ye

The circulation of fluids is important to Chinese Medicine and quite easy to understand. Western medical professionals have a concept of interstitial fluid draining into the lymph system and thus returning to the circulation. Problems will arise if this event is prevented, perhaps by mechanical blockage or congestion in the lymph nodes. The TCM idea is similar, but described in different terms.

Figure 2.5 shows the basic circulation of the Jin Ye fluids. It is intimately connected with the flow of Qi around the body, and the Qi provides the energy for much of it. Air enters the Lungs and is transformed into a clear fluid that is sent downwards, through the body to the Kidneys. The Kidneys separate the impure from the pure, and provide the Yang energy for the pure fraction to rise back up to the Lungs. The impure fluid is sent to the Bladder for excretion as urine. The constant cycle of energy involving the Lungs and the Kidneys is responsible for the movement of fluid generally within the body. Additional energy is provided to the Lungs by the Spleen, which in turn requires energy from the Kidneys.

Thus there are two constant cycles for fluids. Fluids ingested by the mouth enter the system via the Stomach and subsequently the Spleen, which handles the pure fraction. The rest continues through the system to the Small Intestine, where solids and fluids are separated for the Large Intestine and the Bladder.

The clinical importance of this lies in the symptoms of late-onset asthma. The typical wheezing present in this condition is due not so much to damage within the Lung but more to lack of Kidney energy to enable the clearance of fluids from the Lung. This Kidney energy is frequently depleted in old age and the respiratory situation will be difficult to control but will certainly respond better to treatment aimed at supporting the Kidneys.

When the circulation of fluids is not regulated, there is often a problem of Kidney Yang not controlling Kidney Yin. Essential heat must not cease;

Figure 2.5 Diagram showing Jin Ye circulation.

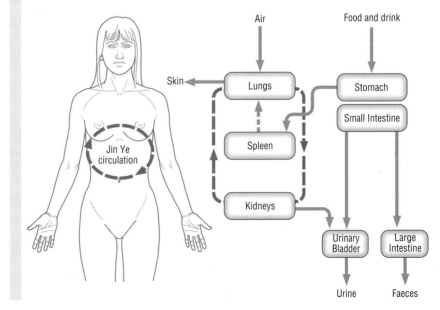

Box 2.2 Differentiation of Jin and Ye

Jin	Ye
Yang	Yin
Thin, clear	Thick
Watery	Sticky
Found superficially under the skin	Found in Zang Fu
Perfuses and warms the tissues and the whole Sanjiao	Not flowing with Qi and Blood
	Functions as moistening lubricant
Flows with Qi and Blood	Found in bone marrow, joints and
Include sweat, tears, saliva and urine	deep Yin areas of the body

if it does, the body cannot remain warm, respiration falters and food cannot be digested. With a deficiency of Kidney Yang the person feels cold and is cold to the touch, and symptoms manifest such as diarrhoea, frequent or incontinent urine, infertility, impotence, premature ejaculation, loss of hearing or ringing in the ears. The Kidney is generally undermined by excessive exercise, sexual activity, work or too little sleep.

Probably the most important organ with regard to the circulation of fluids is the Spleen. If the Spleen is underpowered, for whatever reason, it will fail in its role to transform and transport food and drink. Dampness, an accumulation of fluid in the Spleen, may result. This is an internal form of the Pathogen Damp and is by definition a secondary byproduct of Spleen Qi Xu and Yang deficiency. The many ways in which the Spleen energy can be compromised are discussed in Chapter 3.

The two types of fluid have different functions and are found in different parts of the body (Box 2.2). Some, the Jin or clear fluids, are familiar to us; the Ye fluid is a concept very specific to TCM and is best thought of as a lubricating type of interstitial fluid.

Sweat

Sweat is just another form that may be taken by the Body fluids and is closely linked with urine in that both vary according to the condition of the other and both are dependent on the general Body fluid status. Although sweat is associated with great physical effort, a high ambient temperature or internal fever, in fact it is discharged through the pores in a continual though imperceptible process.

TCM theory considers sweat to be the fluid of the Heart. A deficiency of Heart Yang Qi can lead to night sweats. The production of sweat is considered to be dependent on Jin fluids being 'steamed out' by Yang energy. This Yang energy is provided mostly by the Kidney. The Yin fluids are derived from the Essence (Jing Qi) and from the ingested food and fluid. Sweating is normal activity and occurs when the clothing is too thick or the weather too hot. Conversely, when the weather is cold the pores in the surface tissues close and the fluid is retained. This fluid passes down to the Urinary Bladder, becoming urine and being excreted, while the Qi is retained and returned to the body circulation. This is the TCM explanation of why the desire to urinate increases in very cold weather.

The above circumstances are all part of normal physiology but the retention of excess sweat can be considered dangerous to health, as is the excessive loss of fluid by sweating. The quality and quantity of sweat is an important diagnostic factor, as is the site of the sweating and the time of day that it occurs. This is a complex subject, beyond the remit of this book to describe. It is covered well in Clavey's book which is recommended as further reading (Clavey 1995).

TCM has a saying: 'Profuse sweating leads to the collapse of Yang'. Pathological sweating, that not in response to activity or unnecessary clothing, leads to a loss not only of Body fluids but also of Wei Qi. If this is severe and prolonged, it can be very dangerous. It is seen in myocardial infarction and in some types of stroke. The sweating can be both a cause and a symptom of the condition.

The following is a brief guide only. If the condition is considered to be a relatively external one, then sweating indicates deficiency, whereas a lack of sweat indicates an excess. If the condition is considered to have become internalized, then sweating may indicate several things: it could be due to Damp Heat, a deficiency of either Yin or Yang, or a simple excess of Yang. A quaintly named condition, 'five palm sweat', where sweating is noted on the palms of the hands, soles of the feet and the chest, indicates a Yin deficiency and is often described in syndrome differentiation.

Tears

When sorrow takes hold of the Heart, the largest vessel (which is imagined in TCM to connect the Heart to the other Zang Fu organs) spasms, causing Lung Qi to rise. As the Lung Qi rises (the reverse of normal Lung Qi movement), the fluids also rush upwards. This cannot be sustained, so repeated rising and falling occurs, giving rise to spasm of the diaphragm in the action of sobbing. The throat is tightened; tears, runny nose and occasionally coughing result.

Tears are often referred to as the fluid of the Liver, because the Liver opens into the eyes. Tears arising from hurt or anger have been termed Liver Yin Rising, although this is not a frequently described syndrome.

Tears from emotional upset are considered normal. They can also be caused by pathological Wind, Heat, Wind Cold invasion or Excess Fire in the Liver or Gall Bladder channels, or by any other condition that forces the upward movement of Body fluid. Liver Blood may fail to rise and nourish the eyes, causing watering of the eyes. This is usually associated with an invasion of Cold.

There is some scientific evidence that there are two forms of tears. The response we make when, for example, the surface of the eye is irritated while cutting up onions is a purely protective response to prevent damage. The tears produced as an emotional response to some psychological trauma, such as grief or sorrow, have a different physiological composition and contain 25% more protein. They also contain traces of hormones, particularly adrenocorticotrophic hormone (ACTH). This makes some sense of the folk wisdom that 'having a good cry will make you feel better'. Possibly this is in part a hormonal response. Laughter and tears have much in common: laughing until one cries is a fairly common phenomenon.

The Metal element in Five Element theory is associated with the emotion of grief. Attachment and detachment can be linked with inspiration and expiration, and thus violent movement of the diaphragm. The Metal element is about bonding and then letting go. When loss occurs, grief is the result. For this reason the Metal element is also associated with tears. Disturbances also tend to occur in the Large Intestine meridian when the patient is unable to let go of an idea or emotion.

Saliva

Saliva is classified into two quite different types (Box 2.3), although it is generally considered as a part of the clear Body fluids, the Jin. Saliva is thought to be produced by the Spleen, which also has the responsibility for the sense of taste. The other form of saliva is linked with the Kidneys and is classified as mucoid saliva. It arises from a flooding of water due to weakness of Kidney Yang and the subsequent rising of this fluid to the mouth. To improve this situation, stimulation of Kidney Yang and support of fluid circulation would be the treatment of choice. This may not be possible with acupuncture alone, and may require the addition of TCM herbal medicine.

There is another type of mucoid saliva produced by Spleen and Stomach deficiency following the overconsumption of cold or raw foods. Treatment for this involves warming of the middle Jiao and supporting the Spleen function of transportation.

Excessive salivation is treated by St 40 Fenglong and Sp 3 Taibai, the source point for the Spleen. If there is a Yin deficiency, the fluids are too abundant and Ren 4 Guanyuan and Ren 6 Qihai can be used to reinforce the Yin. The type of dribbling found in young children is said to arise from Stomach Heat, and this could be due to inappropriately spicy food or parasitic accumulation.

The acupuncture treatment of xerostomia, or lack of saliva, has been investigated by List et al (1998). Electroacupuncture proved to be a successful treatment modality for this relatively rare condition, although the authors noted that the tissue in the salivary glands needed to be viable. Unfortunately, some cytotoxic drugs can induce xerostomia artificially.

Box 2.3   Types of saliva

Xian	Tuo
Watery in nature	Mucoid in nature
Fluid of the Spleen	Fluid of the Kidneys
Spleen opens to the mouth	Produced from beneath the tongue;
Spleen Qi Xu leads to drooling	the internal branch of the Kidney
Dry mouth results from Spleen	channel runs to the base of the
Yin Xu, which in turn could	tongue
be caused by Stomach or	
Heart Fire	

Mucus	Nasal mucus is said to be the fluid of the Lungs. It is entirely normal and functions as a moisturizing agent of the nasal membranes. If the usual descending and spreading function of the Lung is impaired, mucus is produced in greater quantities and serves as a sign of Lung pathology. The obvious example here is the common cold – an invasion of Lung tissue by the Cold or Wind Pathogens, resulting in a runny nose.
Urine	The amount of urine produced by the body depends on the amount of available fluid. TCM theory agrees with modern physiology in that urine is viewed as a waste product arising from the metabolism. The excretion of urine is controlled by the Urinary Bladder, but obviously the Kidney is closely involved and other Zang Fu organs such as the Spleen, Lungs, Sanjiao and Small Intestine have a part to play in the transformation and transportation of this fluid. The Kidneys receive some of the fluid constituting urine from the Lungs, a proportion is returned as vapour, and the rest is passed to the Bladder for excretion (see Fig. 2.5).
	The power of the Urinary Bladder to contain the urine is directly dependent on the strength of Kidney Qi. Weakness of Kidney Qi can lead to pathological frequency or incontinence. Night incontinence, enuresis or bed-wetting is caused by a Kidney deficiency manifesting only at night, when Yang Qi is generally weaker. Weakness of Kidney Qi can also cause other urinary problems such as incomplete emptying of the bladder and constant dribbling of urine. Generally a deficiency in Kidney Yang causes an increase in the amount of urine, and a deficiency of Kidney Yin will result in decreased urine production. Weakness of Kidney Yang is also apparent in lower-body oedema.
	Retention of urine is considered to be the result of Damp Heat in the Bladder. Urinary tract infections are generally regarded as being due to Damp Heat, but the trigger can be either an external Pathogen or internal Heat. Pale, dilute, copious urine indicates a Cold pattern, and dark, concentrated urine denotes a Heat pattern. Figure 2.6 indicates the origin and normal direction of the Jin fluids.
Water pattern diseases	The most commonly encountered of these is oedema. The water may accumulate in the upper Jiao producing puffiness of the face, in the middle Jiao producing a feeling of bloatedness in the epigastrium, and in the lower Jiao as frank oedema that demonstrates 'pitting'. Cellulitis can be considered as a form of this type of oedema.
	Water within the tissues that is not moving or part of the immediate circulation is sometimes termed 'dilute Phlegm' or 'Phlegm turbidity'. The tendency to slow down or become sticky is part of this manifestation of Damp. Examples of this are the thinner forms of mucus expectorated from the lungs; clear, frothy phlegm vomited from the stomach; and oedema of the limbs where the body looks swollen but there is no evidence of pitting. Phlegm is capable of congealing and becoming quite solid. This can take the form of gallstones, kidney stones, arthritic bone deformities and atherosclerosis (described below in the section on the Bi syndrome).

Figure 2.6 Origin and normal direction of the Jin fluids.

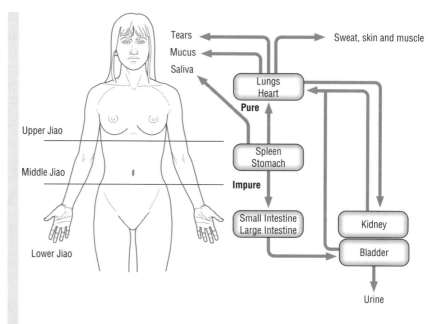

The meridians themselves become involved in this process and may exhibit superficial oedema in the interstitial spaces just below the skin. This area is controlled mainly by the Lung, which is used clinically to decrease this type of superficial fluid stagnation.

Remobilization of the stagnant fluid is achieved by treating the Spleen, the Lungs and the Kidneys, as the Kidneys are responsible for providing the Yang energy to the Spleen to accomplish normal function. Some authorities claim that it is possible to treat cellulite in this way, but the results are at best equivocal. It is generally thought that cellulite is only a symptom of a more serious internal slowing of fluid circulation, and this also should be addressed.

Different points are used for predominantly Yang-type or Yin-type oedema (Box 2.4), although acupuncture needles should never actually be inserted into a seriously oedematous area. If this occurs, inadvertently, the loss of some Body fluids must be expected because the fluid is being held under pressure in the interstitial spaces of the tissues. Care must be taken to avoid any possibility of infection, and a dry dressing applied immediately.

Box 2.4 Points for oedema

YIN	YANG
UB 20 Pishu	UB 22 Sanjiaoshu
UB 23 Shenshu	UB 13 Feishu
St 36 Zusanli	Sp 9 Yinlingquan
Ren 6 Qihai	Ren 9 Shuifen
Sp 6 Sanyinjiao	LI 4 Hegu
UB 39 Weiyang	St 37 Shangjuxu

| **Breast milk** | Although obviously a Body fluid, there is little information available about breast milk; however, there is a strange convention in Chinese Medicine that breast milk is transformed menstrual blood. It is said to be transformed from the Qi and Blood of the Ren and Chong channels, moving up to produce breast milk and down to form the menstrual flow. A long labour can lead to a depletion of Qi and insufficient milk. To restore Qi, the best points are St 36 Zusanli and Sp 6 Sanyinjiao, and GB 41 Foot Linqi and Ren 17 Shanzhong can be used to clear the obstruction. Local points are not advisable. |

| **The relevance of these theories to current practice** | The evolution of the TCM theories of Qi, Blood and Body fluids is an interesting one, which in some ways is still continuing. Readers who wish to pursue these ideas further in their Chinese context should read Professor Yan's book, *Ageing and Blood Stasis*. This excellent and scholarly book explores the ancient TCM theories in order to support the idea that Blood stasis is the root and cause of all the processes implicit in ageing (Yan 2000). |

However, it is self-evident to a Western medical practitioner that blood (or plasma) pooling in the tissues is going to lead to problems. Whether the pooling is, in fact, caused by the invasion of a Pathogen blocking the meridians and smaller collaterals is not really the issue – that was a convenient and logical way of explaining things 2000 years ago.

We look at stagnation differently now. It may arise because there is heart disease with the heart muscle not beating so strongly, perhaps because its own blood supply is diminished (coronary heart disease), the patency of the valves may be compromised (endocarditis) or the lumen of the blood vessels may be narrowed (arteriosclerosis); there may be pathologically high or low blood pressure. The list of causes is long and they do not all involve the heart. Trauma may have a part to play – damage to tissues by external trauma producing easily understandable haematoma. Stagnation may also arise from failure of the muscles to function correctly, or even at all, as in the case of paralysis where the problem lies with damage to the nerve. Less serious than paralysis perhaps, but causing insidious and long-term damage and a great deal of pain, is overuse or inappropriate use of muscle groups, for whatever reason. Repetitive strain injury is a good example of TCM stagnation.

We cannot dismiss the TCM ideas out of hand. The language may be archaic and the search to find things written 2–3000 years ago to justify modern thought is often overzealous, but nevertheless the links between supposed cause and effect were observed meticulously. The Chinese doctors observed the symptoms of chronic heart disease and surmised, quite correctly, that the heart was failing in its function of pumping the blood around the body. That they attributed this to 'Phlegm obstructing the Heart Orifices' is only semantics, as the points that they selected over many, many years of trial still appear to have some value (Ballegaard et al 1993).

What is more fascinating is that their idea that an 'uprush of Liver Wind', taking with it Qi and Blood, was the cause of Windstroke or stroke.

This, on the surface, may seem like just another quaint and outdated idea, but the symptoms leading to diagnosis of Liver Wind and Fire correlate very well with modern ideas about high blood pressure, considered to be one of the main risk factors for stroke (Juvela et al 1995). They also correlate rather well with the idea of a relatively sedentary, self-indulgent lifestyle with excessive consumption of alcohol, believed by both medical paradigms to be damaging to the liver (Gill et al 1986).

Three major groups of disease with clear links to the Qi and Blood theories are discussed in the last part of this chapter: Bi syndrome, cardiovascular disease and stroke. They will be listed in brief by their TCM titles under the syndromes in Chapter 8 with suggested points for treatment, although the research references are given at the end of this chapter.

Bi syndrome

It may seem odd to insert one of the most important TCM syndromes into this chapter but Bi syndrome has a vital connection with the general health and circulation of the Body fluids. As explained previously, the Body fluid is in a constant state of movement, whether Blood flowing in blood vessels or the interstitial fluid moving between the structures and under the skin, or the more precisely defined Jin Ye fluids.

When pathogenic factors invade the body, they enter the most superficial meridians, particularly the Urinary Bladder and Small Intestine, and cause a general slowing of the flow. This affects both Qi and Blood. When fluids are slowed they tend to thicken, stagnate and become sticky. This process is the beginning of the formation of what is defined in TCM as Phlegm.

Each of the external pathogenic factors (Fig. 2.7) produces characteristic symptoms, and this leads to the different classifications of Bi syndrome, which is also sometimes called painful obstruction syndrome.

Wind invasion

Wind invasion is characterized by mobility; the resulting pain tends to be acute and to move randomly from one area of the body to another. The muscles and joints are sore, but the quality of the pain can change quickly, sometimes manifesting as numbness or at other times as a sharp pain.

As Wind is a Yang Pathogen, it tends to affect the upper part of the body, often typified by an upward movement. The symptoms can appear and disappear very suddenly. This type of Bi is known as Wandering Bi or Migratory Bi.

The patient usually expresses a fear of wind or describes increased discomfort in windy weather. It is rare that only Wind is involved; there are usually elements of Damp and Cold as well, but Wind is predominant.

Figure 2.7 External pathogenic factors.

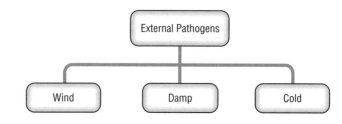

There may be sweating due to the opening of the pores by the invading Wind. Box 2.5 gives suggested acupuncture points for Wind Bi.

Cold invasion

Cold invasion is characterized by severe pain and limitation of movement, and is often called Painful Bi. It is usually unilateral. The pain is often described as deep and 'gnawing'. The Cold is perceived as being capable of freezing the tissues, contracting and blocking the meridian. Any blockage of the meridian produces pain. The pain with Cold has a constant site, and is frequently accompanied by loss of joint movement, mainly due to the accompanying blood stagnation.

This type of pain is always improved by warmth and movement but made worse by cold and rest, and is described as being worse in cold weather. Although an accepted physiotherapy treatment for some arthritic conditions, cryotherapy is not recommended for the pain produced by this type of pathogenic invasion. See Box 2.6 for suggested acupuncture points.

Damp invasion

Damp invasion is characterized by soreness and swelling in the muscles and joints with a feeling of heaviness and numbness in the limbs. It is worse in damp weather. It generally has a slow onset. It is sometimes referred to as Fixed Bi, because it is very localized. Where Wandering or Wind Bi tends to affect the upper part of the body, this tends to sink to the lowest level as liquid would. There is a feeling of heaviness, tiredness and inertia in the limbs, and the affected parts are often swollen. The pain is heavy and dull in nature and onset is gradual. The skin is often affected, becoming thickened and slightly discoloured. The patient feels worse when the weather conditions are humid, damp or foggy. Box 2.7 suggests some acupuncture points.

Box 2.5 Suggested points for Wind Bi

- UB 12 Fengmen
- Du 14 Dazhui
- UB 18 Ganshu
- GB 31 Fengshi
- UB 17 Geshu

All points to clear Wind except UB 17 and UB 18, which nourish Blood in order to expel the Pathogen.

Box 2.6 Suggested points for Cold Bi

- St 36 Zusanli
- Ren 6 Qihai
- UB 10 Tianzhu
- Du 14 Dazhui
- Du 3 Yaoyangguan
- UB 23 Shenshu

Use moxibustion as a source of heat.

Box 2.7 Suggested points for Damp Bi

- Sp 9 Yinlingquan
- Sp 6 Sanyinjiao
- GB 34 Yanglingquan
- St 36 Zusanli
- UB 20 Pishu

All points clear Damp and aid the movement of Qi.

Heat Bi

Heat Bi can be the invasion of the body by an external Heat Pathogen or it can arise from an invasion by the other Pathogens (Wind, Cold and Damp) that has already occurred. It presents a complex picture when arising as a superficial syndrome because it often involves symptoms characteristic of the other Pathogens. Some authorities describe this situation as the result of Wei Qi opposing invading Pathogens.

The patient will have red, swollen and painful joints. There will be marked loss of movement, as in acute inflammatory arthritic conditions. The patient is also likely to show some signs of systemic illness, with fever, a hot sensation in the affected tissue, irritability, nervousness or restlessness, thirst and a dry mouth. Further heat of any kind makes the patient uncomfortable.

There is a TCM saying: 'Better Cold than Heat'. This is a useful guide to treatment priorities: it is nearly always better to clear Heat first. This is primarily because it is more difficult to clear Heat than to provide Heat. Also, if the Cold condition is treated first by applying Heat, perhaps in the form of moxibustion, the Heat condition would be made worse, perhaps increasing the pain. Box 2.8 gives suggested acupuncture points.

All the forms of Bi syndrome discussed so far represent an acute type of condition, with the potential for leading to an Excess internal syndrome (Fig. 2.8).

Bony Bi

Bony Bi is the end result of the slowing and congealing of the Body fluids and subsequent Phlegm in the joint spaces. The deformity of the joints that results is seen as an accumulation of solidified Phlegm. There is often severe pain and a marked loss of range of movement. The patient complains of heaviness and numbness in the affected limb. Bony spurs around the joint margins can be seen on radiography.

This situation is strongly linked with the Kidney. The connection between Kidney and bone formation is cited, but also this type of Bi syndrome takes a long time to evolve and is usually associated with the advent

Box 2.8 Suggested points for Heat Bi

- LI 11 Quchi
- LI 4 Hegu
- Du 14 Dazhui

Use meridian endpoints, Spring, Well and Stream points.

Figure 2.8 Progression of Bi syndrome from external to internal.

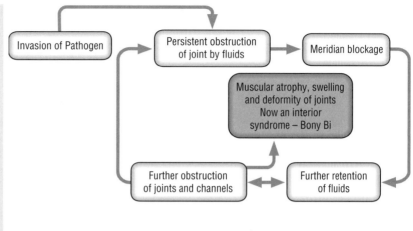

Box 2.9 Suggested points for Bony Bi

- St 40 Fenglong
- UB 23 Shenshu
- UB 11 Dashu
- GB 39 Xuanzhong

These points are used to clear Phlegm and to strengthen Kidney and bone.

of old age and general weakening of Kidney energies. It may be complicated by osteoporosis. Box 2.9 gives suggested points.

The preceding forms of Bi syndrome are those that the average physiotherapist would be most likely to treat in normal practice. However, it must be understood that the changes leading to these joint problems and observed symptoms are not confined only to the joints. Bi syndrome can be interpreted as a blockage of Qi and Blood capable of attacking any body system. This is often seen as a progression from the involvement of a tissue to the involvement of one of the major Zang Fu organs (see Ch. 3).

The Zang Fu links obey the laws of TCM:

- Tendon Bi can lead to problems with the Liver.
- Vascular Bi can lead to Heart problems.
- Muscle Bi will have an impact on the Spleen.
- Skin Bi will affect the Lung.
- Bony Bi is closely linked with Kidney Bi.

Tendon–Liver Bi

This is of particular interest to physiotherapists as it is always linked to pain and weakness in muscles and joints. These joints tend to flexion contracture as in Dupuytren's contracture, resisting passive extension. Previous physical trauma may contribute to this condition, as in the case of chronic whiplash syndrome. Frequent urination may be a symptom, along with a marked increase in appetite. The patient often complains of a feeling of cold within the tendons. Sciatica is sometimes considered as a form of Tendon Bi. There may be a degree of irritability and other mental symptoms indicating the involvement of the Liver.

Local points will be most successful to warm and free the channels and to relax the tendons, but distal points, particularly Shu Stream points (see Ch. 5) are also helpful. The Liver will need support: UB 18 Ganshu or GB 34 Yanglingquan.

Vascular–Heart Bi

This is most commonly identified by numbness and pins and needles, accompanied by pain and soreness in the affected area. The pain itself is stabbing and fixed, often worse at night – typical of that caused by Blood stagnation. The pulse will be weak or may even disappear, indicating the blockage and resulting emptiness of the blood vessels. This form of Bi syndrome has been compared to arteritis in Western medicine.

The fact that Vascular–Heart Bi is linked to general circulatory disturbances means that there may be accompanying symptoms such as skin changes, light rashes, and a feeling of fullness in the body giving rise to general unease and malaise. As the Shen or spirit is disturbed by the involvement of the Heart, there may be marked anxiety and distress, continuous sighing and overbreathing. This may lead to a form of late-onset asthma.

This problem is linked directly with smoking and an overindulgent lifestyle. The link made between smoking and arterial disease in Western medicine is too obvious for comment here. Internal Heat produced by the excess food and alcohol may be responsible for the decrease of Yin and Qi, leading to easy invasion by the Wind, Cold and Damp.

The following points may be used to relieve Blood stasis: LI 4 Hegu, LI 10 Shousanli, SJ 6 Zhigou, Ren 12 Zhongwan, Sp 10 Xuehai, Sp 6 Sanyinjiao, St 36 Zusanli, St 40 Fenglong. Some of these points could be added to the local points used for the painful joint.

Muscle–Spleen Bi

The characteristic signs of Muscle Bi are stiffness and coldness in the muscle group. It is not really the function of the muscle, rather the muscle bulk, that is affected. This means that there may be a degree of muscle atrophy and loss of strength. There will be generalized weakness and easy fatigue with only small effort, with excessive sweating. The Zang Fu function of the Spleen is to maintain muscle bulk from the transformation of food, so there is a direct TCM link to the digestive process and the patient may also have symptoms of indigestion. Overindulgence at the table is implicated as a partial cause of the Spleen problems. The Spleen symptoms may also include shortness of breath, a tight feeling in the chest, an occasional productive cough, loss of appetite and poor digestion. Examination of the tongue is helpful; the characteristic tooth-marked body of the tongue will indicate the involvement of the Zang Fu.

The selection of Jing River points will be important as these points give rise to an overflow of Qi into the so-called 'muscle sinews' or 'tendino-muscular meridians'. As in the other categories, use local and distal points to the affected joints.

Skin–Lung Bi

The characteristic symptoms of this syndrome are a cold sensation and often numbness of the skin. The link with the Lung (the skin is governed by the Lungs), may mean that there is shortness of breath, manifested in rapid superficial panting. The Wei Qi, produced by the Lungs, should circulate just below the skin; this is prevented in Skin Bi. This syndrome is thought to occur more commonly when the patient is grieving or seriously worried about something.

Points to support the Lungs and strengthen the Wei Qi could be useful with Yintang to raise the spirits. The cause of the grief or anxiety should be addressed, if possible.

Bone–Kidney Bi

The characteristic symptoms of soreness and pain in the joints are usually accompanied by stiffness and lack of mobility. Patients occasionally complain of heaviness in the affected limb. Kidney energies are said to decrease with advancing age, so the fact that the joints and the spine tend to become stiff and limited in movement, resulting in the need to walk with some kind of artificial aid in this syndrome, tallies quite clearly with the universal picture of old age. This will be described in more detail in Chapter 3.

As is the way with most medicine, although some symptoms may be collected together in clear groups to form the syndromes, patients rarely present with such a clear pattern. Rheumatoid arthritis is one such situation – a well known collection of symptoms with a complex Bi picture.

Rheumatoid arthritis

This condition is a good example of a Bi syndrome and can usefully be subdivided into two types of Bi: Cold Damp Bi and Damp Heat Bi.

Cold Damp Bi is characterized by stiff swollen and aching joints, with early morning stiffness in particular. These joints are improved by heat and warmth, and worse in cold or wet weather. There is usually a feeling of heaviness and coldness. There is no redness or heat in the joints. The tongue is pale and swollen, with a thin white greasy coating. The pulse may be slippery and thready.

Damp Heat Bi is characterized by swollen, stiff, painful joints that are red and warm to the touch. The pain is often described as 'burning'. The patient may display signs of mild fever, lethargy and loss of appetite. The tongue may be slightly red with a greasy yellow coating. The pulse may be rapid and slippery, or thready and wiry.

These two types of Bi may exist independently or may coexist in different joints in the same patient. All the acupuncturist can do is try to isolate the predominant pattern and attempt to treat that first. Better still, try to select points that have a dual action and will expel all types of Pathogen.

Research

Research into the effect of acupuncture on rheumatoid arthritis has been dominated by one study of poor quality that used a single point (Liv 3 Taichong) as treatment (David et al 1999). The authors have claimed that this trial was set up to test the possibilities of achieving the conditions of a good randomized controlled clinical trial using acupuncture. However, as the study was published in a reputable journal, it has had a wide circulation among medical practitioners who did not appreciate the very limited quality of the acupuncture intervention. The single point, Liv 3, was used, with an insertion time of only 4 minutes and a total of five treatments. As the results for the efficacy of this form of acupuncture were predictably bad, there has been quite a lot of resistance from doctors to the use of acupuncture by physiotherapists in this field.

Scientific acupuncturists, chiefly Tukmachi (2000), have responded with direct criticism of the acupuncture protocol, pointing out that the solitary use of Liv 3 has only a single anecdotal evidence source, that treatment has been shown to be most effective at 30 minutes (Thomas 1995), that clinical experience indicates that five treatments will not be sufficient, and that the full range of acupuncture techniques including moxa and electro-acupuncture were not considered. All parties have agreed that further work is necessary, but the damage is done.

Cardiovascular disease

TCM theories tend to complexity in this field, and some attempt will be made here to rationalize them and relate them to Western categories of disease. The original causes of the disharmonies and imbalances are understood very much in Western terms, and are summarized below (Fig. 2.9.)

The only unusual factor in the collection of causes is cold weather or the Pathogen Cold. This is not thought to affect the Heart directly, but could certainly be considered to affect the peripheral circulation, closing down superficial vessels and thus obstructing Qi and Blood. The link between the emotions and heart disease has long been suspected by folk medicine, acknowledging the pathogenic effect of a 'broken heart', but perhaps only recently has the concept of 'bodymind' gained acceptance and highlighted this sort of influence on disease processes.

The syndromes tend to polarize into those of Excess or Deficiency, as in Box 2.10. Chest Painful Obstruction is the collective term used for the syn-

Figure 2.9 TCM causes of cardiovascular disharmony.

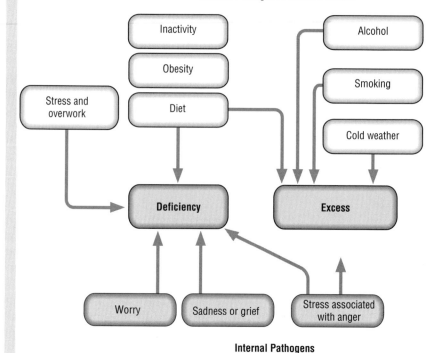

Box 2.10 TCM patterns of cardiovascular disharmony

Excess		
Stagnation of Qi and Blood in chest	Liver Yang rising	Stagnation of Qi
Stagnation of Phlegm in chest	Liver Wind stirring	Stagnation of Blood
Stagnation of cold in chest	Liver Fire	Obstruction of channels by Phlegm
		Obstruction by internal Damp Heat
Angina	**Hypertension**	**Peripheral vascular problems**
Heart Yang Xu	Kidney Yang Xu	Qi Xu
Kidney Yang Xu	Liver and Kidney Yin Xu	Blood Xu
Spleen Yang Xu	Heart Yin Xu	Yin or Yang Xu
Liver Yin Xu		
Deficiency		

(Acknowledgements to C. Donellan)

dromes listed in the bottom left-hand corner of Box 2.10. These all give rise to Phlegm and Blood stasis, similar to that discussed in the preceding section on Bi syndrome, as the Qi does not warm or move the Blood. This in turn manifests as angina-type pain. Western medical practitioners have been interested in the effect of acupuncture on angina pain, and Richter et al (1991) published a randomized crossover study which showed that acupuncture used at traditional points was of additional benefit to a group of patients with angina pectoris.

Palpitations are an important symptom in TCM, indicating the type of heart disease present. A weak constitution, prolonged illness or overstrain may result in a deficiency of Qi, Blood, Yin and Yang. A lengthy state of apprehension or worry may cause poor nourishment of the Heart due to the consumption of Heart Blood. The consequence of either of these factors will be a Deficiency-type palpitation. On the other hand, stagnation of Heart Qi, causing a disturbance of Phlegm Fire, or an accumulation of internal Phlegm Heat due to poor Spleen function, can result in disturbance of the Heart by these pathogenic combinations. There will tend to be an excess type of palpitation with irritability, anxiety and dream-disturbed sleep.

Heart Qi Xu is characterized by occasional palpitations and shortness of breath. The patient is usually very pale and lacking in vitality. Heart Qi Xu is often caused by long chronic illnesses, particularly those involving long-term blood loss such as very heavy periods (menorrhagia). There will be a forceless pulse and a pale tongue. At the same time, because of the link between the Heart and the emotions, emotional distress can also lead to a deficiency of Heart Qi.

Stagnation of Heart Blood may also cause palpitations and is usually identified by a purplish tongue and lips, and a thready, hesitant pulse with missed beats.

Box 2.10 shows how these TCM syndromes fit in with regard to the major Western classification of heart disease.

Figure 2.10
Differentiation of Heart
disease.

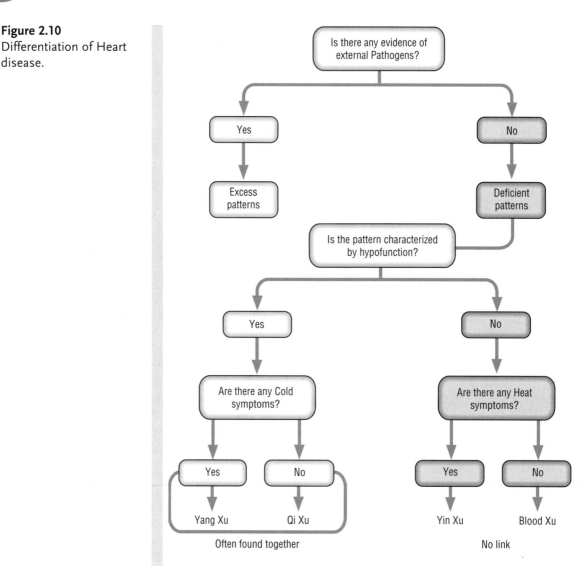

The diagnostic pattern for establishing the basis for the Heart disease is interesting. The differentiation between Yin and Yang and between Deficiency and Excess (Fig. 2.10) is important, and follows the algorithm given by Li & Zhao (1993), which can then be related back to Box 2.10.

While interesting from a theoretical point of view, this type of TCM differentiation is unlikely to fall within normal physiotherapy practice, as physiotherapists are more actively involved in rehabilitation processes. Acupuncture treatment in cardiac pathologies should never be undertaken without the agreement of the patient's physician.

Stroke or Windstroke

There are many factors involved in a stroke or, in TCM terms, Windstroke. The causes are mostly associated with the Liver but the sequelae or aftereffects have much to do with stagnation of Blood and Qi.

The different categories of Windstroke are shown in Box 2.11. That affecting the collaterals, viewed as very superficial damage, is usually only

Box 2.11 Differentiation of Windstroke

Structures affected				
Collaterals	**Channels**	**Yang organs**	**Yin organs**	**Sequelae**
External Wind	Internal Wind	Internal Wind	Internal Wind	Qi Xu
Weak Wei Qi	Liver and Kidney Yin Deficiency			Blood stasis
Numbness in extremities, minimal motor impairment Mild facial paralysis	Hemiplegia Facial paralysis Stiff tongue	Coma Hemiplegia Constipation Retention of urine	Coma Hemiplegia Cold limbs Double incontinence	Conscious Hemiplegia, hemiparesis Facial paralysis Speech problems

transient and equates well with a transient ischaemic attack (TIA) in Western medicine. The main symptoms are likely to be numbness in the extremities with some transient signs in the facial muscles. These events are seen as precursors of major stroke or as warning events in both medical paradigms.

Internal Wind, arising from the Liver, is a more serious problem and affects the channels, leading initially to headache, dizziness and difficulty remaining upright. This may ultimately result in hemiplegia in the limbs and some paralysis of the face. The facial paralysis is often identified in TCM by clear deviation of the mouth with a stiff tongue, causing difficulty with speech.

The Yang organ type is also caused by Internal Wind and is characterized by heat with loss of fluids and subsequent constipation and retention of urine. Owing to the Yang nature of this manifestation, there may be brief loss of consciousness and spasm in some of the muscles, followed by paralysis.

Liver and Kidney Yin Deficiency cause the Yin type of Windstroke. This is indicated by a sudden loss of consciousness with weak, slow breathing, cold limbs and weak muscles. The muscles tend to flaccidity (decreased tone), rather than to spasm and increased tone. The loss of muscle tone affects the sphincters, leading to double incontinence. There may also be a vertex headache.

Sequelae are understood very much as in Western medicine, with hemiparesis or hemiplegia associated with facial palsy and speech problems. The appetite is generally poor with a resulting sallow complexion.

Whatever the cause of the Windstroke, most patients are expected to progress to the sequelae stage unless they are unfortunate enough to suffer a massive Yin-type attack.

TCM treatment depends on the perceived cause of the stroke. Much treatment may be undertaken to prevent stroke from ever happening, with the deficiency of Yin in both Liver and Kidney being tackled along with support for the Spleen, and advice on diet and lifestyle.

Physiotherapists are rarely in a position to prevent this kind of neurological catastrophe, but are much concerned with the treatment and rehabilitation of the patient after it has occurred. The consensus of opinion in

TCM terms seems to be that an energetic policy, stimulating the points on the Yang meridians, is most successful (Box 2.12). The aim is to remove the stagnation of Qi and Blood. Electroacupuncture is often added, as is scalp acupuncture. Stimulation of both Spleen and Stomach is useful to aid digestion, and points for the Kidney and Liver are sometimes used to prevent recurrence.

The resulting paralysis may not affect both limbs, so the points used to free the channels should be used only where necessary. The points selected to support the major Zang Fu organs should be used in all cases.

Some authorities recommend the use of points on the unaffected limb, others use them bilaterally, and there seems to be no clear guide as to which is better. From the point of view of a stimulus to the nervous system, it seems logical to treat only the affected side. It also seems logical to add electroacupuncture using a current of 2 Hertz in order to produce a muscle twitch.

Research

Research into the effect of acupuncture on stroke recovery has not shown it to be any better than placebo or normal physiotherapy (Johansson et al 2001, Sze et al 2002). Early papers were very positive (Hu et al 1993, Sallstrom et al 1995), but it seems that, as the research question is refined and the protocols become tighter, the effect of acupuncture in this situation diminishes (Gosman-Hedstrom et al 1998, Hopwood 2003, Johansson et al 2001, Sze et al 2002).

It may be that acupuncture was never point specific for stroke sequelae, and the wide variety of points chosen in previous research protocols – all of which seemed to have a positive effect – may support this idea. The general neurohumoral effects of acupuncture treatment may actually be more important than the TCM theories in this context. Acupuncture may still have some value as an additional form of neuromuscular stimulus when used in conjunction with physiotherapy in the later stages of recovery (Hopwood 1996).

It would seem reasonable to use acupuncture when the diagnosis indicates the risk of Windstroke, bearing in mind the known effects on the sympathetic and parasympathetic nervous systems. There has been no

Box 2.12 Acupuncture for Windstroke sequelae

GB 20 Fengchi ⎫
LI 15 Jianyu ⎪
LI 11 Quchi ⎪
LI 10 Shousanli ⎬ Arm
LI 4 Hegu ⎪
SJ 5 Waiguan ⎭

GB 31 Fengshi ⎫
St 31 Biguan ⎪
St 36 Zusanli ⎪
Sp 10 Xuehai ⎬ Leg
GB 39 Xuanzhong ⎪
GB 43 Xiaxi ⎪
Liv 3 Taichong ⎭

research of any quality looking into the prevention of stroke with acupuncture. It is always difficult to prove a negative, and setting up a trial would pose enormous problems. However, as high blood pressure is known to be one of the risk factors in stroke, it would be interesting to record the long-term effects of acupuncture treatment to lower blood pressure in a cohort of patients known to be at risk of stroke. The points used to clear Blood and Qi stagnation should be effective.

General research

Research supporting the concept of Qi is hard to find (Box 2.13). Most modern researchers would be unwilling even to mention the word, and previous studies have stipulated only that 'acupuncture' was used for the treatment group. In an attempt to assess acupuncture by using a selection of points that could be expected to work clinically, given the empirical clinical evidence available, more recent research advice now stipulates that the type of acupuncture being used must elicit 'DeQi', or the sensation of the arrival of Qi, at the acupoint. This is included in a document recently published, the STRICTA guidelines, which recommend what constitutes good acupuncture practice in the context of research (MacPherson et al 2002). The emphasis on DeQi is important because it is now clear that the stimulation of three different types of nerve fibre contributes to this sensation, whether or not the concept of Qi is invoked (see Fig. 9.4).

A number of researchers have claimed that they obtained 'needling sensation' as part of the acupuncture protocol, and this is to be applauded.

Box 2.13 Experiencing the phenomenon of Qi

A useful experiment that can be carried out by any acupuncturist may convince them that there is a phenomenon that does not lend itself to easy explanation. First, insert needles along a meridian, perhaps LI 11 and LI 4 in the arm or UB 40, UB 57 and UB 60 in the leg. Then place the middle finger of the left hand gently against the lower needle, LI 4 or UB 60. Keeping the finger approximately 2 cm above the skin surface, trace the course of the meridian down to the other hand. Do not let the two fingers touch, but repeat the movement of the right hand several times.

A slight sensation may be felt by both the operator and the patient. The operator may feel a thickening of the air just above the meridian. This has been described as feeling as though someone is blowing gently against the fingertip; it indicates a disturbance of some sort in the flow of Qi in the meridian. The patient may be able to link the sensation to an old injury of some sort – perhaps an old fracture or contusion. Often, if the area is treated as an 'AhShi' point or trigger point, with the insertion of single needle it can be much improved.

At other times, the movement of the fingertip will serve to disperse the discomfort. It is hard to say in Western terms what is happening here. To therapists familiar with the feel of a low-frequency electric current, such as that from a TENS unit, it is like a very weakened version.

CASE HISTORIES

Case study 2.1
Late-onset asthma

- Elderly woman, slightly overweight, sedentary lifestyle
- Anxious about getting short of breath on exertion. Normal blood pressure. No heart signs. Has been prescribed salbutamol and beclomethasone to control the symptoms
- Tongue pale with 'frilled' edge
- Low back pain, some knee pain; possible early osteoarthritis of the knees

Using salbutamol four or five times per day. Asked to record how often this is needed

- Aim of treatment: to support the Kidney and improve Lung function
- Points:
  —Ren 17 Shanzhong
  —Kid 3 Taixi
  —Du 4 Mingmen
  —UB 23 Shenshu
  —UB 17 Geshu
  —Sp 6 Sanyinjiao

Ren 17 used only once. Other points used bilaterally. Moxa could have been used on Back Shu points, but proved unnecessary.

- Within six treatments, the use of salbutamol decreased to once daily as 'insurance'
- Patient asked to consult doctor about changing dose of beclomethasone. Discharged.

Case study 2.2
Stroke

A 59-year-old woman with a left-sided stroke caused by a thrombosis 5 years ago. Discharged after a period of inpatient rehabilitation. Treated by community physiotherapist every 2 weeks, working on increased central control and mobilizing the right hand and forearm. No hand activity at present. Being taught weight transfer techniques. Previous treatment during the year after the stroke by a professional acupuncturist was unsuccessful.

Aim of physiotherapy: to decrease high tone in pronators and flexors, and to increase potential extensor ability. Acupuncture introduced twice weekly to attempt this.

Treatment 1 employed points: LI 11, LI 10, LI 4 and Baxie 15 min. DeQi felt at all points. Activity with supination, pronation, and wrist and finger extensors.

Results: Flicker of activity with facilitation in wrist extensors. Nil noted in fingers. Some activity in triceps with shoulder protraction. Subjectively, the patient reported a 'buzzing' feeling in her arm for 2 hours afterwards, and the friend who carried out the daily exercises said the arm was looser the following morning.

Nine further treatments followed. The points were not changed. The patient continued to get a strong 'buzzing' response afterwards. The physiotherapist reported more potential for movement but no functional changes, and further commented: 'The improvements noted (right scapular stabilization, some mid-range shoulder medial and lateral rotation, mid-range elbow extension, supination and pronation, wrist extension and flickers of finger extension) were remarkable as they had not been observed in the 4 years since her stroke, despite continuous good-quality neurophysiotherapy input.'

(Thanks to P. Bulley)

References

Ballegaard S, Muteki T, Harada H et al 1993 Modulatory effects of acupuncture on the cardiovascular sytem: a crossover study. Acupuncture and Electro-Therapeutics Research International Journal 18: 103–115.

Clavey S 1995 Fluid physiology and pathology in Traditional Chinese Medicine, 1st edn. Melbourne: Churchill Livingstone.

David J, Townsend S, Sathanathan R et al 1999 The effect of acupuncture on patients with rheumatoid arthritis: a randomised, placebo-controlled crossover study. Rheumatology 38: 864–869.

Gill JS, Zezulka AV, Shipley MJ et al 1986 Stroke and alcohol consumption. New England Journal of Medicine 315: 1041–1046.

Gosman-Hedstrom G, Claesson L, Klingenstierna U et al 1998 Effects of acupuncture treatment on daily life activities and quality of life. Stroke 29: 2100–2108.

Hopwood V 1996 Acupuncture in stroke recovery: a literature review. Complementary Therapies in Medicine 4: 258–263.

Hopwood VA 2003 An investigation into the effects of acupuncture in stroke recovery. PhD thesis, University of Southampton.

Hopwood V, Lovesey M, Mokone S 1997 Acupuncture and related techniques in physiotherapy, 1st edn. London: Churchill Livingstone.

Hu HH, Chung C, Liu TJ et al 1993 A randomised controlled trial on the treatment for acute partial ischaemic stroke with acupuncture. Neuroepidemiology 12: 106–113.

Johansson B, Haker E, von Arbin M et al 2001 Acupuncture and transcutaneous nerve stimulation in stroke rehabilitation. Stroke 32: 707–713.

Juvela S, Hillbom M, Palomaki H 1995 Risk factors for spontaneous intracerebral haemorrhage. Stroke 26: 1558–1564.

Lawson-Wood D, Lawson-Wood J 1973 The Five Elements of acupuncture and Chinese massage, 2nd edn. Bradford: Health Science Press.

Li X, Zhao J 1993 Patterns and practice. Seattle: Eastland Press.

Maciocia G 1989 The foundations of Chinese Medicine, 1st edn. Edinburgh: Churchill Livingstone.

MacPherson H, White AR, Cummings M et al 2002 Standards for reporting interventions in controlled trials of acupuncture: the STRICTA recommendations. Acupuncture in Medicine 20: 22–25.

Richter A, Herlitz J, Hjalmarson A 1991 Effect of acupuncture in patients with angina pectoris. European Heart Journal 12: 175–178.

Sallstrom S, Kjendahl A, Osten PE et al 1995 Acupuncture therapy in stroke during the sub-acute phase. A randomised, controlled clinical trial. Complementary Therapies in Medicine 23: 2884–2887.

Sze FK, Wong E, Yi X, Woo J 2002 Does acupuncture have additional value to standard poststroke motor rehabilitation? Stroke 33: 186–194.

Thomas M 1995 Treatment of pain with acupuncture: factors influencing outcome. PhD thesis, Karolinska Institute, Stockholm.

Tukmachi E 2000 Acupuncture and rheumatoid arthritis. Rheumatology 39: 1153–1165.

Waley A (trans.) 1934 Tao Teh Ching. G. Allen & Unwin.

Yan D 2000 Ageing and blood stasis, 2nd edn. Boulder, CO: Blue Poppy Press.

Zhang YH, Rose K 2001 A brief history of Qi. Brookline: Paradigm.

Further reading

Clavey S 1995 Fluid physiology and pathology in Traditional Chinese Medicine. Melbourne: Churchill Livingstone.

Zhang YH, Rose K 2001 A brief history of Qi. Brookline: Paradigm.

Zang Fu – the TCM organ system

KEY CONCEPTS

   ꙮ Zang Fu organs are defined by their function.
   ꙮ All are concerned with producing, refining or moving Qi, Blood and the Body fluids.
   ꙮ Some of their functions do not correspond with what is understood by Western medicine.
   ꙮ They are damaged by internalized Pathogens.
   ꙮ They are damaged by strong emotions.
   ꙮ It is important to understand the functional links between Zang Fu organs in order to see the TCM patterns of disease.
   ꙮ These links partly inform Five Element acupuncture.
   ꙮ Five Element correspondences can help diagnosis.
   ꙮ There has been little research in this field.

Introduction

The Zang Fu organs are perhaps the most fascinating aspect of the theory of Traditional Chinese Medicine (TCM). The ancient Chinese medical practitioners did not have the advantage of meticulous dissection and careful histological studies to help them understand the body. Gross functions could be understood but the complexity and subtlety of human physiology could only be guessed at by observation, trial and error when administering herbs or acupuncture. Nonetheless, when used to define treatment protocols, the observations made in the past still appear quite valid.

Many of these ideas originated in a martial society and the metaphors for function and control tend to sound like elements of campaign. Each organ will be described in turn and the links to the others discussed. Disease patterns generally involve more than one organ at a time. The primary focus may be identifiable from the associated symptoms, but, unless the practitioner has a good working knowledge of all the Zang Fu characteristics and connections, the secondary foci and possibly the origins of the problem may be hard to determine. Chinese Medicine defines disease as disorders within these Zang Fu relationships rather than as a single failing organ.

Five Element acupuncture also depends on an understanding of the physiological characteristics of the organs. It is a complex subject and so is considered only briefly in this book, but it allows a holistic approach to the

Box 3.1   Zang and Fu organs

Zang organs (Yin)	Fu organs (Yang)
Heart (Xin)	Small Intestine (Xiao Chang)
Lung (Fei)	Large Intestine (Da Chang)
Liver (Gan)	Gall Bladder (Dan)
Spleen (Pi)	Stomach (Wei)
Kidney (Shen)	Urinary Bladder (Pang Guan)
Pericardium (Xin Bao)	Sanjiao
(Extra Uterus)	(Extra Brain)

mind and body of the patient recognizing, as it does, the many links between physiology and the emotions.

The emotions are frequently regarded as pathological factors but, while emotional disharmony may give rise to Zang Fu imbalance, disease affecting the Zang Fu may in turn result in emotional disturbance. The emotions with the greatest effect will be described, but it is worth bearing in mind that emotions are not so easily defined and some oversimplification is inevitable.

In general the Zang organs tend to be predominantly Yin in character and are considered to be solid, whereas the Fu organs are predominantly Yang and thought to be hollow in nature (Box 3.1). The Zang organs are given more emphasis in syndrome differentiation and are involved in the processing of substances. The Fu organs are principally involved in storage and are thought to interact directly with the channels. These are only generalizations, however, and, as in most TCM, whether an organ is more Yin or more Yang depends on the current comparison – none is purely one or the other.

Zang organs

Heart (Xin)

The Heart is the emperor within the body and as such has control over everything. It is said to govern all the other organs and is pictured as a benevolent and enlightened ruler. It regulates the flow of Blood and Qi, and governs the Blood in two ways. Some TCM authorities claim that the final transformation of the food Qi into Blood takes place in the Heart. However, the majority see it as a pump and responsible for the circulation of Blood in the vessels, as understood in Western medicine. This gives it responsibility for the innate health of the vessels too. The Heart propels the Blood through the tissues, communicating with every part and suffusing the body with consciousness and feeling.

The relationship between the Heart and the Blood is important and determines the strength of the constitution of an individual. Tongue diagnosis can give an indication of the relative strength of the constitution. The presence of a clear crack down the centre would alert a TCM practitioner to the possibility of a deficiency of Heart Qi or energy.

The state of the blood vessels and general circulation reflects the strength of the Heart Qi, as does the condition of the Heart pulse. As the Heart controls the blood vessels and circulation, a 'rosy and lustrous' complexion is a sign of health. Deficient Heart energy leads to a very noticeable bright, white complexion.

Blood and Body fluids have a common origin, so sweat is considered to be controlled by the Heart and to be found in the spaces just under the skin. If there is a lack of fluid within the circulation, it can be replenished from this source. If there is too much heat within the body it is 'steamed off' and discharged through the pores. Whatever the true physiology, Heart points appear to have a clinical influence on problems of hyperhydrosis.

In addition to the clear links with the mechanism of circulation, the Heart also houses the mind or Shen. This involves five particular functions:

☯ mental activity
☯ consciousness
☯ memory
☯ thinking
☯ sleep.

The term 'Shen' is also used sometimes to indicate vitality. The involvement of the Heart with all of the above means that it must be considered when treating mental illness and, indeed, Ht 7 Shenmen is a useful point to calm and relax a patient, or to treat insomnia or depression. 'Shenmen' translates as 'gateway to the spirit'. The Heart has a strong influence over sleep patterns. If the Heart is deficient in energy, the mind is said to have no residence and it will float at night causing disturbed sleep or excessive dreaming, should sleep come at all.

The connection between the Heart and the emotions is well understood in folk legend in most countries, but there is little scientific proof that this could have any foundation. However, there are some interesting ideas in a recent paper (Rosen 2001) in which the internal memory of the heart cells with regard to physiological process is recognized and discussed. Rosen (2001, p 468) suggests that the heart does remember 'making use of mechanisms similar to those in other systems that manifest memory, the brain, the gastro-intestinal tract and the immune system.'

The emotion of joy is most closely associated with the Heart. Joy is said to slow down the Qi and actually affects the Heart in this way. As the Heart controls the mind or spirit, and hence the emotions, it follows that an excess (i.e. over-joy or extreme anxiety) will damage the balance of Qi in this Zang Fu organ. Excess joy is said to disturb the Xin Qi so much that the Shen becomes confused and scattered. Over-joy is quite a violent emotion and a sudden laughing fit is thought in TCM to be able to trigger a heart attack.

The concept of a 'broken heart' is far from alien to TCM. When the Heart is overwhelmed by strong emotion, usually in this case shock or sorrow, the Shen is able to break free and thinking becomes disordered and confused; the resulting anxiety will be evident in the abnormal circulation. The impaired circulation will lead to stagnation of the Blood, blood pressure decreases and the patient will show signs of heart disease, angina or chest pain. Shock and fright have an opposite effect on the Heart and are said to cause the Shen to contract.

The most extreme disharmonies of the emotions arise from imbalances within Xin (Heart) and Gan (Liver), and it is sometimes difficult to differentiate between a lack of *joie de vivre* caused by Xin deficiency and the sorrow and melancholy caused by Depression of Gan Qi.

A further disharmony that will give rise to confusing symptoms is that between the Heart and the Kidney. This is often considered in terms of Yin and Yang or of Fire and Water. The Water aspect of the Kidneys must control the Fire aspect of the Heart, but if the Yin aspect of the Kidney energy is deficient then it will not control and cool the Heart Fire, which then flares up causing symptoms such as insomnia and irritability.

A useful comparison for TCM function of the Heart is with that of the cerebral cortex – an integrative function, giving rise to the capacity for individual thought and memory. This is further expressed through speech, the voice and facial expression.

Lungs (Fei)

The Lung is characterized as a very diplomatic foreign minister, conducting affairs of state and determining foreign boundaries, thus effectively governing the relationship between the inside and outside of the body. The Lungs are the most external of all the organs, having direct contact with the outer air. Because it is so susceptible to pathogenic invasion, the Lung is sometimes referred to as the 'tender organ'.

The Lungs control respiration and are responsible for the intake of clean air, which they convert into 'Clear Qi'. Together with the Qi produced from substances that are eaten and drunk, this goes to make up the Post-Heaven or renewable Qi within the body. The rhythm of the Lungs sets the rate for all other body functions, starting with the first breath taken by the newborn baby. The Qi from the Lungs passes down through the Sanjiao and is linked with that of the Kidneys, which rises, forming a sort of circular motor that effectively controls the water circulation within the body (see Ch. 2). The emptying of the Lungs, expiration, slows the movement of Qi, whereas the act of filling them, inspiration, speeds it up. Some teachers compare the activity of the Lungs to that of the parasympathetic system – an inhibitory action – but it could be argued that they are just as likely to be involved in a sympathetic mode.

The Lung controls the condition of the hair and also the state of the pores. The skin is sometimes referred to as the 'third lung'. If the skin is in poor condition, the pores may remain more open than usual, allowing the invasion of exogenous Pathogens. The Lung is also said to produce and control the Wei Qi, or Defensive Qi. This is the first line of defence against pathogenic invasion of the body and circulates in the spaces just underneath the skin. The link with the Kidneys and water circulation coupled with the control of pore size means that it also has an effect on sweating, together with the Heart.

The Lung opens into the nose and is considered to be the most external organ. It is vulnerable to the external Pathogens Wind and Cold. The common cold is said to be an invasion of a combination of Wind and Cold. The sense of smell and the loudness of the voice are dependent on Lung health. A husky voice and a runny or blocked nose are therefore not surprising as common cold symptoms.

The Lung houses the Corporeal Soul or Po. It is particularly sensitive to grief or sadness, and often affected by bereavement. It is associated with the pain of loss, of letting go, sorrow, loneliness, anxiety and melancholy. The effect of sorrow on the Lung can result in a lack of desire to face the world. Sadness of this kind tends to produce stagnation of Zong Qi in the chest and this in turns inhibits the function of both the lungs and the heart. This could result in the subsequent stagnation of Blood throughout the body. Treatment of Lu 7 Lieque may have a powerful release effect in constrained emotional conditions. The link between sorrow and the function of the Lung has been suggested as the reason why many recently bereaved elderly patients contract fatal chest infections while still grieving.

Liver (Gan)

The Liver is responsible for the smooth movement of Qi and Body fluids throughout the body. The Liver is involved in the process of digestion, providing energy for the transportation of the Gu Qi produced by the Stomach and Spleen. It is also responsible for the direction of Qi flow. The Qi from each organ has a characteristic direction of flow, fitting it into the TCM physiological pathways. This means that the Liver is the source of endurance in times of mental stress or physical exertion. If the Liver Qi is weak, the person is easily exhausted, finding it difficult to get out of bed in the morning.

Liver Qi should flow freely in all directions. If Liver Qi is constrained it is said to invade the Stomach, Spleen or Lung. 'Liver invading Spleen' is fast becoming a common modern syndrome, perhaps because of the combined effect of unsuitable diet and stress on the Liver triggering off a chain reaction throughout the Zang Fu. The Liver functions as a gentle regulator of the Spleen and Stomach, and thus as a regulator of digestion. In addition the bile, under the control of the Liver, can aid in the digestive process.

Storage of Blood is seen as integral to Liver function. The Liver releases Blood for the start of menstruation and continues to do this regularly, in appropriate quantity, throughout the fertile life of the female. Menstrual problems, such as amenorrhoea and dysmenorrhoea, are primarily treated by restoring Liver function. The Liver has an influence on the even movement of Blood around the body in both sexes. Stagnation is often seen as a result of poor Liver function, because Blood and Qi flow together and Qi is said to clear and smooth the channels to allow the accompanying blood flow.

The Liver controls normal muscle tone in the body. Disturbance of this function leads to muscle twitching or spasm, or even to convulsions. This may be described as the result of an 'insufficiency of the Yin and Blood in the Liver', resulting in malnutrition of the tissues. The Liver is also said to influence the muscle tendons. The fingernails are considered by TCM to be extensions of the tendons, and the condition of the Liver can be deduced from their state. Dry, flaky and ridged nails are indicative of an energy deficiency in the Liver.

A link with the eye means that the condition of the Liver can also be detected through examination of the 'white of the eye'. Conversely, it also means that Liver points can be used to treat eye problems, particularly those of an inflammatory nature. (Liv 2 is a useful emergency point.) The fluids most closely associated with the Liver, apart from Blood, are the tears. The syndrome 'Stirring of the inner Wind of the Liver' can cause poor vision, night blindness and abnormal movements of the eye.

Failure of the free-flowing function of the Liver may be associated with both frustration and depression and with outbursts of uncontrolled anger.

The Liver requires a calm internal environment, with an even disposition. It is very sensitive to being obstructed in any way and the function is easily upset. It is interesting that the English language equates being 'liverish' with being irritable.

Blazing Gan Fire is linked with severe and violent outbursts of rage. Feelings of irritation and moderate anger are also associated with Liver imbalance and are often ascribed to Deficient Liver Yin or Hyperactive Liver Yang, both of which cause the even tenor of life to become a little more bumpy. The Liver is often compared to an irascible Major General, efficient in command of the troops (or Qi) but with a short fuse where temper is concerned.

Stagnation of the Liver Qi, often produced by anger, can also have a profound effect on the Stomach and Spleen Qi.

Spleen (Pi)

The Spleen is an interesting organ from a TCM point of view but has never excited much enthusiasm in Western medicine. It occupies the very last pages in *Gray's Anatomy* and has always been regarded as generally superfluous to requirements. Splenectomy is not regarded as a life-threatening situation, although antibiotics are required to maintain health afterwards, and the Spleen has been classified with the appendix almost as an optional extra.

The Spleen is said to store Blood and to have some blood-manufacturing properties but the overwhelming importance in the digestive process as perceived by TCM is not recognized in Western medicine. Interestingly, the Spleen has been observed to increase in size during digestion, although no conclusions appear to have been drawn from this.

In TCM the Spleen is regarded as the minister of agriculture, able to control and regulate the production and distribution of essential nourishment. The Spleen is said to govern transformation and transportation. It is the main digestive organ in TCM and responsible, along with the Stomach, for the breaking down or transformation of ingested food and drink and its subsequent transportation to the other sites in the body where it will be utilized. The Spleen is said to incorporate and then distribute Nutritive Essence in order to diminish or augment body mass. It is responsible for forming and reconstituting the internal milieu, gathering and holding together the substance of the body.

Overeating can damage the Spleen; being continually full slows the metabolism and assimilation of nutrients. Food will sit undigested in the stomach, uncomfortably inflating the abdomen with stagnant fluid and gases. Lacking sufficient energy from the food ingested, the possible gain from this new food decreases steadily. This leads to a form of weight increase that could be described as more mass than energy.

Retarded indigestion engenders an urge for a quick fix of sugar and starch. Hence a frequent symptom of Spleen imbalance is the craving for sweet foods or chocolate. This organ is closely involved with the control of the fluid balance throughout the body, so the Spleen channel is frequently used when there is a local excess of fluid (oedema), particularly in the legs. The Spleen itself is said to prefer dryness; this means that it is adversely affected by the Western habit of excessive consumption of icy, sweet drinks and forced to use too much energy in the breakdown of uncooked foods such as salads.

The Spleen controls or supervises the Blood, keeping it in the blood vessels and preventing bleeding. If the Blood seeps from the vessels, causing superficial bruising with no perceived cause, this is thought to be a weakness of Spleen Qi failing to keep it within the vessels. If the Spleen fails in this role, the walls of the blood vessels may become fragile and even collapse, and marked extravasation occurs with unexplained bruising appearing on the body surface. Blood may also appear in the stools, which are characteristically loose in any Spleen syndrome. Deficient Yang Qi in the Spleen will also adversely affect the formation of Blood.

The Spleen exerts a control over all rising Qi, and Spleen energy holds all organs in their proper place in the body. It could also be said to have a centralizing and uplifting effect. In practical terms this is said to explain why Spleen points are used to control prolapse, particularly of the uterus or rectum. Spleen points are very useful when treating haemorrhoids.

The Spleen opens into the mouth, and the lips indicate the general state of the Spleen, which should be a healthy red colour. Spleen Qi deficiencies are indicated by pale, thin lips. The associated Body fluid is saliva, which is described as protecting the mouth cavity and helping in the digestive process.

The Spleen has a direct influence on the muscle bulk as the transformation and transport of food substances help to maintain this. It adjusts the quantity of pure fluid or essence produced by the digestive process and released into circulation, a function rather like providing additional fuel when the tank is emptying. Hence, Spleen points are recommended where there is evidence of muscle wasting. In addition the control exerted over the water content of the tissues affects the muscle bulk.

The Spleen houses thought and is associated with the act of thinking. If the balance is wrong, then excessive or obsessive worrying will be the signs with general lack of energy and lassitude as the result. There is an obvious link here with the Heart. The Spleen influences our capacity for thinking, studying, concentrating, focusing and memorizing, while the Heart actually does it. The Spleen is damaged by long periods of intensive study or chronic anxiety, and several Spleen syndromes are made worse by comfort eating, overdependence on chocolate etc., which of course is brought about in the first place by low-grade stress.

Some scholars have also suggested that the Spleen has a connection with compassion and the emotion of caring, but this link may be perceived just because, at a time when the Spleen is overwhelmed, the capacity for these emotions is lost.

Symptoms of Spleen Qi deficiency include a disinclination to talk, a low indistinct voice, sallow or pale complexion, and general lassitude. Another symptom associated with imbalance in the Spleen is loss of the sense of smell and, associated with this, the sense of taste. There may also be chronic diarrhoea due to excessive Dampness. Swelling or oedema in the lower part of the body, particularly the legs and ankles, is common. Strengthening the Spleen always accompanies a similar treatment for the Stomach and is frequently used to invigorate Blood and the circulation and to expel the Pathogen Damp.

Kidney (Shen)

The Kidney is characterized as a minister of the interior who conserves natural resources, storing them for use in time of need, growth, crisis or transition. It is of fundamental importance in TCM and said to be the Root of Life. The Shen Kidney stores Jing or Essence, which is derived from each of the parents and established at conception. This in turn controls the Yang aspects of sexual potency. The Yin and Yang of the Kidneys serve as the foundation for that of the rest of the body. Kidney Yin is the fundamental substance for birth, growth and reproduction, whereas Kidney Yang is the motive force for all physiological processes. Although, according to the Five Element theory, the Kidneys belong to Water, they are also said to be the source of Fire in the body. This is called Fire of the Gate of Vitality.

The Pre-Heaven Essence determines constitutional strength, vitality, etc. It is also associated with individual creativity and is the basis of sexual life; impotence and infertility can be linked with it. The Kidneys store Post-Heaven Qi or Essence, the refined essence extracted from food through the transforming power of the internal organs. Kidney Essence is the original material substance that forms the basis of all other tissues. It is compared to the genetic information encoded in DNA. Essence is finite, and the length of life is dependent upon the quantity and quality. After birth, through childhood and youth, through maturity and old age, all the normal development and ageing processes are associated with the Kidney Essence. When it is abundant, the body has the facility to develop and grow. The changes associated with old age are all symptomatic of Kidney deficiency: loss of hair, blurring of vision, low back pain, tinnitus and loose teeth.

As it is the origin of both vitality and endurance, the Kidney is important in many ways. It represents our own personal link in the continuous chain of existence. It is ultimately responsible for the instinct to procreate and thus survive. If Kidney Qi is abundant, a long and vigorous sex life is expected as it supports the reproductive organs, material and activity.

The Kidneys belong to Water and so govern the transformation and transportation of Body fluids in many ways. They act like a gate that opens and closes to control the flow of fluids in the lower Jiao or lower third of the body cavity. This flow is regulated by the Kidney Yang, which in turn controls Kidney Yin. All forms of Body fluid are derived from the synthesis of acquired and inherited body Essence. This includes tears, saliva, mucus, urine, sweat, cerebrospinal fluid, synovial fluid, plasma and semen.

If too much fluid accumulates in the lower Jiao, it stagnates giving rise to swelling at the knees and ankles, gravitational oedema, abdominal bloating and, occasionally, puffiness beneath the eyes. The build-up of fluid will have a direct effect on the Lungs and eventually the Heart, leading to further swelling in the upper part of the body.

Because of this involvement in the circulation of water, the Kidneys have a more direct effect on the functions of the Lung. They are said to control and promote respiration. If the Kidney energy is low, the necessary energy to 'steam' the pure fluids and send them back up to the Lung will be lacking. The connected descent of the heavier fluid down to the Kidney will not occur, with a build-up of fluid in the Lung tissues for a different reason. This type of accumulated fluid causes wheezing and is identified as late-onset asthma.

The Kidneys are said to open into the ear, making Kidney points useful for the treatment of deafness and tinnitus. TCM associates deafness with the idea of extra thick bone being laid down in the ear, this therefore being under the control of the Kidney. The growth of the hair is dependent on Essence and Blood, and its loss is a result of poor supply. The whitening of the hair in the elderly is connected to the state of the Kidney Essence. There is a saying: 'The function of the Kidney reflects in the glossiness of the hair'. This is interesting because the Lung is also credited with playing a part in the condition of the hair. Perhaps this just serves to emphasize the connection between these two Zang organs.

Fear is the emotion most strongly associated with the Kidneys. It is closely linked to the desire for self-preservation and consequently encompasses true terror. The basic physiological responses, fight or flight, are involved and the other Zang Fu organs are brought into play. The type of fear that immobilizes or paralyses involves weakness of Dan (Gall Bladder) and, when linked with anger, involves Gan (Liver). If caused by worry, the Spleen may be involved; if a result of anxiety, the Lung also shows symptoms.

Pericardium (Xin Bao)

The Pericardium is closely related to the Heart; traditionally it was thought to shield the Heart against the invasion of external pathogenic factors. It is also known as the Heart Protector. The ancient manuscripts, most particularly the Spiritual pivot, do not grant the Pericardium true Zang Fu status, describing the Heart as the master of the five Zang and the six Fu. The Heart is considered to be the dwelling of the Shen, and no Pathogen can be allowed past the barrier of the Pericardium in case the Heart is damaged and the Shen departs and death occurs.

The Pericardium displays some of the characteristics of Xin Heart but is of far lesser importance in that it only assists with the government of Blood and housing the mind.

The points on the channel are often used to treat emotional problems, having a perceived cheering effect. They are also frequently used for their sedative effect. The meridian is also used in treatment of the Heart but is considered to be a gentler form of therapy than the use of Heart points.

In effect, the Pericardium is considered as the active mechanism of the Heart, the physical pumping activity, while the Heart itself is more involved with containing the spirit and maintaining full consciousness.

In spite of this lesser importance in Zang Fu terms, the meridian is a very useful one with many internal connections and wide-ranging physiological effects.

Fu organs

Small Intestine (Xiao Chang)

The Small Intestine does not differ greatly in function from what is understood in the West, but the description of the connections is rather different. The Small Intestine receives food and drink from the stomach and separates the clean or reusable fraction from that which is dirty. The clean part is then transported by the Spleen to all parts of the body. The dirty or turbid part is transmitted to the Large Intestine for excretion as stools and to the

Bladder to form the urine. This means that the Small Intestine has a direct functional relationship with the Bladder and it influences urinary function. The Small Intestine thus plays a minor part in the Jin Ye or body water circulation.

The Small Intestine is paired with the Heart and is said to have an effect on dreams, although it is not so strong as the Heart itself. The Small Intestine is linked with the Heart through the purification of the substances that enter the Blood, thus protecting the Shen or spirit. The traditional pairing with the Heart is rather tenuous and really evident only when Heat from Fire in the Xin Heart shifts downwards into the Small Intestine and disturbs the lower Jiao. This relationship is relevant only in the psychological sense. The Small Intestine is said to have an influence on judgement, and on making the best choices.

Large Intestine (Da Chang)

The digestive function of the Large Intestine, as described in TCM, is similar to that understood in Western medicine. In some Chinese texts it is described as 'passing and changing', referring to what happens to the faecal matter. However, many of the normal functions of the Large Intestine are also ascribed to the Spleen. The most important action is the reception of food and drink from the Small Intestine, and the reabsorption of a proportion of the fluid. The remainder goes to make up the faeces and is excreted.

The Large Intestine is the final part of the digestive system and will reflect any imbalances occurring in the other organs of digestion in terms of quantity or quality.

Deficient Yang energy in the Spleen is also called Deficient Energy in the Large Intestine because both tend to result in the same symptoms. This means that the Large Intestine is part of the fluid balance mechanism of the body. The Large Intestine is linked to the Lung both interiorly and exteriorly via the meridians, and can therefore have an influence on the Lung–Kidney water cycle. The Lung is said to disperse water while the Large Intestine absorbs it. Equally the Lung takes in air while the Large Intestine discharges gas. If there is Heat in the Lung the faeces will be dry, and when the function of the Lung is weak the faeces tend to be loose. Simple stagnation of food in the Large Intestine or constipation can give rise to a degree of breathlessness.

If the Large Intestine is functioning poorly, the mind becomes unclear and muddled. It is as though the failure to eliminate the waste leaves feelings of staleness and lifelessness. Many elderly patients suffering from constipation will describe the effect of it in just this way. Optimal functioning of the body requires elimination of that which is no longer of use both physically and psychologically.

Gall Bladder (Dan)

The main function of the Gall Bladder is perceived to be that of assisting the Spleen and Stomach in the process of digestion. The bile from the Gall Bladder is discharged into the Small Intestine under the control of the Liver. If this flow is impaired, the digestion process is affected and there will be loss of appetite, abdominal pain and distension with diarrhoea.

This Fu organ is closely connected to the Liver. In TCM terms it is thought that Gan, the Liver, produces the bile and Dan, the Gall Bladder, stores it. The Gall Bladder is not always included in the list of Fu organs and is sometimes termed a 'curious organ' because it is hollow and secretes a pure fluid (making it more Zang than Fu). It has much in common with the pancreas and, as the pancreas is not mentioned in the Zang Fu, is sometimes regarded as serving in that capacity too.

The Gall Bladder is said to be responsible for making decisions, whereas the Liver is responsible for smooth planning. Both are affected by the emotional Pathogen anger and irritability. A deficiency in Gall Bladder energy leads to timidity, indecision or procrastination. The Gall Bladder is said to give an individual courage and to increase their drive and vitality. A man with a serene character and firmness of resolve was considered most appropriate for combat by Eastern philosophers, and he might be referred to as 'having a large Gall Bladder' or a 'thick Liver' and regarded as most valuable in a military sense.

A graphic illustration of the interconnectedness of the Zang Fu organs comes from Dey's translation of Zhang Cong Zheng in his book on treating schizophrenia (Dey 1999, p 9):

> when the Liver constantly plans, and the Gall Bladder is constantly indecisive, by being bent over without stretching, and holding anger that is not discharged, the Heart blood grows dryer by the day. Spleen humor does not move and phlegm then confounds the orifices of the Heart, forming Heart Wind.

(Heart Wind or Phlegm misting the orifices of the Heart is described in Chapter 8.)

The Liver and Gall Bladder are so closely linked that it is difficult to regard their disharmonies individually; the balance of energy within the Liver obviously has a bearing on the storage and release of bile, and the subsequent symptoms of poor digestion may result in jaundice, hepatitis or cholecystitis.

The TCM genesis of jaundice is interesting. It is thought to be due to an overflow of stagnated bile constituents into the Blood due to gallstones, inflammation of the biliary tract or liver abscess. In severe cases of jaundice, convulsion or coma may occur. This is assumed to be due to the acidic salt from the Gall Bladder invading the central nervous system.

Stomach (Wei)

The Stomach is the most important of the Fu organs and has a vital role in digestion. Together with the Spleen it is known as the root of Post-Heaven Qi. Digestion was understood by the ancient Chinese to be a rotting or fermenting process in which the Stomach was described graphically as the 'chamber of maceration'. This process prepares for the action of the Spleen, which then separates and extracts the refined Essence from the food and drink. It has also been compared to a bubbling cauldron.

After the transformation process that takes place in the Stomach, the food passes into the Small Intestine for further breakdown and absorption. The Stomach is always considered as the true origin of acquired Qi, or Gu Qi, and is vital for a healthy constitution. For this reason it is often necessary to tonify Stomach Qi when any disease process is present. The most commonly used acupuncture point is St 36 Zusanli, often described as a boost to the system or Qi metabolism.

The Stomach has a similar role to that of the Spleen in transporting food Qi to all the tissues, most particularly the limbs. Weak muscles and general fatigue may indicate a lack of Stomach Qi.

The state of the Stomach may be seen quite clearly in the tongue coating, which is formed as a byproduct of the rotting process. A thin white coating is normal. Absence of a coating implies impaired function and a yellow coating indicates Heat in the Stomach.

The Stomach sends transformed food down to the Small Intestine and is described as having a descending function. If this is absent or impaired, the food stagnates, leading to fullness, distension, sour regurgitation, belching, hiccups, nausea and vomiting. Vomiting is often described as 'rebellious Stomach Qi'. Under normal conditions the Liver Qi has a hand in this smooth downward flow, so it often needs to be treated alongside the Stomach in digestive disorders.

In order to perform the ripening and rotting task assigned to it, the Stomach requires large quantities of fluid to dissolve the valuable parts of the food. It is, of course, itself a source of fluid, but it works best when damp and is damaged by dryness and the Pathogen Heat. Eating large meals late at night depletes the fluids of the Stomach and sets up disharmonies right through the system.

As it is easily damaged by Heat, the Stomach is susceptible to Excess patterns, such as Fire or Phlegm Fire, and may eventually produce mental states similar to mania. Mild cases are likely to suffer from confusion and severe anxiety.

The Stomach and the Spleen are so closely interlinked in physiology and function that they are always treated together. While the Stomach controls the downward movement of the less pure elements in the food, the Spleen governs the upward movement of the clear fraction, linking with the Lung. Any type of illness pattern that involves the malabsorption of food and subsequent diminishing Qi production requires both Stomach and Spleen points to be stimulated. This is often apparent in any type of wasting disease in which muscle bulk diminishes visibly.

The link between digestion and the mental state has often been considered in the West, and common sense tells us that one affects the other. It is rare to see this link considered from the Chinese perspective, however, and an article by McMillin et al (1999) throws some light on the sympathetic and parasympathetic nerve connections that serve to reinforce the Zang Fu attributes.

Urinary Bladder (Pang Guan)

The Urinary Bladder holds few surprises. It secretes and stores urine, using energy from the Kidney, and releases it when appropriate. It is closely involved in the circulation of fluid around the body, receiving fluids separated by the Small Intestine and transforming them into urine. Energy in the lower Jiao, particularly that of the Kidney ensures the maintenance of clear water passages.

The Urinary Bladder tends to be susceptible to the Pathogen Heat, producing the painful symptoms of cystitis if this occurs. Incontinence of urine is directly attributable to the Bladder, but is usually caused by deficient Kidney Qi. The Urinary Bladder is also said to have control of the urethral, anal and cervical sphincters, regulating the discharge of all Body fluids in this area.

The Bladder is thought to be linked to negative emotions such as jealousy and the holding of long-standing grudges. Another saying associated with the Urinary Bladder is: 'When the Bladder is deficient one dreams of voyages'.

Sanjiao

The Sanjiao, or Triple Burner, is a fascinating concept peculiar to Chinese Medicine; it demonstrates the essential holistic concept of the physiological body. It is an explanation of the predominant functions in distinct areas of the trunk, and TCM theory demonstrates the interconnectedness of everything. It is a uniquely Chinese concept and is the subject of much speculation. The word Sanjiao means 'three chambers' or 'three spaces'.

To understand the Sanjiao one needs to reconsider the circulation of Qi, Blood and Body fluids (see Ch. 2). The upper Jiao is said to contain the Lungs and Heart, and is known as the 'chamber of mist'. It is clearly defined as being the portion of the trunk above the diaphragm. The middle Jiao is just below, between the diaphragm and the navel, and contains the Spleen and Stomach. This region is particularly concerned with the digestion and absorption of food. It is known as the 'chamber of ripening and rotting' or sometimes the 'chamber of maceration'. As the predominant direction of Stomach Qi is downwards and that of the Spleen is upwards, it is clear that the middle Jiao acts as a kind of junction. The lower Jiao contains all the other organs, even the Liver and Gall Bladder, although true anatomical location is somewhat inaccurate here. Of major importance physiologically, however, are the Kidneys and Bladder, giving the region the general name of 'drainage ditch' and controlling the storage and excretion of water.

The Sanjiao is really the summary of the physiology of the Zang Fu organs, and points on that meridian can be utilized in coordination of function, particularly fluid circulation. Figure 3.1 shows the contents of the three Jiaos with the predominant direction of Qi flow. In fact, all the Zang Fu organs are interlinked in some way, either by the fluid circulation or Qi production, so any diagram can become very complex once every factor is taken into account.

The Sanjiao has a very close link with the Kidneys, both Yin and Yang aspects. As it controls water metabolism, the Sanjiao relies on Kidney energy to accomplish this.

Extraordinary organs

The extraordinary organs are those about which there has been some doubt: either they were not really identified in the ancient writings or they did not fully qualify in their assigned classification. Also not everybody had them!

The Uterus (Zi Gong)

The basic function of the Uterus was perceived as that of nurturing the fetus. The energies of the Kidney, Liver and Spleen largely accomplish the function of the Uterus in coordination with the Chong and Ren channels (see Ch. 4). The menstrual cycle is a complex physiological process in TCM, relying on a Yin–Yang division between Blood and Qi energy.

Figure 3.1   The Sanjiao.

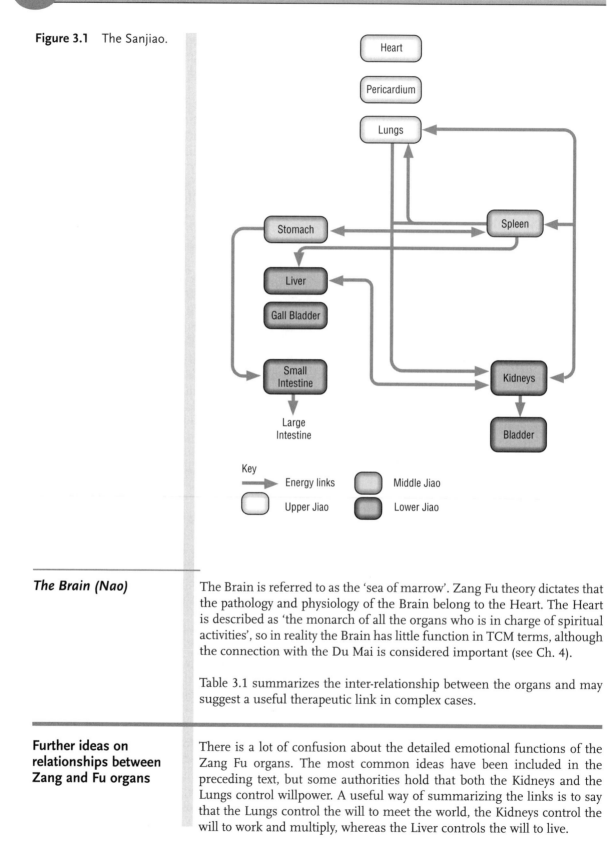

The Brain (Nao)

The Brain is referred to as the 'sea of marrow'. Zang Fu theory dictates that the pathology and physiology of the Brain belong to the Heart. The Heart is described as 'the monarch of all the organs who is in charge of spiritual activities', so in reality the Brain has little function in TCM terms, although the connection with the Du Mai is considered important (see Ch. 4).

Table 3.1 summarizes the inter-relationship between the organs and may suggest a useful therapeutic link in complex cases.

Further ideas on relationships between Zang and Fu organs

There is a lot of confusion about the detailed emotional functions of the Zang Fu organs. The most common ideas have been included in the preceding text, but some authorities hold that both the Kidneys and the Lungs control willpower. A useful way of summarizing the links is to say that the Lungs control the will to meet the world, the Kidneys control the will to work and multiply, whereas the Liver controls the will to live.

Table 3.1 Inter-relationship between Zang Fu organs

		Key links
Zang organs		
Liver	Kidney	☙ Both situated in lower Jiao, interdependent ☙ Kidney stores Essence, Liver stores Blood ☙ Liver smoothes Qi flow ☙ Kidney stores Qi ☙ Deficiency of Kidney Essence fails to nourish Liver ☙ Liver Fire damages Kidney
Spleen	Kidney	☙ Kidney stores Pre-Heaven Qi ☙ Spleen transforms Post-Heaven Qi ☙ Kidney provides warmth (Yang energy) ☙ Spleen supplies Kidney ☙ Interdependent
Lung	Kidney	☙ Lung controls respiration but needs Kidney energy ☙ Kidney controls water metabolism but needs descending Lung function ☙ Interdependent
Heart	Kidney	☙ Heart lies in the upper Jiao, controls Blood and is Yang ☙ Kidney lies in the lower Jiao, controls Essence and is Yin ☙ The Yang of the Heart should descend to nourish the Kidney Yin ☙ The Heart houses the mind ☙ The Kidneys connect with the Brain and control thinking ☙ Interdependent
Spleen	Liver	☙ Liver smoothes Qi flow ☙ Spleen controls transformation and transportation ☙ Liver stores Blood ☙ Spleen produces Blood ☙ Spleen keeps Blood flowing in vessels ☙ Combine to produce normal Blood circulation ☙ Liver imbalance can seriously disturb Spleen function leading to less Blood for the Liver to store
Lung	Liver	☙ Liver controls smooth flow and direction of Qi ☙ Liver is internally connected to the Lung ☙ Liver Qi should move upward while the Lung Qi moves downward ☙ Liver stagnation can cause a form of asthma

Continues

Table 3.1   cont'd

		Key links
Lung	Spleen	☙ Linked in Qi production and water metabolism ☙ Lung produces Clean Qi from inspired air ☙ Spleen transforms ingested food into Qi ☙ Interdependent ☙ Lung is the upper source of water and Spleen is regarded as the pivot ☙ Lung points are used for water problems in the upper part of the body ☙ Spleen is used for similar problems in the lower body
Heart	Spleen	☙ Heart circulates Blood ☙ Spleen controls transformation and transportation ☙ Food essence from the Spleen is required for new Blood manufacture ☙ Heart circulates Blood ☙ Spleen keeps the Blood in the vessels ☙ Interdependent
Heart	Liver	☙ Heart circulates Blood ☙ Liver regulates Blood (particularly in females) ☙ Interdependent
Heart	Lung	☙ Heart circulates Blood ☙ Lung produces Zong Qi, which links with the Heart ☙ Lung energy supports the function of the Heart ☙ Zong Qi deficiency causes both stagnation of Blood and prevents Lung energy from supporting it, resulting in palpitations, cough and shortness of breath
Fu organs		☙ The relationship between the Fu organs is less important. They share a similar general function with regard to the transforming and transportation of water and food ☙ The Sanjiao is the most influential because it contains the Fu organs and controls the circulation of Body fluids in and around them
Zang and Fu organs		☙ Echoes the Yin and Yang relationship throughout the body, the Zang organs being predominantly Yin and the Fu organs predominantly Yang ☙ Internal and external connections are said to link them with the meridians and with one another

There is also some argument about the relative realms of control of the Spleen and Liver. They are both said to control the muscles, but perhaps the idea that the Spleen controls the actual muscle bulk, the connective tissue, and the Liver controls the function, including the tendons and 'sinews', makes better sense in view of their respective Zang Fu physiology. The word 'sinews' is a difficult one for physiotherapists; it appears sometimes to mean the muscle itself, on other occasions the surrounding tissues. It appears to take no account of defined anatomical muscle boundaries. At other times it is used for the tendons themselves and also, possibly, the ligaments. Although the ideas are from different medical paradigms, it is reasonable to bring in the concept of myotomes, dermatomes and sclerotomes to explain sinews and the areas of influence ascribed to the meridians (see Ch. 6).

The idea that different organs within the body can throw everything else out of balance and produce disease irrespective of medical diagnosis is not a new one. The predominance given by any culture to certain aspects of ill-health is endlessly fascinating. According to Lynn Payer (1990), each country appears to emphasize certain organs or illnesses. For example, the French are very concerned with their livers and blame ailments from dandruff to hay fever on a *crise de foie*.

Payer found that the French attributed 80% of their headaches and migraines to liver crisis, a conclusion happily supported by TCM theorists. West Germans, on the other hand, tend to emphasize the heart and so use six times more heart drugs per capita than the French or the British. One of the most frequent diagnoses in Germany is *herzinsufizienz* (literally, cardiac insufficiency), which is not actually recognized as a problem elsewhere. This emphasis results in very different levels of medical drug consumption. For instance, the Germans have 85 listed drugs for the treatment of low blood pressure (hypotension), whereas for a US doctor it could almost be seen as malpractice to treat such a desirable condition.

Nonetheless, the meticulous observation of the Zang Fu characteristics can be useful in modern medicine and will enrich any type of acupuncture practice. The emotional aspects of the Zang Fu are of much greater importance when considered with the Five Element framework, because it is believed that the typical psychological characteristics for each element can by manipulated by acupuncture.

Five Element acupuncture

The Chinese thought that these matters were of great importance too and evolved Five Element acupuncture. Having travelled to China with the express wish of studying this, I discovered that it was not practised at all in Nanjing where I did some of my early training. In fact, I think that Five Element acupuncture is probably taught rather better in the West now, having been refined over the past 30–40 years. It has evolved, or returned to its roots, depending on your point of view, to be a complex and subtle tool for holistic treatment with a strong emphasis on the emotional subtext of the patient's symptoms. The Five Element or Five Phase type of acupuncture is based on philosophical teachings that, following on from the ideas on Qi and Yin and Yang, held that all known substances could be divided into five groups according to their affinities. Once designated, the behaviour of these substances, organs or emotions could be explained by clear interactive processes or patterns. Thus disease had a remedy, if only the ideal balance could be restored.

The elements are Wood, Fire, Earth, Metal and Water. These substances were considered to be in a relationship that was constantly redefining itself. They were not viewed as static or immutable, which is why the word 'phase' is sometimes used, rather than 'element'. This means than attribution of all other substance to Wood, Fire, Earth, Metal and Water is done on the basis of their perceived properties, and comparison is made by means of similes and allegories. This process can of course be endless and there are many lists of correspondences to be found in TCM textbooks.

It is probably helpful to include yet another here (Table 3.2). To Western practitioners this comparison and listing seems quite arbitrary, but it does allow a logical framework to be imposed on very disparate symptoms when they are confronted in a clinical setting, and sometimes the clues given by season and pathogenic factor can identify a syndrome.

The Zang Fu organs are considered as two groups of five in this framework, with the Pericardium and Sanjiao being collected with Heart and Small Intestine under the Fire category. When considered from a Zang Fu perspective this makes some sense as both could be said to be rather nebulous in substance but powerful because of their many connections. The correspondences listed in Table 3.2 indicate very clearly both the element and the main Zang Fu organs involved in the disease. The characteristics are described below.

Wood

The colour is green and there may be a visible tint to the complexion in liver disease. Wind is the Pathogen associated with Wood, and the symptomatology will reflect this with mobile symptoms and involvement of both the Liver and Gall Bladder channels.

Fire

The tongue and the activity of speech are associated with Fire. Four organs/meridians are clustered under the Fire label: Heart, Small Intestine, Pericardium and the Sanjiao. High fever, excessive thirst and coughing blood are all symptoms associated with Fire. Heart conditions of the Hot, Shi type are typical with a florid complexion and severe anginal pain. These patients dislike hot weather and respond poorly to overexcitement.

Earth

There are some interesting parallels with nutrition to be drawn here. The internal emotion is depression and the common response to depression is 'binge' eating of sweets and chocolates, thought to be very damaging to the Spleen. Stomach and Spleen syndromes are often accompanied by internal Damp and are worse in damp weather. Earth is broadly associated with everything below the navel in the human body. Patients may complain of heaviness in the limbs and a dull ache in the joints.

Metal

The associated structure is the nose and the tissues are skin and mucous membranes. The link with the Lung and the sense of smell is clear. Grief affects the Lung, and frequently causes associated skin disease.

Water

This element is envisaged as black, cold and salty, like the sea, and linked to the Kidneys, winter and the need to store energy. Dark blue/black shadows under the eyes often denote a Kidney disturbance.

Table 3.2 Five Element correspondences

	Wood	Fire	Earth	Metal	Water
Internal correspondences					
Zang	Liver	Heart	Spleen	Lung	Kidney
Fu	Gall Bladder	Small Intestine	Stomach	Large Intestine	Urinary Bladder
Sense organ	Eye	Tongue	Mouth	Nose	Ear
Tissue	Tendon	Vessel	Muscle	Skin and Hair	Bone
Fluid	Tears	Sweat	Saliva	Mucus	Urine
Emotion	Anger	Joy	Meditation	Melancholy	Fear
Sound	Shout	Laugh	Sing	Cry	Moan
Motion	Walking	Observing	Sitting	Lying	Standing
Activity	Speaking	Salivation	Swallowing	Cough	Yawning
Faculty	Active awareness	Transcendent awareness	Passive awareness	Subliminal awareness	Primal awareness
	Hun	Shen	Yi	Po	Zhi
External correspondences					
Season	Spring	Summer	Late Summer	Autumn	Winter
Development	Germination	Growth	Transformation	Reaping	Storing
External Pathogen	Wind	Heat	Damp	Dryness	Cold
Colour	Green	Red	Yellow	White	Black
Meat	Sheep	Chicken	Beef	Horse	Pork
Taste	Sour	Bitter	Sweet	Pungent	Salty
Orientation	East	South	Centre	West	North

The basic theory uniting the elements follows the normal laws of growth and development together with those of motion and change. The first idea to be applied is that each of the elements will have a generating or supporting effect on at least one of the others. This is sometimes called the inter-promoting or Sheng cycle. Wood produces Fire, Fire generates Earth (perhaps easier to visualize as ash), Earth itself produces Metal (found in the earth) and Metal generates Water (visualize water condensing on cold metal) (Fig. 3.2).

The elements have a controlling function upon one another and this is called the Ko cycle, or the restraining or interacting or overacting relationship. The ideas are quite simple and logical. Water will put out Fire, Fire will melt Metal, Metal can be used to cut down Wood, Wood will invade Earth and, finally, Earth can block the flow of Water (Fig. 3.3).

These actions of one element on another are described in terms of either family relationships or governmental command. That most commonly described is that of Mother and Son (Fig. 3.4) to explain the

Figure 3.2 The Sheng or generating cycle.

Figure 3.3 The Ko or controlling cycle.

Figure 3.4 Zang Mother–Son (Sheng cycle).

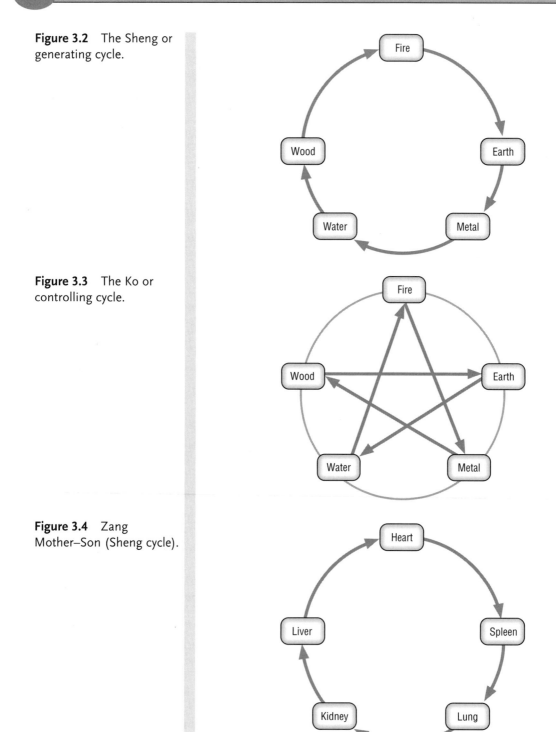

generating cycle; thus the Mother of Fire is Wood. As an example, Liver is the Mother of the Heart or, conversely, the Heart is the Son of Liver.

The Sheng or generating cycle is related to the Zang Fu organs in the following way. The Kidney Essence nourishes the Liver, which stores

Blood. This in turn supplies or nourishes the Heart. The Heart energy warms the Spleen, which then transforms and clarifies food essence to supply the Lung. Finally, the Lung provides the descending energy to maintain and supply the Kidneys.

The organs of the body are not always in a state of optimal balance and this is echoed in the concept of the Anti-Ko or counteracting cycle. Elements may at times become so strong that they are able to reverse the Ko or generating cycle.

The logic of this reverse cycle (Fig. 3.5) is rather more difficult to see but it can be interpreted simply as a reversal of the natural order of things. Of course, it has far-reaching effects on the acupuncture treatment to be utilized.

The application of acupuncture depends on knowledge of the Antique points, (see Ch. 5), in particular the classification of points below the knee or elbow according to their Five Element designation. Once a diagnosis has been made, according to the Eight Principles, the appropriate stimulus to the Mother and Son points needs to be decided.

In simple terms, if more energy is required in a deficient or Xu condition, the Mother point of the element should be tonified. The tonification point of a meridian is always that of the Mother of the element. If there is an Excess – too much energy – the Son point of the element should be sedated or dispersed, although convention holds that it is always better to tonify rather than sedate (Fig. 3.6).

Of course, this can become much more complex and can be a fascinating study. Fitting into the simple, basic pattern is the metaphor of the Mother and Son extended into chains of governmental control. In this pattern all the elements have a job to do and some kind of power that can be invoked by acupuncture. Now it becomes important to be aware of some external factors, for instance the season in which the symptoms are occurring. The corresponding seasons were listed previously, in Table 3.2.

In any season, the organ of that season will be dominant: it will rule the other organs and be 'emperor' for that short time. Figure 3.7 provides a rough guide to the apportioned power with respect to each of the others.

Figure 3.5 Anti-Ko cycle.

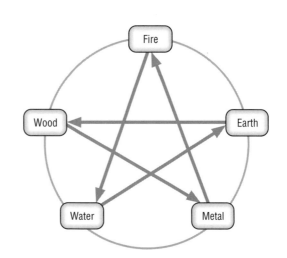

Figure 3.6 Zang Fu organs and the Ko cycle.

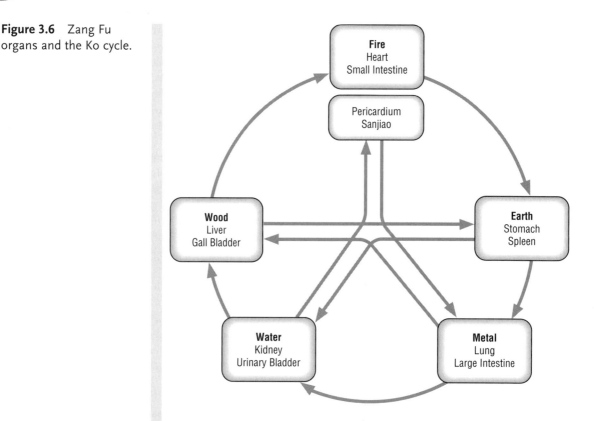

In the right season, the organ of that season will be dominant or full of energy. The metaphor here is that of the rule of an emperor having the most power, preceded by his mother, who is now drained of energy, having nourished him; his son, the next in line, awaits, full of energy for the next season. There is an enemy, who must be dominated by the emperor for obvious reasons, and an adviser whose task it is to advise the emperor but who could step in as a regent should the emperor fail in his duties. While quite fanciful, there are helpful ideas in this metaphor that could be used to help select a full treatment protocol.

Figure 3.7 The emperor in his season.

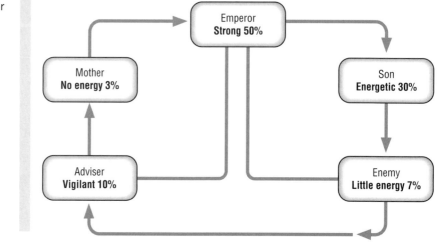

Five Element application to diagnosis and treatment

If a patient is suffering from a heart condition that has been identified as an Excess, it could be the result of a lack of control from the Kidney, which is itself deficient. Using the Ko or controlling cycle, one could simply tonify the Kidney by needling the Yuan source point, Kid 3 Taixi. This would suppress the Heart activity. Alternatively one could draw energy around the Sheng or generating cycle to increase the control of the Kidney over the Heart, which would involve using the Metal point on the Kidney meridian, Kid 7 Fuliu.

It becomes apparent that it is necessary to have a good working knowledge of the Antique points and their designation according to the Five Elements in order to utilize this form of acupuncture. The characteristics of these points are described in Chapter 5. It takes some time to learn and become expert in selecting the correct points. In order to detect the changes in Zang Fu energy one can assess the state of the organ by the symptoms manifesting, but use of pulse diagnosis is much more accurate. Indeed, I would consider it vital, as it will offer immediate feedback to the treatment, because changes in the force or quality of a specific pulse can be felt straight away. Use of Five Element diagnosis without a competent understanding of the pulse characteristics is not really recommended.

Zang Fu research

There is little available in mainstream medical research to substantiate the ancient Chinese ideas of Zang Fu physiology. That is not to say that there is no basis for some of the ideas, however. As has been emphasized throughout the descriptions in this chapter, the observation of some of the minute functions of body physiology by the ancient masters was amazingly accurate. If this was so, perhaps we can take some of the other statements as being at least possible to prove?

For instance, for many years the spleen was thought to be of little importance by the Western medical profession. It could be removed when damaged without having a serious effect on the patient. The functions described in this chapter seem of considerable importance and very far from what we think we know about this organ. In this case, more studies are needed. Clinically, treating points on the Spleen meridian would appear to have a profound effect on oedema in the leg, although one of the most effective, Sp 6 Sanyinjiao, could be claimed as a general Yin point because it lies on all three Yin channels – Spleen, Kidney and Liver.

I am not aware of any research along these lines, although an interesting attempt was made to investigate whether the acupoint Sp 6 itself was more painful when needled in women than in men (Janovsky et al 2000). No statistically significant difference between the sexes was demonstrated, although the theory that the regular menstrual flows influenced by the TCM physiological function of the three organs in question – Spleen, Kidney and Liver – might sensitize that particular point was a reasonable one.

The hypothesis that the Heart in some way controls the mind would seem to be one of the more outrageous TCM ideas, now that we are beginning to understand the intricacies of the brain. There is certainly, as yet, no research evidence to convince us of any link, although a speculative article has been written, mentioned above, discussing a kind of cellular memory apparent in heart tissue (Rosen 2001). However, there is considerable anecdotal evidence of a link provided by recipients of a donated heart. Several cases have been described in the popular press where recipients have found themselves craving for unlikely foods or inappropriate pastimes. One elderly woman found herself inexplicably drawn to a combination of baseball, riding fast motor cycles and consumption of large amounts of beer – a far cry from her lifestyle before the heart replacement operation! Apparently, when she tracked down the family of her donor she discovered that the unfortunately deceased young man had had these very interests. These stories, while entertaining, remain firmly in the realm of anecdote.

A recent controlled study on the effect of acupuncture on the cardiac autonomic nervous system in patients with minor depression or anxiety disorders showed statistically useful results in favour of acupuncture at specific points (Agelink et al 2003). When treating mental disorders such as schizophrenia, the use of Ht 7 Shenmen is recommended for feeble-mindedness and tendency to manic laughter, and Pe 6 is suggested to open the orifices of the Heart, together with other points to sweep Phlegm clogging the system. A good clinical text dealing with this is *Soothing the Troubled Mind* (Dey 1999).

Kidney disease has been linked with osteoporosis, corroborating the TCM theory. Metabolic bone disease is associated with alterations in calcium and phosphate homeostasis. Calcium salts are not freely soluble in body fluids, and increased levels of either calcium or phosphate, or both, can lead to the deposition of calcium salts in the soft tissues. Disorders in the normal process can result in a change in bone structure, and may contribute to the ease with which fractures occur. In osteoporosis, destruction exceeds production, and the transfer of calcium across the lumen of the kidney is vital (Mankin & Mankin 2003). Osteoporosis is clearly linked to end-stage renal failure, complicating the process of dialysis (Adams 2002).

References

Adams JE 2002 Dialysis bone disease. Seminars in Dialysis 15: 277–289.

Agelink MW, Sanner D, Eich H et al 2003 Does acupuncture influence the cardiac autonomic nervous system in patients with minor depression or anxiety disorders? Fortschritte der Neurologie-Psychiatrie 71: 141–149.

Dey T 1999 Soothing the troubled mind. Brookline, MA: Paradigm.

Janovsky B, White AR, Filshie J et al 2000 Are acupuncture points tender? A blinded study of Spleen 6. Journal of Alternative and Complementary Medicine 6: 149–155.

Mankin HJ, Mankin CJ 2003 Metabolic bone disease: an update. Instructional Course Lectures 52: 769–784.

McMillin DL, Richards DG, Mein EA, Nelson CD 1999 The abdominal brain and enteric nervous system. Journal of Alternative and Complementary Medicine 5: 575–586.

Payer L 1990 Medicine and culture – notions of health and sickness. London: Gollancz.

Rosen MR 2001 The heart remembers: clinical implications. Lancet 357: 468–471.

Further reading

Maciocia G 1989 The foundations of Chinese Medicine. Edinburgh: Churchill Livingstone.

Ross J 1984 Zang Fu, the organ system of Traditional Chinese Medicine. Edinburgh: Churchill Livingstone.

The extra meridians – the deepest level

KEY CONCEPTS

- ☯ The extraordinary vessels lie deeper than the basic meridian system.
- ☯ They do not have a direct relationship with the internal organs.
- ☯ The Du, Ren and Dai Mai are all singular.
- ☯ They act as storage reservoirs for Qi.
- ☯ They also drain off excess energy.
- ☯ Use of the extraordinary vessels can add a refinement to an acupuncture treatment and allow the use of fewer acupoints.
- ☯ Use of these vessels addresses very complex symptomatology.

Introduction

The origin of the extraordinary vessels is quite obscure. They are not specifically mentioned in the oldest Traditional Chinese Medicine (TCM) literature, the Nanjing, but are assembled in later versions, often being linked with the more superficial Luo vessels. The vessels as envisaged in current acupuncture practice are strictly storage vessels, serving both as a reservoir for Qi and as an emergency valve to drain off excess Qi. They all begin on the lower legs or trunk and ascend the body, with the exception of the Girdle vessel, Dai Mai. None is found on the upper limbs. Pirog (1996) makes the comparison with the vascular structure of a tree trunk, pumping the reserve energy upwards.

The extra vessels are not used in every patient treatment; they are almost a kind of back-up system and are usually used when the patient is responding only slowly (or not at all) to use of the regular meridians. They lie deeply in the tissues, close to the bone, and do not have a circulation in the same sense as the other meridians, each being described as a closed system. They are commonly brought into a treatment protocol as reservoirs of energy, or Qi, and tapped from one of the regular meridians when there is a deficiency condition, Xu, either within the meridian itself or in the connected Zang Fu organ. They can also be used as an energy sink, however, when there is a need to absorb energy quickly and the regular channels will not be able to contain it – a Shu condition.

With the exception of the Ren Mai and Du Mai, the extra vessels do not have their own acupuncture points but serve as a way of 'joining the dots' between the points already located on the regular channels, to redirect the flow of Qi. These vessels do not have Transport or Antique points in the same way as the regular channels. They are brought into action by the stimulation of their designated confluent point or opening point.

It is said that there are only eight of these extra vessels because they were an attempt to redefine the body in terms of a three-dimensional object. Thus, they will deal with the anteroposterior plane, interior–exterior dimension, superior–inferior and right–left. Each of the extra vessels corresponds with one of these planes.

Anterior–posterior	Ren, Du
Interior–exterior	Chong Mai, Dai Mai
Right–left	Yin Chiao Mai, Yang Chiao Mai
Superior–inferior	Yang Wei Mai, Yin Wei Mai

Each of the extra vessels has corresponding symptoms, which enable the practitioner to select the appropriate treatment. They are used in conjunction with ordinary acupuncture points, but enable a considerable reduction in the total number of points used. If the underlying theories are well understood, it is often possible to treat a wide pattern of symptoms by using a pair of these meridians only.

The extraordinary meridians are not connected to the Zang Fu organs in the same way as the regular meridians, but are considered to have an impact on the central nervous system, the hormonal system, the genitalia and the formation of blood cells. The two most commonly used are the Du and Ren meridians; these have much in common with the 12 regular meridians as they have their own distinct pathway with named points. They have alternative names:

☯ Du or Governor vessel
☯ Ren or Conception vessel.

Irrespective of Western custom, I prefer to use the original Chinese terms, Du and Ren, mainly because they are much less easy to confuse when abbreviated and written hastily. These two meridians serve as a central energetic axis for the body, dividing it into Yin and Yang hemispheres, anterior and posterior.

Du Mai

This meridian starts from the right kidney, runs downward to the perineum to Ren 1 Huiyin and then to Du 1 Changqiang, just behind the anus. From there it ascends in a straight line up the centre of the spine, passing up over the head and ending at Du 28 Yinjiao, on the inner surface of the upper lip. It is said to have a secondary branch in the lower abdomen linking it with the Ren Mai.

This is an essentially Yang meridian and is said to govern the other six Yang meridians. The character Du translates as 'controller' or 'governor'. It is associated with the central nervous system in modern Chinese acupuncture, but this idea is difficult to confirm in the TCM writings. The answer may lie in the original ideas on the contents of the skull, these being deemed to have most in common with the marrow of the long bones and to be connected to the kidneys. While the Heart housed the mind and spirit, the Kidney was also associated with consciousness and thought. The Du Mai is nonetheless regarded as having an influence over mental illness and problems with the central nervous system including paralysis, seizures, Windstroke and Parkinson's disease. The Chinese say: 'The Du Mai belongs to the Brain and joins it with the Kidney'.

Du Mai is most closely associated with the Taiyang, or most superficial meridians, particularly the Small Intestine, which comes quite close at SI 15 Jianzhongzhu. Excess energy in the meridian will cause stiffness and rigidity of posture, an exaggerated military bearing, while a lack of energy will bring about a slumped body posture.

It is generally recommended for any pain located centrally in the spine and is incorporated into routine pain relief for musculoskeletal acupuncture when the referred pain is improving and centralizing, particularly after mobilization. The points that lie at the same level as the Back Shu points on the UB channel also have some influence on the associated organs; for example, Du 4 Mingmen lies at the same level as UB 23 Shenshu, the Back Shu point for the Kidney.

The Du Mai is seen as a source of general support, not just that of the spinal column, and Du points, particularly Du 20 Baihui are used in cases of organ prolapse such as haemorrhoids or prolapse of the uterus. As the energy contained within it is predominantly Yang in nature, the Du Mai may be used to supplement Yang Qi. Another major point of the Du Mai is Du 26 Renzhong, which moves stagnation of Qi and Blood, and is used widely as a resuscitation point for patients. This point is used to revive a sleepy or fainting patient and has a strong sensory effect. It is also used for acute back pain where the spine is laterally deviated and fixed, and the patient cannot even lie on a bed for treatment. Needling this point and encouraging the patient to walk up and down for about 10 minutes can be very effective in relieving this type of muscle spasm in the clinic.

> The opening point for the Du Mai is SI 3 Houxi.

Ren Mai

The Ren and Du meridians are seen as complementary in terms of energy and, indeed, some authorities have regarded them as a single vessel, with a closed energy circulation. It has been suggested that Ren Mai originates in the womb, but the first external point is Ren 1 Huiyin, in front of the anus. From here it runs up the anterior midline to the neck and lower jaw to the centre of the mentolabial groove, passing through St 4 Dicang and bilaterally entering the eyes at St 1 Chengqi.

Ren Mai controls the six Yin channels and the anterior aspect of the body. It is the key to illnesses affecting the female reproductive system and to the treatment of women in general. The upper branch supplies the face and eyes, and can be used in facial paralysis or trigeminal neuralgia. Ren Mai regulates the Yin energy throughout the Sanjiao, acting as a drain when the Yin energy is abundant and as a reservoir that can be tapped when in short supply. When the Ren Mai absorbs excess energy, it also absorbs the Pathogens, neutralizing them.

The Ren Mai is the first choice for any kind of stagnation, making it influential in both respiratory and gastrointestinal disorders. It has a close relationship with the Lungs. The opening point is Lu 7 Lieque, which can be used in all 'sticky' Lung conditions such as emphysema, bronchitis, chronic congestive disease and congestion of the mucous membranes found in some types of sinusitis. Perhaps surprisingly, it is suggested for some skin conditions – those arising from any form of stagnation. It is also useful when there is a problem with the distribution of Body fluids throughout the Sanjiao.

The Ren Mai is linked with female fertility, and the Chinese claim that it is in charge of pregnancy. The following quote from the *Su Wen* (Chapter on Innate Vitality, Familiar Conversations section) indicates the transition from potential fertility to menopause:

A woman starts her period at the age of 14, when Ren Mai is unblocked and the pulse at Liv 3 Taichong is full. She is then capable of having a child... At the age of 49 Ren Mai is empty and the pulse at Liv 3 is forceless. Menstruation is exhausted and she cannot have a child.

There are particular points along the meridian that have defined functions: Ren 2 Qugu and Ren 3 Zhongji for urinary problems, Ren 3 and Ren 4 Guanyuan for genital conditions, and Ren 6 Qihai – the 'sea of energy' – for general debility. Ren 9 Shuifen is used for general fluid regulation, Ren 12 Zhongwan for gastric disturbances, Ren 17 Shanzhong for lung conditions and Ren 22 Tiantu for acute asthma.

The Ren Mai can be chosen as the main meridian for treatment if there is a lack of the Yin substances such as Yin Qi and Blood in the Kidney or Liver. It is also frequently selected to treat lung conditions.

The opening point for the Ren Mai is Lu 7 Lieque.

Chong Mai

The Chong Mai has two alternative names: the Penetrating or Vital vessel. It is regarded as the main store of Ancestral energy. It is paired and originates from the Kidneys, specifically the adrenal glands, and in the usual descriptions descends to the genitals and splits into two branches, an anterior and a posterior branch (Fig. 4.1). The anterior branch follows the Ren channel to Ren 4 Guanyuan, where it connects with the Kidney meridian at Kid 11 Henggu. From Kid 12 Dahe, a branch resurfaces and runs up the anterior chest wall to the neck and face where it circles the lips. The posterior branch is described as ascending in front of the spine. The meridian is also, less commonly, said to have a lower branch, leaving the main channel at St 30 Biguan, running down the medial aspect of the lower limb as far as Kid 4 Dazhong, where it divides, with one branch following the Kidney meridian and the other passing to Liv 3 Taichong.

The lower branch of the Chong Mai is said to join the three Yin meridians of the lower limb, perhaps in the region of Sp 6 Sanyinjiao, and the meridian has a link with both Spleen and Stomach function. The reason for the opening or master point being given as Sp 4 Gongsun is that, although the course of the Chong Mai relates it to the Kidney meridian, it is closer functionally to the Spleen.

Figure 4.1 Chong Mai. (Redrawn with kind permission from Low 1983.)

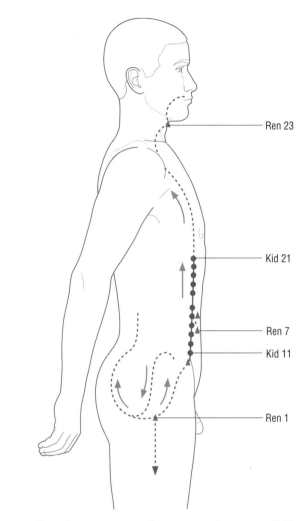

Ren 23

Kid 21

Ren 7

Kid 11

Ren 1

The meridian is sometimes known as the 'sea of blood', perhaps because of a primitive attempt to map arterial circulation, basing it on the abdominal aorta and noting that the extended branches cross several pulse points. This name may also arise from the connection with the uterus and menstruation. Low (1983, p 154) quotes a charming translation from the *Ling Shu* (Ch. 65), explaining the difference between the Chong Mai in men and women:

> *The Yellow Emperor asked: 'Does the fact that women have no beard or moustache mean that they have no blood or energy?'*
>
> *Chi-Po replied: 'The connective (Chong Mai) and Conception (Ren) meridians are both originated from the womb, and they travel upwards along the spine and are the sea of meridians. Their superficial branches travel along the abdominal region and upward to meet at the throat, and then separating from each other to link with the lips and mouth. When their blood and energy are in abundance, their skin will be hot and full of muscles: when their blood alone is in abundance, it will penetrate into the skin and they will grow fine hair. Now, the physiological characteristics of women are such that that they will have an excess of energy but a*

deficiency of blood, because their blood is periodically draining (namely, they have menstruation) with the result that the Chong Mai and the Ren meridian become incapable of nourishing the mouth and lips which explains why women do not have beards or moustaches.

This meridian is also sometimes referred to as the 'sea of the twelve meridians' because it is said to have so many internal connections, particularly in the chest and abdomen. The main symptoms of the Chong Mai are pains in the heart, tightness and discomfort in the chest, and abdominal swelling with intestinal gas pushing up against the diaphragm. The patients often suffer from abdominal pain after eating with audible peristalsis, borborygmus. There may be other symptoms, such as vomiting or palpitations with bradycardia. Treatment is aimed at 'flushing' the system and reversing rebellious Qi. The combination of Sp 4 Gongsun and Pe 6 Neiguan is often effective.

In spite of the quote from the Yellow Emperor from the *Ling Shu*, the Chong Mai does not appear to be particularly concerned with symptoms affecting the genitals, although it can be used when menstruation is decreased or abnormal. It is used in general cases of Blood deficiency. The Chong Mai is particularly useful when symptoms include stagnation of Blood and is often used in conjunction with the linked extraordinary meridian, Yin Wei Mai (described below). It is similar in use to the Liver meridian, perhaps explaining why the linked point Liv 3 Taichong can be so effective in many conditions. The Chong Mai is quite similar in function to the Ren meridian but has a more direct effect on digestion and Blood stagnation and rather less on the Kidneys and Lungs.

> The opening point for the Chong Mai is Sp 4 Gongsun.

Dai Mai or Girdle vessel

This meridian is singular and runs around the abdomen just like a belt; it is, in fact, the only meridian with a horizontal trajectory (Fig. 4.2). It is said to bind all the meridians that ascend or descend the trunk, providing support to them while having no clear direction of flow.

The Dai Mai receives energy from the Liver and the Gall Bladder, and probably from the Kidney. There are Liver and Gall Bladder points along its course and it is linked with GB 26 of the same name, Daimai.

Low (1983) suggests that the integrity of this vessel is maintained by the energy in the Stomach meridian. The concept of a support system, or even a corset, is confirmed by the characteristic symptoms. The patient feels as though 'sitting in water' and complains of a bloated abdomen and a stretched or sagging waist. The Dai Mai is particularly associated with congestion or stagnation in the lower abdomen in female patients, and there may be accompanying leucorrhoea. It is clearly indicated as a supportive structure in late pregnancy, and some authorities claim that injuring the Dai Mai can cause abortion. It can be used to treat headaches when these are associated with the Liver or Gall Bladder.

It is an interesting paradox that most symptoms directly associated with the Dai Mai directly concern the lower part of the body, whereas the indication for GB 41 Zulinqi, the opening point, are all to do with the upper

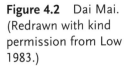

Figure 4.2 Dai Mai. (Redrawn with kind permission from Low 1983.)

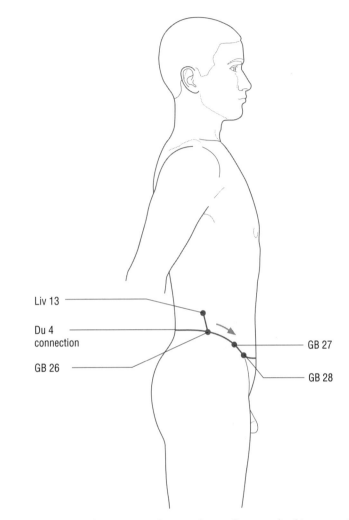

body; indeed, even the name indicates this – 'foot overlooking tears'. It has been suggested that the Dai Mai really does work like a belt cutting the body in two, and that sometimes it needs to be loosened to allow the two halves to communicate more freely. If the Yang remains in the head and the Yin becomes dominant in the lower body, the resulting symptoms would include headaches, dizziness and visual symptoms, with cold and weakness in the lumbar area, gravitational oedema, cold legs and chronic leucorrhoea.

The theoretical basis of the extraordinary meridians may seem rather obscure and not particularly relevant to modern acupuncture, but the following quotation from Pirog (1996, p 199) is illuminating:

It may well be that modern, urban life with its continuous stimulation of the sympathetic nervous system, has altered the appearance of some cases of Yang vacuity. Excessive use of the eyes (for driving, reading, operating computers, watching television) combined with a continuous sense of urgency tend to agitate the mind and keep the energy focused in the head. Meanwhile a lack of exercise and a general 'couch potato' body posture cause the back and lower limbs to deteriorate. The resulting modern stress disorder bears little resemblance to the Yin vacuity patterns that are typically called upon to explain spirit disturbance and 'rising Fire' symptoms in historical Chinese medicine.

Loosening of the girdle by using GB 41 Zulinqi and the coupled point SJ 5 Waiguan, allowing the Yang Qi to flow freely back to the Kidneys, may be helpful for these patients and prevent the slow development of more serious stagnation and heat conditions. Of course, lifestyle advice is always useful.

> The opening point for the Dai Mai is GB 41 Zulinqi.

Yang Chiao Mai and Yin Chiao Mai

These two vessels form a balanced pair starting from the lateral or medial aspects of the heel and running up the Yang or Yin aspects of the lower limb (Figs 4.3 & 4.4). The Yang Chiao Mai is considered to be a secondary vessel to the Urinary Bladder meridian, whereas the Yin Chiao Mai is considered to be secondary to the Kidney meridian. Both of these meridians are involved in fluid metabolism. The character 'Chiao' in this context translates as the motion of lifting up the feet. For this reason they are also often called the Yang or Yin Heel vessels. The implication is that they are mostly to do with motion and balance, and therefore influence the muscular structures of the lower limb. The Yin Chiao Mai is also linked to the general health of the female reproductive organs.

The Yang Chiao Mai starts from UB 62 Shenmai, runs up to UB 61 Pushen at the ankle and then up the outside of the leg to UB 59 Fuyang and GB 29 Femur Juliao. It then passes laterally up the trunk to SI 10 Naoshu, over the shoulder to LI 15 Jianyu and LI 16 Jugu, up the lateral aspect of the neck to St 4 Dicang and St 3 Nose Juliao and, passing through UB 1 Jingming, terminates at GB 20 Fengchi.

The Yin Chiao Mai starts at Kid 2 Rangu, ascends the medial aspect of the leg, passing through Kid 6 Zhaohai and Kid 8 Jiaoxin, running up to the inguinal ligament. It then enters the genitalia and runs from there up the anterior abdominal and thoracic wall to the clavicular region. It then reappears on the surface to run up the neck to St 9 Renying and finally to UB 1 Jingming, where it connects with the UB meridian.

There is an intriguing TCM theory of reciprocal muscle activity inherent in the theory linking these two meridians. If there is excess in the Yang Chiao, the muscles on the lateral aspect of the lower limb tend to become tight, while the muscles on the medial aspect of the limb tend to slacken, and vice versa with excess in the Yin meridian causing cramping on the medial aspect of the limb. Although this does indeed occur, careful palpation is needed to detect it, as there is rarely a gross inequality of muscle tone.

There is also an effect on vision, allowing the therapist to distinguish between the effects of the two meridians. Excess in the Yang Chiao causes red, irritated eyes unable to close, whereas an excess in the Yin channel means that the patient is sleepy and has difficulty opening the eyes at all. These meridians are also traditionally associated with epilepsy; fits occurring during the day are said to be due to excess in the Yin Chiao Mai, whereas those at night indicate excess in the Yang Chiao Mai. (Normal pat-

Figure 4.3 Yang Chiao Mai. (Redrawn with kind permission from Low 1983.)

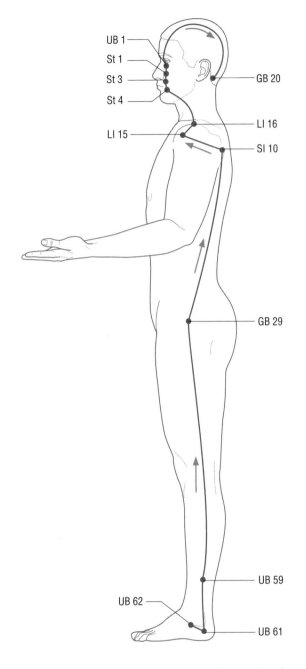

terns are general predominance of Yang energy during the day and of Yin energy during the night.)

These two meridians are considered to be able to help harmonize the spirit and to encourage the movement of energy up towards the head.

Yang Chiao Mai is recommended for use in rheumatoid arthritis, where red, swollen and hot joints indicate an excess of Yang. The technique is to drain the meridian. If a single Yang Chiao Mai is affected, this will lead to a unilateral stiffness and the patient will tend to lean towards the affected side – recognizable symptoms of the sequelae of stroke.

Figure 4.4 Yin Chiao Mai. (Redrawn with kind permission from Low 1983.)

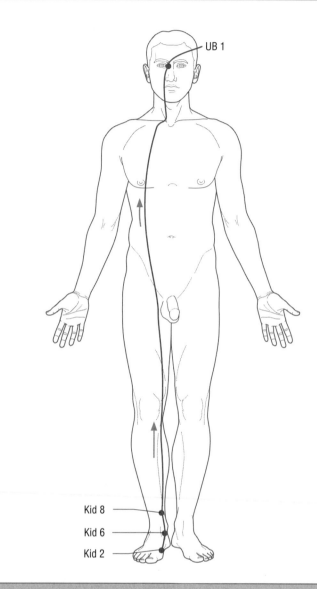

UB 1

Kid 8
Kid 6
Kid 2

The opening point for the Yang Chiao Mai is UB 62 Shenmai. The opening point for Yin Chiao Mai is Kid 6 Zaohai.

Yang Wei Mai and Yin Wei Mai

This is another commonly used pairing.

In this final pairing of extraordinary vessels, the character 'Wei' in Wei Qi was not understood in quite the same way, meaning less of an activity, more a state of readiness. The function of the Yang Wei Mai was to tie together all the Yang meridians, thus maintaining the integrity of the pathways – 'lacing it up tight' (Pirog 1996), and the Yin Wei Mai is seen in a similar way. Some authorities therefore refer to them as the Yin or Yang Regulating vessels. The Yin Wei Mai is seen as essentially controlling the interior and the Yang Wei Mai the exterior.

The Yang Wei Mai is considered as a secondary vessel to the Urinary Bladder; it starts at UB 63 Yinmen and ascends the lateral aspect of the leg through GB 35 Yangjiao, through the lateral area of the abdomen and chest to SI 10 Naoshu (Fig. 4.5). It then travels through SJ 15 Jianliao, GB 21 Jianjing and up through a number of GB points, St 8 Touwei and finishes at Du 15 Yamen. Connections with the Gall Bladder, Stomach, Small Intestine, Sanjiao and Du meridians are evident.

Problems within this meridian tend to be superficial, often manifesting as skin conditions such as acne or boils. As the Yang Wei Mai is sometimes

Figure 4.5 Yang Wei Mai. (Redrawn with kind permission from Low 1983.)

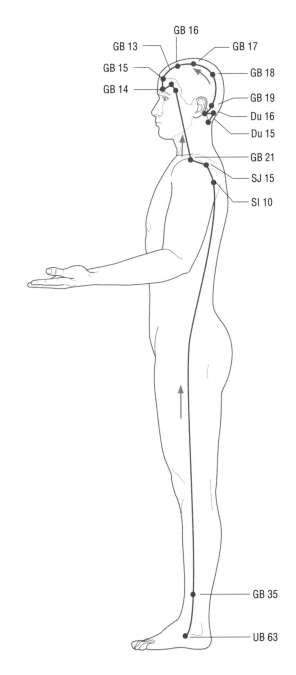

described as a network winding around the body supporting the muscles and keeping them tight, a lack of energy will cause low muscle tone, perhaps muscle weakness and hypermobility of the joints. A relaxation in function also predisposes the surface tissues to invasion by pathogenic factors, most particularly Wind. This means that the opening point, SJ 5 Waiguan, is used generally to augment defensive Qi and expel the Pathogen Wind.

Yin Wei Mai, like Yin Chiao Mai, is considered as a secondary vessel to the Kidney; it starts at Kid 9 Zhubin and ascends to the abdomen and Sp 13 Fushe. It runs upwards through Sp 15 Daheng, Sp 16 Fuai and Liv 14 Qimen. It then runs centrally to Ren 22 Tiantu and finishes at Ren 23 Lianquan (Fig. 4.6).

This meridian has a much deeper effect than its companion, the Yang Wei Mai, and displays symptoms in the main Zang Fu organs. These can include pain in the heart region, a heavy sensation in the chest and difficulty with respiration, pain in the genitalia, stomach problems, diarrhoea

Figure 4.6 Yin Wei Mai. (Redrawn with kind permission from Low 1983.)

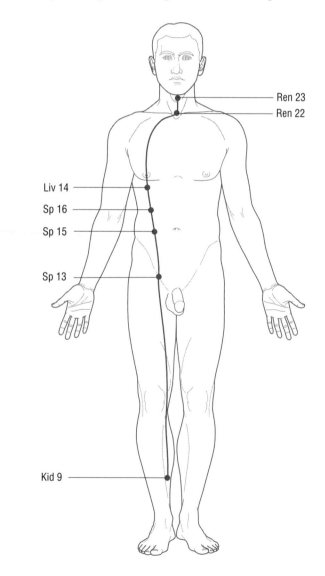

and rectal prolapse. It is also associated with mental symptoms such as fear and depression. According to Low (1983, p 164):

> *Classically, when Yin Wei is affected the patient is easily angered, groans with anguish and complains of pains in the heart. It has in fact been said that if Yin Wei is affected there must be some cardiac discomfort present. Yin becomes blood, blood belongs to the heart, thus the heart becomes painful.*

The TCM texts suggest that the two regulating vessels work best when they work together; failing to connect will cause a loss of willpower and a weakening of physical strength.

> The opening point for the Yang Wei Mai is SJ 5 Waiguan and that for the Yin Wei Mai is Pe 6 Neiguan.

Paired extraordinary meridians (Table 4.1)

Dai Mai and Yang Wei Mai

This pairing is frequently used in women's health, most commonly for menstrual disorders, particularly those involving a cyclical tendency to migraine. It can also be used for an excess of superficial energy. This combination is chosen when the symptoms are predominantly lateral and involve rising Yang or weakness of the abdominal wall or back. Basically, their use causes Yang to descend, and supports or binds the external structures.

Du Mai and Yang Chiao Mai

This pairing is commonly used for neurological problems affecting the spinal nerves or the brain. It is also used for joint problems in the head, neck and back, and tends to be selected more frequently for male ailments. These meridians are said to store and then redistribute Yang energy.

Chong Mai and Yin Wei Mai

These are often used when there is a thyroid problem. These two meridians have an effect on the deeper structures and are used in heart disease to regulate both spiritual and physical aspects. They can also be used in digestive problems involving the Spleen or counterflow of Qi. They will move

Table 4.1 Use of the paired extraordinary meridians

Coupled meridians		Paired points	
Dai Mai (hormonal influence)	Yang Wei Mai (CNS influence)	GB 41	SJ 5
Du Mai (CNS influence)	Yang Chiao Mai (hormonal influence)	SI 3	UB 62
Chong Mai (hormonal influence)	Yin Wei Mai (CNS influence)	Sp 4	Pe 6
Ren Mai (CNS influence)	Yin Chiao Mai (hormonal influence)	Lu 7	Kid 6

Blood stasis and treat Blood deficiency, and can be used for gynaecological problems.

Ren Mai and Yin Chiao Mai

This is another pairing that is frequently used for women's health problems, and also any problem involving Yin energies. These meridians have an effect on water metabolism throughout the Sanjiao. There is also an emphasis on symptoms arising near the anterior abdominal wall and those arising in the throat and lungs. The Ren Mai is always considered for abdominal disorders.

It is not always necessary to needle both components of an extraordinary meridian pair; as this form of treatment can be profound, decide which answers the predominant symptoms and use only that component at the first treatment. If there is little or no response, use the full pair the next time.

When using the extraordinary meridians in pairs there is a convention that not all four points need to be used, just a diagonal pair. The most important key point need be needled on only one side: the left side for male patients and the right side for female patients. The secondary point is then needled on the opposite side. Remove needles in the reverse order. It is debatable whether this ordering really makes any difference to the result – authorities are divided over it – but using fewer, well chosen needles is always a good idea.

Body points can also be used at the same time; the actual treatment points may well be selected first, with the extraordinary vessel chosen to support the treatment aims. It is preferable only to use points that are actually on the meridian selected, although other points with a clear theoretical TCM connection can be considered.

Use in physiotherapy

Extraordinary meridians are an interesting concept, uniting large areas of TCM theory and enabling a more subtle and economical use of acupoints. The practitioner is not likely to want to access this additional resource with every treatment – nor should they. These meridians are most appropriate when the situation is a chronic one and is perhaps not resolving with more orthodox acupuncture treatment. Use of the extraordinary meridians usually calls upon the body's reserves. Not all patients can respond to this. Care must be taken with patients who are suffering from long-term debilitating diseases: the Kidney energies are not infinite. However, use of the Chong Mai and Dai Mai in particular can sometimes produce good results in patients presenting with long-term joint pain but who appear to have general low-grade health problems.

There is some discussion about the effect of acupuncture on the hormonal system generally and on the pituitary in particular. Most of the clinical effect seems to depend on needling UB 1 Jingming, which is not recommended to any but the most adventurous acupuncturist.

Low (1983) writes about the use of these meridians, suggesting that a boost of cortisone can be achieved by tonifying the following points when it is desirable to wean the patient off oral steroids:

- ☯ Kid 2 Rangu
- ☯ Sp 2 Dadu
- ☯ GB 39 Xuanzhong

- GB 25 Jingmen
- A 'special point' between C3/4
- UB 23 Shenshu.

Low also recommends this formula for use in rheumatoid arthritis or asthma. While interesting clinically, and quite widely used, there does not appear to be any research evidence for this combination of points, although acupuncture has been shown to increase the concentration of adrenocorticotrophic hormone (ACTH) (Nappi et al 1982). This occurs as a consequence of stimulating the pituitary, usually through the needling of UB 1 Jingming, and could be responsible for an increased release of corticosteroids from the adrenal cortex.

CASE HISTORY

Case study 4.1

Female, 66 years old, recent hospital discharge after serious gastrointestinal problem diagnosed as 'diverticulitis'. Has had heavy doses of antibiotics and remained in hospital for several weeks 'under observation' with a high temperature. Now lacking in energy, sleepy and generally uncomfortable. Suffers from chronic asthma. Shooting pains in right hip, and tingling and numbness in both feet. Nothing indicating back problems. No appetite.

Impression: Spleen Qi Xu, underlying undefined deficiencies, maybe Kidney Yin?

Treatment 1 points

- SJ 5 Waiguan and GB 41 Zulinqi, to relink top and bottom Qi
- GB 34 Yanglingquan and GB 43 Xiaxi for right hip pain
- Sp 6 Sanyinjiao for poor lower leg circulation (skin condition too fragile for this point, so Sp 10 substituted)
- Yintang to lift spirits
- Needles retained for 20 minutes. See in 1 week.

Treatment 2
Claimed to have been completely 'wiped out' by treatment; spent 3 days sleeping. Now a little brighter. Some pain relief, less tingling.

Repeated points using Sp 6 Sanyinjiao as skin was much improved. Needles retained for only 10 minutes.

Treatment 3
Similar response; drowsy for 4 days, but now much better. Pain mostly gone, much brighter in herself. Feels she had a healing crisis. A general Qi boost now given:

- Kid 3 Taixi
- Sp 6 Sanyinjiao
- St 36 Zusanli
- Yintang
- Needles retained for 20 minutes.

Continues

Case study 4.1   cont'd

Treatments 4 and 5
Much better, normal appetite, bright, attentive, out walking. No further pain.
Discharged.
    The initial work with the extraordinary meridians may have been too
strong, but certainly produced results in this woman.

References

Low R 1983 The secondary vessels of acupuncture. New
    York: Thorsons.

Nappi G, Facchinetti F, Legnante G et al 1982 Different
    releasing effects of traditional manual acupuncture
    and electroacupuncture on propriocortin-related
peptides. Acupuncture and Electro-Therapeutics
    Research International Journal 7: 93–103.

Pirog JE 1996 The practical application of meridian style
    acupuncture, 1st edn. Berkeley, CA: Pacific View
    Press.

Meridian acupuncture – linking the layers

- Acupuncture meridians lie just under the skin.
- Simple meridian acupuncture is very effective for pain.
- Most of it is based on a need to get the Qi circulating freely.
- The Antique points play a vital part in the intelligent use of meridian acupuncture.
- Each meridian has a characteristic clinical pattern.
- It is important to understand the links with the underlying Zang Fu organs.
- Reasons for point selection are many and varied.

Introduction

Meridian acupuncture is the most common form of acupuncture currently in use. It is what is taught in most basic courses and frequently claimed by 'scientific' medical practitioners or physiotherapists to be only for pain relief. A brief examination of the traditional acupuncture theories about the activity of the points should convince a student that it would be impossible to confine the effects only to the relief of pain. All current scientific investigations also tend to confirm this. While some of the pain relief mechanisms are understood, if only partly, many others are still puzzling, linking with complex sympathetic and parasympathetic responses as they do.

Notwithstanding our patchy comprehension of the *modus operandi*, the principles of meridian acupuncture are easy to understand and use clinically. A lot of meridian acupuncture is derisively termed 'formula' or 'cookbook' acupuncture, but this is to underestimate the effects produced. The best acupuncture is simple. Indeed, a popular saying among acupuncturists is that an acupuncture master uses only one carefully chosen point to treat the patient. Perhaps that is asking too much, but certainly the homeopathic adage 'less is more' holds true for acupuncture, and the most effective treatments seem to be those involving only three or four points.

The meridian network is invisible and difficult to sense, although some practitioners and patients are able to describe the movement of Qi along the meridian as a sort of tingle, or warmth. It is difficult not to view this as wishful thinking, although I have convinced myself, my patients and many of my students that there is something to be felt. Certainly some talented practitioners claim to be able to sense blockages within the meridians and to 'move the Qi' without contacting the patient at all. I am not aware that any-one has come up with a satisfactory explanation for this phenomenon yet.

However, this state of affairs may soon be changed. Some researchers investigating the effects of acupuncture needling on the brain with functional magnetic resonance imaging have shown some very interesting links (Cho et al 1999, Wu et al 1999), described in Chapter 1. This work is dramatic and has no real explanation as yet. It is difficult to establish precisely which structures are carrying the stimulus. The work by Darras et al (1992) was also mentioned in Chapter 1, and has been an additional piece of intriguing evidence for acupuncturists – although by no means a vindication.

The meridians shown in all the illustrations are channels in which the Qi flows, and the acupoints on the meridians are sites where the flow of Qi may be influenced. Simple meridian acupuncture is based on the use of distal and proximal points to control pain or some other local manifestation of imbalance. Pain itself is said to be caused by a blockage of the flow of Qi in the meridians or between the internal organs. All the meridians have the name of one of the Zang Fu organs (see Ch. 4) and influence that organ to a greater or lesser degree. Particular points on the meridian are considered to have a stronger effect on the internal organs than others (see Antique points below).

Internal links or collaterals from the external channel network are postulated by Traditional Chinese Medicine (TCM), but the course of these remains impossible to prove. The linking is according to Zang Fu theory and also to the perceived clinical applications of the meridians. For example, the Liver meridian is said to have a collateral link to the throat area leading to its use to treat the symptom 'plum stone throat' in which the patient feels that something has been swallowed and lodged uncomfortably in the throat.

As the health of the body and its pain-free state depend on the smooth flow of Qi around the meridians, any blockage will cause a problem. Blockage or slowing is usually considered to be caused by the invasion of Pathogens. Pathogenic invasion is often implicated in rheumatic or arthritic conditions, termed Bi syndrome by the Chinese. The external or exogenous Pathogens implicated are Wind, Cold and Damp (see Ch. 1). Heat is also listed, but this tends to be less of a problem with regard to invasion from the exterior. It usually occurs after one of the other Pathogens, or a combination of them, has entered and slowed the flow of Qi and fluids. This slowing tends to produce a stickiness or thickening in the fluids, ultimately giving rise to Phlegm. Phlegm itself turns into an internal form of Heat.

Endogenous Pathogens can also cause damage to the flow of Qi and fluids. These are described in detail elsewhere, but consist predominantly of overjoy, overthinking, anxiety, grief, fear and anger. These are normal emotions but present in an excess or pathological form; they act on the Zang Fu organs, disturbing the normal physiological balance (see Ch. 3).

Treatment of pain

The following strategies are commonly used to select points for the treatment of pain (Table 5.1).

Local points

Local points are chosen because they are on the meridian in the near vicinity of the pain. The meridian may, of course, not run precisely over the spot, so it may be necessary to select two points as near as possible to the

Table 5.1 Choosing points for meridian acupuncture

Method	Comment
Local point(s)	Selected according to pain site
Distal point(s)	Selected according to the meridian(s) chosen
Adjacent points	Points on nearby meridians when it is not possible to select one running across the area
Extra points	Points not on a meridian but local to the pain
Influential points	Points with a specific link to a body area or function
Antique or Transport points	Selected according to the quality of the Qi energy found at different levels in the meridian or according to Five Element theory
Zang Fu links	Chosen according to Zang Fu physiology
Luo or connecting points	Chosen to access energy from the Yuan point of the coupled meridian
Xi Cleft point	Chosen to treat acute disease on the corresponding meridian
Influence on pathogenic factors	Chosen to expel a specific invading Pathogen
According to Eight Principle diagnosis	Allows logical identification of problem category
The Four Seas	Regulation and coordination
According to pulse diagnosis	Indicates system under stress
According to tongue diagnosis	Indicates system under stress
According to links with the extra meridians	Selected more for the action of the meridian than for the actual anatomical site
Treat the opposite side	Aim for energy balance

locus of the pain. These points are used to collect or concentrate the energy where it is most needed.

Distal points

The distal points are to be found on the extremities on the same meridians. They are not usually the very last points, the so-called Tsing points, because these are relatively uncomfortable to the patient, but often points situated at the wrist or ankle, or occasionally the elbow or knee. It is customary to use UB 40 Weizhong, located behind the knee, when treating low back pain. It is said that the local points stabilize or collect the energy, whereas the distal points are used to encourage movement and circulation of the Qi.

The Chinese recommend the use of the two types of point on the selected meridian: those local to the pain and those situated distally. To take a common example, when treating a case of tennis elbow, the usual site of pain lies under the course of the Large Intestine meridian. The most obvious points to use would be LI 11 Quchi or LI 10 Shousanli as local points. The distal point is usually selected on the same meridian, and in this case would be LI 4 Hegu. This type of treatment is commonly used and fits quite well with the idea of using a sensory stimulation in an area with the same spinal nerve supply, following dermatomes and myotomes.

Although it is difficult to prove that these are the best points to use in this type of case, some useful work has been done in Sweden to check the accepted wisdom of the optimal dose of acupuncture (Lundeberg et al 1988). Experimental tooth pain was treated by needling only local acupoints, only distal acupoints, or a mixture of the two. The combination was significantly more successful than the other two methods, indicating that the accepted form of meridian acupuncture could be supported by research. Lundeberg et al demonstrated that the optimal time for acupuncture treatment was 20 minutes, although Lundeberg has since said that as the optimal time for the development of a placebo effect is 30 minutes, this should also be taken into account.

Adjacent points

Adjacent points are also considered when the meridians do not lie over the area – not all problems locate themselves conveniently beneath a line of acupuncture points. That said, there are few places on the body where it is not possible to find a relevant acupoint. Adjacent points will be selected on neighbouring meridians, usually of the same Yin or Yang polarity.

Extra points

Extra points are those that have a defined anatomical location but do not lie on one of the meridians. They will frequently supply a local point when the pain location does not coincide with a meridian. These points are named and have defined actions and indications. There are exceptions to this rule; for instance, the extra point Yintang is plainly on the Du meridian, lying as it does directly above the nose, between the inner ends of the eyebrows – in the position of the 'third eye' of some cultures. It is not clear from the literature quite why it is considered as an extra point because it has been in use for some hundreds of years. Another exception to the rule is Shiqizhuixia (known by students as the sneeze point!), which also lies on the Du meridian just below the spinous process L5.

Influential points

The Influential or Hui points are designated acupoints that are thought to have a particular sphere of influence. They are frequently added to a prescription in order to boost some aspect of that treatment. Some of the links are clearer than others. The main groups are listed in Table 5.2.

The influence of GB 39 on 'marrow' is slightly controversial. The original TCM theories do not recognize either the brain or the nervous system as such; however, many acupuncture authorities use GB 39 to influence the

Table 5.2 Influential points

Name	Location	Action
UB 11 Dashu	1.5 cun lateral to the lower border of the spinous process of T1	Influence on bone. Used in all bone diseases and bony Bi syndrome
Ren 12 Zhongwan	On the midline of the abdomen 4 cun above the umbilicus	Influence on the Fu organs. Used for gastrointestinal problems, vomiting, diarrhoea, etc.
GB 34 Yanglingquan	Just below the head of the fibula, anterior to the neck	Influence on muscles and tendons. 'Physical therapy' point
Lu 9 Taiyang	At the wrist joint in the depression between the radial artery and the tendon of abductor pollicis longus	Influence on blood vessels. Used when the pulse is weak generally
GB 39 Xuanxhong	3 cun above the lateral malleolus, posterior to the shaft of the fibula	Influence on 'marrow'
Liv 13 Zhangmen	On the lateral side of the abdomen, below the free end of the floating 11th rib	Influence on the Zang organs. Benefits both the Spleen and the Liver
Ren 17 Shanzhong	On the midline of the sternum, between the nipples, level with the 4th intercostal space	Qi and respiratory function. Meeting point of Qi
UB 17 Geshu	1.5 cun lateral to the lower border of the spinous process of the 7th thoracic vertebra	Used for all Blood problems, circulation, stagnation, deficiency, etc.

Cun, often defined as the Chinese inch, is a proportional measure corresponding to the width of the first distal interphalangeal joint of the patient.

nervous system and it is considered almost obligatory in the treatment of hemiplegia, and occasionally recommended as a point for preventing stroke.

Low (2001) considers that there are at least a further six points with some claim to being considered 'influential points':

- Sp 6 Sanyinjiao – for all gynaecological conditions and for the three Yin channels on the lower limb
- Sp 8 Diji – for the uterus
- UB 60 Kunlun – for general pain

☯ UB 57 Chengshan – for anal conditions, haemorrhoids

☯ St 39 Xiajuxu – poor circulation in the lower limb

☯ Sp 3 Taibai – reduces and resolves dampness.

It is certain that each acupuncturist develops their own list of Influential points – those that seem particularly felicitous in their use with clearly defined categories of damage or imbalance. The list could be very long.

Antique or Transport points

The Antique points are groupings of points on each of the regular meridians that lie below the elbow or knee. They are remnants of an older belief about the circulation of Qi. Originally it was thought that Qi entered the body from outside – so-called 'cosmic Qi'. It entered at the extremities, the fingers and toes, and then flowed along the meridians into the body (Fig. 5.1). This idea predates that of the 24-hour enclosed Qi circulation (Fig. 5.2) in which the Qi concentration can be located by the practitioner at any time during the day or night; the new Qi, the Post-Heaven Qi, is transformed from food, drink and air.

It is said that in ancient China at an early stage in Chinese Medicine, doctors were not allowed to view the whole body of their female patients but just an arm or a leg from behind a screen. It is perhaps fortunate for acupuncture that this group of points includes some of the most powerful and effective points.

The rather charming metaphor underpinning the Transport points is that the quality of Qi present in the meridian changes its character as it

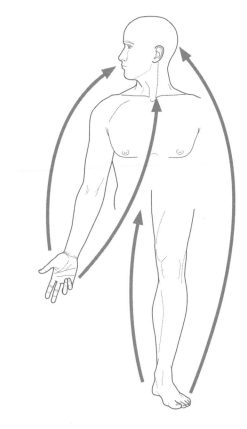

Figure 5.1   Qi flow supporting Antique Qi points. (Redrawn with kind permission from Hopwood et al 1997.)

Figure 5.2 Modern theory of self-contained Qi flow. (Redrawn with kind permission from Hopwood et al 1997.)

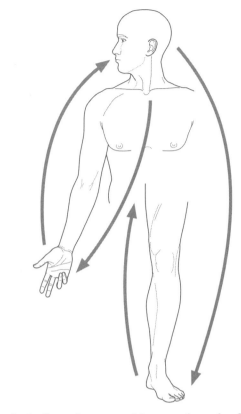

flows into the body from the extremities, much as the flow of water in a river (Fig. 5.3). It is important to note that these points all have a designated element – Wood, Fire, Earth, Metal or Water – and that correct use of these is vital in Five Element acupuncture (Fig. 5.4) (see also Ch. 3 for Five Element theory).

Jing Well points

The Qi enters at these points, sited right at the tips of the extremities in most cases (fingers and toes), the Kidney being the exception. The Qi, although vigorous, is not easily obtainable as bleeding is required to extract it at these points; comparison is made with dipping a bucket into

Figure 5.3 Antique or Transport points.

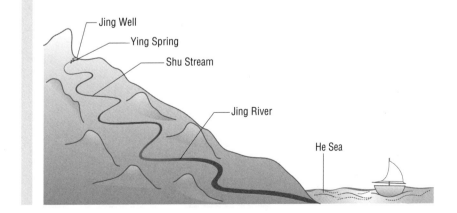

Figure 5.4 Five Elements and Antique points.

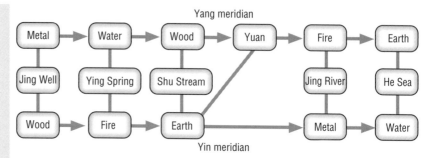

a well. If a bucketful is removed, more will come, but obtaining the water requires initial effort. These points are recommended for use in local stagnation and in cases of pathogenic Heat. Use of these points is not generally popular with physiotherapists or patients, because they are quite painful, but they have a place in hot, febrile, acute situations (Table 5.3). In TCM they are bled – a single drop allowed to escape after needling – in order to clear pathogenic Heat from the channel. Bleeding any point is not encouraged by the Acupuncture Association of Chartered Physiotherapists in the UK.

Ying Spring points

The metaphor describes a small but strong mountain spring. Unlike the Well points, the Qi flows freely and constantly, needing no encouragement. There is sufficient power in the flow to clear Pathogens from the channel but, because the channel is narrow, it is rare for Pathogens to enter at this level. These points are situated on the borders of the palms and soles where the skin changes colour, and they are associated with visible signs of heat, flushed face, red eyes, sore throat, etc.

These points are more comfortable to needle and are often used in preference to the Jing Well points because their properties are similar. They are sometimes used in Bi syndromes to relieve the pressure of exogenous Pathogens. In Yin meridians they should be used alone or together with the Shu Stream point. Similar use is recommended on Yang meridians to influence visceral patterns. See Table 5.4.

Some well known points for draining excess Heat are found at the Ying Spring level: St 44 Neiting, Liv 2 Xingjian and Lu 10 Yuji. Pe 8 Laogong can also be used to clear Heat, but it is preferable to use only a light touch, not a needle.

Table 5.3 Jing Well or Tsing points

Normal flow to extremities	Normal flow from extremities	Therapeutic uses
Lu 11	LI 1	To treat disease of Zang organs
St 45	Sp 1	Mental illness
Ht 9	SI 1	Sudden emotional change
UB 67	Kidney 1	Stifling sensation in the chest
Pe 9	SJ 1	Sudden severe pain
GB 44	Liv 1	

Yin meridians: Wood; Yang meridians: Metal.

Table 5.4 Ying Spring points

Normal flow to extremities	Normal flow from extremities	Therapeutic uses
Lu 10	LI 2	Febrile diseases
St 44	Sp 2	Changes in skin colour, flushed
Ht 8	SI 2	cheeks
UB 66	Kid 2	Inflamed mucous membranes
Pe 8	SJ 2	Accelerates flow of energy in the
GB 43	Liv 2	meridian

Yin meridians: Fire; Yang meridians: Water.

Shu Stream points

These are different in character to the previous points; the flow of Qi is now established and substantial, with a clear direction. The Shu Stream points are considered as a balancing point for the energy in the channel. On the Yin meridians the Shu Stream point and the Yuan Source point are identical. This means that there is one less point in this group on Yin meridians. The Yang meridians have a separate Yuan Source point that is associated with Fire, not Wood. The function of the Yuan points on the Yang meridians has been hotly contested; the use of the designation 'Yuan Source' indicates the favourite theory that these points can be used to access the Source Qi of the meridian. The most commonly used Yuan point is LI 4 Hegu. It has also been suggested that this additional point on the Yang meridians offers a further barrier to pathogenic invasion and can be utilized in Bi syndromes, particularly those involving fluctuating symptoms (e.g. rheumatoid arthritis). Pirog (1996) offers two other ideas: (1) the Yang meridians are generally longer and need an extra transportation point and (2) the contrast of five Yin points as opposed to six Yang points has its roots in Chinese astrology.

Shu Stream points are used for spleen diseases accompanied by a heavy sensation in the body or heavy painful joints. This is most often associated with Spleen Qi Xu. As the syndrome also diminishes the normal physiological function of the Spleen, transformation and transportation dampness tends to collect in the body and the Shu Stream points are used for this (Table 5.5).

Table 5.5 Shu Stream and Yuan Source points

Shu Stream	Yuan Source	Therapeutic uses
Lu 9	Lu 9	Bi syndrome
LI 3	LI 4	Chronic pain
St 43	St 42	Wind and Damp pathogenic invasion
Sp 3	Sp 3	Damp stasis
Ht 7	Ht 7	
SI 3	SI 4	
UB 65	UB 64	
Kid 3	Kid 3	
Pe 7	Pe 7	
SJ 3	SJ 43	
GB 41	GB 40	
Liv 3	Liv 3	

Yin meridians: Earth; Yang meridians: Wood.

The points on the meridians connected to Zang organs tend to be widely influential and are frequently included in prescriptions.

Jing River points

There is abundant Qi at the Jing River points, which are capable of strong action. Their name indicates that, like untamed rivers, they are capable of bursting their banks and flooding the surrounding countryside, or being used for controlled irrigation. They are frequently used to influence the musculotendinous meridians, situated mostly in the surrounding muscle tissue (see Ch. 6). The Qi nourishes and protects bones and sinews, so Jing River points are used for tendon or joint pain.

This influence on muscle tissue means that they are also used in cases of paralysis or spasm, and for the more complex or chronic Bi patterns. In Yang meridians Jing River points can be used to treat febrile diseases such as malaria. They are said to be useful when illness is reflected in the voice (Table 5.6).

He Sea points

The He Sea (or Ho) points are situated just below the elbow or the knee joint, and are the last points on each limb where the Qi can be said to be close to the surface. After the He Sea point, the Qi goes deeper into the tissues and, although it can still be accessed for superficial and local treatment, will not have much effect on the Zang Fu organs.

The He Sea points all have a strong physiological effect. They are said to regulate the flow of Qi between the distal parts of the meridian and the inner body. They are used to access the Zang Fu energy or to treat the Zang Fu organs. Two at least, LI 11 Quchi and St 36 Zusanli, have a strong immune effect. St 36 is generally used as a tonic for the whole digestive system, and many of the He Sea points can be used in a similar way.

The He Sea points are used in the treatment of Bi patterns, muscle spasm and paralysis (Table 5.7). On Yin meridians they are used for urinary symptoms, and on Yang meridians they tend to be used to irrigate the joints and tendons in the same way as the River points on the Yin meridians.

Each of the Fu organs has a He Sea point in the three Yang channels of the foot. These are called the Lower He Sea points; the most well known of

Table 5.6 Jing River points

Normal flow to extremities	Normal flow from extremities	Therapeutic uses
Lu 8	LI 5	Asthma, wheezing
St 41	Sp 5	Cough, sore throat
Ht 4	SI 5	Change in voice
UB 60	Kid 7	Lockjaw
Pe 5	SJ 6	Paralysis
GB 38	Liv 4	Spasm
		Tendon or joint pain

Yin meridians: Metal; Yang meridians: Fire.

Table 5.7 He Sea points

Normal flow to extremities	Normal flow from extremities	Therapeutic uses
Lu 5	LI 11	Stomach disorders
St 36	Sp 9	Allergies
Ht 3	SI 8	Imbalances in Fu organs
UB 40	Kid 10	Immune disease
Pe 3	SJ 10	Shoulder pain (St 38)
GB 34	Liv 8	

Yin meridians: Water; Yang meridians: Earth.

these is St 38 Tiakou, which, because of its link with the Large Intestine meridian, is use to treat chronic shoulder pain.

Zang Fu links

The Zang Fu links tend to be similar to those of the named meridians. Knowledge of the Zang Fu characteristics will inform intelligent therapeutic combination of points (see Ch. 3). This rationale for point selection also depends on use of the Eight Principles and, if practised, on pulse diagnosis. The links are also important when Five Element acupuncture is used.

Luo points

Luo points are acupoints where a meridian diverges to connect with the Yuan point of the coupled meridian. They are indicated when there is disease of the paired or externally–internally related meridian. They can be used singly, or coupled with the Yuan points in what is described as a 'host–guest' combination. The Yuan point is selected from the meridian that was diseased first (the host), and the second meridian Luo point is the guest. For example:

- For diseases in the Lung meridian, take Lu 9 Taiyang as the Yuan point and LI 6 Pianli as the Luo point.
- For disease in the Large Intestine meridian, take LI 4 Hegu as the Yuan point and Lu 7 Lieque as the Luo point. Lieque can thus be said to have an action on the shoulder or the elbow via this Luo connection. This is often a very useful technique in 'real life' when pain does not confine itself to the course of a single meridian but seems to be spread across the area of influence of both Yin and Yang channels.

The Luo points can also be used to influence the Luo vessels when excess or stasis is observed, for instance in visibly congested superficial varicosities.

Xi Cleft points

These points may be used to treat acute diseases in the respective related organs. They are thought to be spaces or clefts where the Qi is accumulated for the corresponding channel. There is one in each of the 12 regular channels and one in each of the four extraordinary channels (Yinwei, Yangwei, Yinqiao and Yangqiao), making 16 in all. It will be seen from Table 5.8 that some of these points are more commonly used than others, perhaps because the distal points on the channels tend to be substituted.

Table 5.8   Xi Cleft points

Channel	Xi Cleft point
Lung	Lu 6 Kongzui
Pericardium	Pe 4 Ximen
Heart	Ht 6 Yinxi
Large Intestine	LI 7 Wenliu
Sanjiao	SJ 7 Huizong
Small Intestine	SI 6 Yanglao
Stomach	St 34 Liangqiu
Gall Bladder	GB 36 Waiqiu
Urinary Bladder	UB 63 Jinmen
Spleen	Sp 8 Diji
Liver	Liv 6 Zhongdu
Kidney	Kid 5 Shuiquan
Yangqiao	UB 59 Fuyang
Yinqiao	Kid 8 Jiaoxin
Yangwei	GB 35 Yangjiao
Yinwei	Kid 9 Zhubin

Influence on pathogenic factors

The pathogenic factors are thought to be the cause of much superficial pain and many disease processes within the body. Many of the commonly used pain points – the eyes of the shoulder and the eyes of the knee, for example – are also defined as those expelling one or two Pathogens. All acupuncturists are likely to have a list of favourite points for this, but Table 5.9 provides a list of the more common ones. The best are shown in bold type. Many treatment choices are ruled by the relative ease of positioning a patient with an appropriate combination of points.

Table 5.9   Points to expel Pathogens

Pathogen	Points
Resolving Heat	**LI 11 Quchi, LI 4 Hegu, UB 40 Weizhong, Sp 10 Xuehai, GB 20 Fengchi, Liv 2 Xingjian** Lu 5 Chize, Lu 9 Taiyuan, St 40 Fenglong, SI 3 Houxi, SJ 5 Waiguan
Resolving Damp	**St 40 Fenglong, Sp 9 Yinlingquan, Sp 6 Sanyinjiao, SJ 5 Waiguan, SJ 6 Zhigou** St 25 Tianshu, UB 12 Fengmen, UB 23 Shenshu, Kid 6 Fuliu
Dispelling Wind	**GB 20 Fengchi, LI 4 Hegu, Du 16 Fengfu, UB 11 Dashu, UB 12 Fengmen, LI 4 Hegu, LI 11 Quchi** Lu 9 Taiyuan, Lu 11 Shaoshang, LI 15 Jianyu, LI 20 Yingxiang
Dispelling Cold	**LI 4 Hegu, Lu 7 Lieque, Sp 6 Sanyinjiao, Ren 9 Shuifen, Du 16 Fengfu** Du 14 Dazhui, Ren 4 Guanyuan, Ren 6 Qihai, GB 30 Huantiao (Wind Damp)

According to Eight Principle diagnosis

This is described in detail in Chapter 1, but the diagram in Figure 5.5 serves to focus on the pairings. However, most patients are not aware that they should conform to this particular theory and tend to present with a mixed bag of signs and symptoms. It is useful to make a list and group the symptoms by their Eight Principle category. Points may then be chosen to complement the predominant symptoms.

Figure 5.5 Eight Principle pairs.

Excess	Hot	Yang	External
Deficiency	Cold	Yin	Internal

Yin and Yang can be used to select the appropriate meridian(s) by following the algorithm in Figure 5.6. It is clear that Yang meridians tend to be chosen to treat external problems or those involving the Pathogens Wind or Heat, the Fu organs, and stagnation of Qi or Blood. Conversely, the Yin meridians are used for the Pathogens Cold and Damp, and for deficiencies in Blood, specific Yin or Yang energy deficiencies, and Essence.

Figure 5.6 Selection of meridians using Yin and Yang.

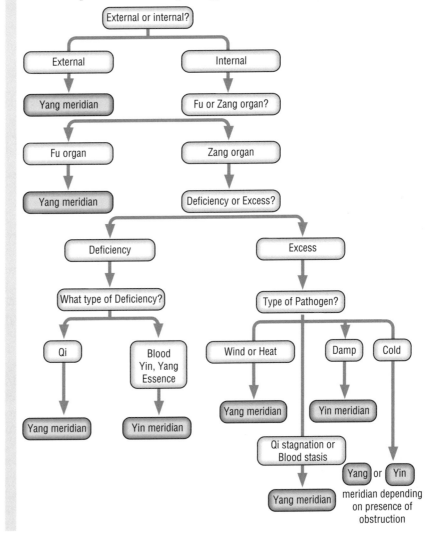

However, all treatments need to be practical and it may be that points are ultimately chosen because of their strategic distance from, or closeness to, the problem and their ease of use in the position adopted by the patient.

The Four Seas

The Seas are points that are held to have connections to wider availability of the substances identified – Energy, Nourishment, Blood and Marrow.

The *Sea of Energy* is held to be the following three points:

- Ren 17 Shanzhong – regulates the Qi associated with respiration
- St 9 Renying – controls ascending Qi, said to be that ascending to heaven
- UB 10 Tianzhu – controls the descent of Qi throughout the body.

The Sea of Energy is used for pain in the chest, red face and dyspnoea. It could also be used to energize the system.

The *Sea of Nourishment*:

- St 30 Qichong – a point of the extra Chong meridian, controls the distribution of Qi throughout the body
- St 36 Zusanli – regulates the digestion, bowels and drainage of the lower part of the body.

The Sea of Nourishment is used for abdominal distension or anger and lack of appetitie.

The *Sea of Blood*:

- UB 11 Dashu – connected to the bones, thought of as the framework for energy flow
- St 37 Shangjuxu – involved in movement of Yang towards Yin
- St 39 Xiajuxu – involved in movement of Yin towards Yang.

The Sea of Blood is used for changes in body sensation, bloatedness or tight feelings.

The *Sea of Marrow*:

- Du 16 Fengfu
- Du 20 Baihui

Both points are associated with the central nervous system.

According to pulse diagnosis

Not all acupuncture practitioners would claim to be expert at pulse diagnosis. This is a diagnostic technique that requires considerable practice to perfect. It is too complex to describe in detail, but allows the expert to pick up clues as to which Zang Fu system may be stressed. The pulse is felt just above the wrist, over the radial artery; three fingers are used, giving three positions. These are then divided into superficial, middle and deep at each fingertip, allowing for many subtle variations. Most acupuncturists should be able to sense the difference between a vigorous and a weak pulse, and further refinement comes only with practice.

According to tongue diagnosis

Tongue diagnosis is useful when facing a complex set of symptoms, but the state of the tongue tends to reflect only conditions of longstanding. Even if used only in the broadest sense, tongue diagnosis can be a useful indication of whether stagnation or pathogenic Heat is present. The practitioner is advised to study the patient's tongue on a regular basis in order to develop a clear idea of the normal parameters and whether changes occur after successful acupuncture treatment.

Links with the extra meridians

Use of the extra meridians is described in Chapter 4. They can be used for several reasons. The most common use is as a source of additional energy in a depleted or seriously ill patient. Extra meridians should not be accessed unless more orthodox treatment is failing. They can also be used to decrease the number of needles used or simply to pull together a disparate or widely spread collection of acupoints.

Using the opposite side

The simple basis for this is that the two sides of the body should be roughly equivalent with regard to Qi energy; where there is a marked imbalance, it makes sense to try to right this. Although there are many ways of restoring balance, the basic principle is to utilize the abundant energy on the healthy side to treat the sick side. This is a useful technique when dealing with phantom limb pain after amputation, or in situations where the patient is unable to tolerate needles on the affected side, as in some forms of reflex sympathetic dystrophy.

Using meridians

If the meridians are envisaged as a reticular formation lying under the skin, the fine details can be mapped and utilized in order to achieve a precise effect in the area where it is required. It is important to be aware of the direction of Qi flow in each individual meridian in order to encourage or increase this effect. Although difficult to prove, most practitioners have at some time or other come across patients who describe a propagated sensation quite accurately in terms of the course of the meridian. However, it must be said that patients also describe sensations associated with needling in quite bizarre patterns, echoing neither the meridian course nor the nerve root distribution. Current thinking suggests that the acupuncture stimulus travels in the muscle fascia, sometimes following the course of a major nerve and sometimes not. Some authorities claim that the acupuncture points and meridians are unnecessary and that most needling can be done in 'zones of influence' (Mann 1992). This may be an explanation for some of the very powerful points, the best example being Liv 3 Taichong, but for the other points – and for acupuncturists who are prepared to use the TCM paradigm to inform their treatment, at least until anything else is proved better – the meridian system will suffice.

Working from the outside

In the following list, structures are ordered from the most superficial to the deepest:

Cutaneous regions
Minute collaterals
Sinew channels
Luo connecting channels
Primary channels
Divergent channels
Extraordinary channels
Deep pathway of the primary and divergent channels

The *cutaneous regions* are regions of skin rather than actual channels, through which the external Pathogens may enter the body. However, it is sometimes possible to perceive the disorder in the underlying channel by palpation for trophic changes in the skin. *Minute collaterals* form a small network of capillary channels just under the skin and also assist with the diagnostic process. Small varicose areas just under the skin will indicate a stagnation of energy in the affected channel. It is thought by some acupuncture historians that these observed areas may have been the origin of acupressure treatment. Pirog (1996) suggests that a smooth implement or stone could have been used as a form of acupressure and that this may have led eventually to the more invasive form of acupuncture that we know now.

Sinew channels circulate on the periphery of the body; they follow the course of the primary channels but are spread wider to take in the areas of muscle along the meridians. They are linked into the meridians by the Jing River points, the Qi at these points being expected to flood the banks and spread over a wider area. It is interesting to note that these channels are considered to originate distally, conforming to the older idea of Qi circulation implicit in the Antique points. Ah Shi points are frequently found in these areas.

The *Luo connecting channels* are still found relatively superficially. They branch from the primary channel at the Luo connecting point, connect with the paired channel, and then follow their own pathway. The *primary channels* are carefully described in all the ancient texts and follow a clear anatomical pathway. *Divergent channels* or collaterals tend to strengthen the Yin–Yang connection. They tend to supply the face and areas not so well covered by the primary channels. They often help to explain the actions of acupuncture points that seem otherwise unconnected to the area of effect.

The *extraordinary channels* or extra vessels lie deepest, below the primary channels. These form an additional network, linking the primary vessels. They have no points of their own, but the energy is accessed by using points from the primary channels. Because of this, there is no real circulation in these channels, which serve as closed-ended reservoirs for Qi.

General functions of channels

Nutritive

Qi and Blood are transported throughout the body in order to nourish the tendons and bones and to improve and maintain joint function. The passage of Qi and Blood within the meridians also helps to maintain the Yin–Yang balance. TCM theory has always considered that Blood passes along the meridians, although this is not susceptible to any kind of proof. It is reasonable to suppose that Qi also passes along blood vessels. Clinically, an area of muscle with a poor circulation is likely to lose bulk and strength.

Protective

Although Wei Qi, which resists the invasion of Pathogens through the skin surface, flows outside the meridians, it is carried within them and some of the resistance takes place in the meridians themselves. This is sometimes manifested as local Heat. Related sense organs may also show these signs, for example excess Heat in the Heart may produce ulceration in the tongue.

Transporting and regulating

The flow of Qi in the meridians regulates deficiency and excess conditions. The exchange of differing forms of Qi between one Zang Fu organ and another, or between different areas of the body, is fundamental to maintaining homeostasis. The meridians could also be said to transmit the needling sensation.

Needling techniques

This is a much vexed question, with books written on the topic and probably as many opinions as there are therapists! It is reasonable to suppose that the manner with which the needle is inserted might have an effect on the subsequent treatment, and this idea is difficult to dismiss when we are still not totally clear about the mechanism of acupuncture.

Beginners will be taught how to make a safe, accurate, painless, efficient insertion. It is the word 'efficient' that is open to discussion. Most schools of acupuncture thought insist that the needling sensation, or DeQi, is produced at most of the points used. As the sensations associated with DeQi do have a basis in the type of nerve ending stimulated, this makes good sense. However, looked at with a scientific eye, it is difficult to justify the differences in technique connected with 'draining, supplying, reducing and tonifying'. This has not stopped whole books being written about it. One of the clearest descriptions of all the techniques can be found in *Acupuncture and Moxibustion* (Auteroche et al 1986). This book contains many good photographs and is probably as close as one can get without practical tuition. Watching an acupuncture master is an instructive experience and serves to reinforce the idea that acupuncture is an art with important individual variations in technique, only some of which can be imitated. (Another useful exercise is to be needled yourself by a number of practitioners.)

I have to state my prejudices here; after many years of acupuncture practice I have not yet been convinced that there is a great deal to be said for the delicate changes in needling technique that distinguish between draining and supplying, although leaving a hole open in order to allow a bleed to happen makes some sense. I favour the approach of Anton Jayasuriya (1967), who claims that the body will take the stimulus it requires from the acupuncture without any additional manipulation of the needle.

Acupuncture needs to accomplish the freeing of Qi or energy in the meridians that are causing the pain or discomfort. Simple insertion of needles at carefully chosen acupuncture points seems to achieve this. Certainly, those sensitive enough to feel the movement of Qi can corroborate this. The only other thing that I can comfortably envisage happening is the 'borrowing' of energy from some other part of the meridian system or organ that is capable of providing it. A word of caution here: if we are considering a closed system, then that also carries the possibility that the quantity of Qi might be finite. It is possible to make too heavy a demand on the system and to exhaust the patient.

All of the above techniques will serve to free the flow of energy in the meridians, particularly when some form of pathogenic invasion or trauma has caused a slowing or sticking in the healthy circulation. Perhaps the technique will actually remove the blockage by dispersing the cause, dispelling or dispersing the Cold, Wind or Damp implicated. On other occasions, we call on the services of a Zang Fu organ – perhaps the Liver to ensure smooth flow. As described in Chapter 1, the Qi and the Blood are believed to flow together in the meridians, so an increased blood circulation can be perceived, perhaps manifested as pinkness of the skin or a slight rise in local temperature, and presumably the Qi will follow this. Although it may not be susceptible to any form of proof, the visible increase in blood supply and change in temperature when treating Sudeck's atrophy lends some credibility to this. Some researchers, particularly Ballegaard et al (1995), have noted a slight rise in temperature.

The actual needling can be described in the following terms.

Supplying, reinforcing or tonifying

- slow insertion
- inserted as the patient breathes out
- obtain Qi and remove the needle
- fast withdrawal
- taken out as the patient breathes out
- no pressure on the hole, allow the Qi to exit.

Sedating, dispersing or reducing

- fast insertion
- inserted as the patient breathes in
- obtain Qi and leave for at least 20 minutes
- slow, gentle withdrawal
- taken out as the patient breathes out
- usual pressure on the point to prevent bleeding.

The 'even' method requires regular stimulation of the needle during treatment to maintain the movement of Qi. A better method of doing this is to apply electroacupuncture, which by its nature tends to be a dispersing agent and requires much less effort on the part of the acupuncturist.

The meridians themselves have certain characteristics that make them more or less appropriate for use in particular conditions or disease patterns. Each one is considered in turn below, and the most important characteristics highlighted.

Urinary Bladder

This is probably the most important single meridian for a physiotherapist using acupuncture. This meridian has the longest course and has 67 individual points. It runs from the inner corner of the eye, up over the head and down the back of the neck, where it divides into two parallel channels at the level of C1. These channels run down the back; the inner line is the location of the important Back Shu points, lying 1.5 cun from the midline, and the outer (with generally less important points in terms of pain relief) is 3 cun from the midline. The inner line is said to have a more physiological effect, because of its links with the Zang Fu organs, and the outer line has a greater effect on the emotions. The Back Shu points lie mostly on the inner line; they are very important in TCM as they are used to tonify the Zang organs.

The channels continue down the back of the thigh, uniting behind the knee. The single channel then continues down the back of the lower leg, terminating at the outer edge of the little toe. The sheer number of points on the meridian and the inclusive nature of its course makes it ideal for musculoskeletal problems.

This meridian is considered to be the most superficial in the body and therefore the most vulnerable to external pathogenic invasion, particularly Cold, Wind and Damp. Many painful conditions arise from this vulnerability, and most end up in physiotherapy outpatient departments. Points frequently used to expel these Pathogens are UB 10 Tianzhu and UB 11 Dashu. However, logically, these points are more useful when the condition is acute. This meridian is considered to be linked to the Small Intestine channel, which is also very superficial, thus forming a superficial protective net covering large portions of both the upper and lower parts of the body.

> The chief signs of a problem within the Urinary Bladder meridian are those associated with the Pathogen Cold in the upper body: headache, stiff neck and aversion to cold. In the lower body the signs are pain in the lower back and along the sciatic nerve. The pain tends to be acute rather than chronic.

Kidney

The Kidney meridian can be used to treat multiple conditions, because the energy or Qi it contains is directly or indirectly vital to most body processes. It has particular relevance to the treatment of urinary and gynaecological conditions, respiratory and musculoskeletal problems, and the treatment of mental health problems and the elderly.

The Kidney meridian has a relatively short external course, totalling only 27 points and lying within the Yin regions of the body, inner lower leg, thigh and anterior aspect of the trunk.

The functions of the Kidney as a Zang Fu organ are closely related to the individual uses of acupoints along the channel. One of the most important functions of the Kidney is to be the 'root' of the Yin of the body. When Yin is deficient, deficiency Heat or uprising Yang is often the result. Deficiency of Kidney Yin leads to a disturbance of the spirit, which in turn can lead to a variety of mental disorders, from mild agitation or poor memory to severe madness. The upward movement of part of the Kidney energy leads to symptoms in the throat, eyes, ears and head generally. Kidney points are thus frequently used to nourish Yin, calm the spirit and reduce internal Pathogens in the upper body. The favourite point for this is Kid 1 Yongquan, which also corresponds to a minor chakra point in Ayurvedic medicine. This point is considered to have an influence on the mental processes of the patient and, when the situation requires it, can be used to 'ground' or calm a hysterical patient. Kid 4 Dazhong supports Kidney essence and is used for dementia.

The Kidney is said to be responsible for willpower and, if the Kidneys are sufficiently strong, the mind will be focused and able to attain the goals it sets for itself.

The Kidney is held to have a powerful effect on the development and condition of the bones. Kid 3 Taixi is frequently added to treatment for osteoarthritis or osteoporosis. This point is considered to influence the bone in the skull as it opens to the ear, so it is frequently used for ear conditions such as otitis media, tinnitus and deafness. Good results are claimed clinically, but not supported by the recent research. The National Institutes of Health in the USA stated recently that the evidence was at best equivocal (NIH Consensus Development Panel on Acupuncture 1998).

The Kidney meridian is used to influence the reproductive organs and the reproductive cycle in the female; Kid 7 Fuliu is frequently used. This point is also used when treating impotence in men and infertility in women. As the Kidney is considered to control development and growth, points may be used to influence the basic constitution of frail patients. The Kidney meridian is also suggested by some authorities for use in fetal development, to be used once in each trimester to purify fetal blood. No research exists to support this, however.

The Kidney is sometimes considered as a gate that controls the flow of water in the body. Thus, the first seven points on the meridian may be used for urinary problems. By the same token, Kidney points are used to control the two lower orifices, preventing leakages, with Kid 1, 2 and 3 being used for urinary retention and incontinence.

The Zang Fu link between the Kidney and the Lungs, described in Chapter 3, leads to a clinically important use of Kidney points when treating late-onset asthma. Congestion of fluids in the chest occurs when the Kidney energy is deficient, so an increase of Kidney Yin and Yang by needling Kid 3 can be effective, and Kid 2 is used for shortness of breath. Local Kidney points on the trunk are also used to ease the symptoms of emphysema, asthma and bronchitis.

> The chief signs of a specific problem within the Kidney meridian are pain in the lumbar region and pain in the sole of the foot.

Liver

This is a relatively simple meridian with extensive internal collateral vessels. These reach to the eyes, throat and nasopharynx via the trachea. Consequently, Liver points may be used to treat eye problems, particularly inflammation (characteristically, redness of the eye), and the rather peculiar TCM symptom of 'plum-stone throat' where a patient complains that the throat feels as though some hard object, perhaps the size of a plum stone, is stuck in it. This is a symptom often associated with stress conditions. As well as a link with the Liver, there are internal connections to the Stomach, Gall Bladder and Lung, and the meridian itself flows through the genital area.

The Liver meridian is used when the flow of Qi in the body appears to be disrupted. The Pathogens that affect the Liver – Wind and Anger – will cause jerky flow of Qi in the meridian and appropriate needling will smooth it out. Anger, depression and weeping can be caused by Liver Qi stagnation. Other symptoms of disharmony include insomnia and dream-disturbed sleep.

More precisely, the Liver ensures the downward flow of Stomach and Lung Qi, and the upward flow of Spleen Qi. It supports the production of bile by the Gall Bladder and ensures the smooth flow through the intestines and uterus. The energy of the Liver is thus important in the digestive process.

One of the Zang Fu functions of the Liver is blood storage; this concerns females perhaps more than males. The Liver stores blood and regulates the volume in circulation. Menstruation and genitourinary symptoms are primarily treated by Liv 8 Ququan, which removes Dampness from the lower Jiao, and also improves urinary function. If the menstrual flow is delayed or deficient, or if it is excessive, points such as Liv 3 and Liv 13 may be used to regulate it.

The influence that the Liver meridian has on the tendons has considerable relevance to physiotherapists. The smooth contraction of the muscles and tendons is under the control of Liver Blood. When this is deficient, muscle aches, spasms, cramps and contractures result, but when it is abundant the muscles and tendons will be supple. Liv 3 Taichong is used to treat this. Paralysis, tic or twitch is thought to be caused either by damage to the Liver by Wind or by internal Liver Wind. Liv 2 Xingxian and Liv 3 Taichong can both be used to subdue Wind.

Liver points are often incorporated in treatment of hemiplegia, again because of the effect of the points on Liver Wind, particularly the type of stroke arising from deficient Liver Yin. Liv 8 Ququan is used to rectify this. Sadly, most physiotherapists see their hemplegic patients only once the stroke has occurred, but these points can be used to help prevent further damage.

The Ethereal Soul, Hun, associated with the Liver is responsible for human kindness and benevolence, and the maintenance of an even and relaxed disposition is important for the smooth flow of Qi within this and the other meridians.

> The chief signs of a problem in the Liver meridian are muscle cramps in the legs, headache, pain and irritation in the eye.

Large Intestine

This meridian is said to have abundant Qi energy and it is possible to 'borrow' from it. As it is a richly connected meridian, linking with the Lung, Stomach, Urinary Bladder, Sanjiao, Small Intestine and Heart, it can be very influential in the body. The link to the Lung is an important therapeutic one, leading to the use of both channels to treat skin problems.

Following the course of the channel, pain problems in the hand, wrist, elbow and shoulder can be treated. This meridian is commonly used for both tennis elbow and periarticular arthritis at the shoulder joint. It can be used to treat rhinitis, sinusitis, hay fever, toothache and headache. LI 4 Hegu is also a useful acupressure point for the emergency treatment of tooth or head pain.

The Large Intestine meridian has an effect on the Zang Fu organs, being used in cases where the Pathogen Heat is found in either the Large Intestine or the Stomach. However, it is noticeable that this meridian is not often recommended for use on the Large Intestine as such, but more often in its capacity as a link to the Liver and Stomach, when it is used more as a source of ready energy.

The Large Intestine meridian is an important source of pain relief. LI 4 Hegu is said to be the strongest analgesic point available and, although it would appear to work best for pain in the upper quadrant, it is used clinically for pain anywhere in the body. It is also commonly used in combination with Liv 3 Taichong, as the 'four gates'. These points are used clinically to calm and relax agitated patients and to deal with global pain, and may have an effect on the limbic system, which mediates pain. MacPherson & Blackwell (1994) reviewed 368 cases in which acupuncture was used to treat rheumatoid arthritis in the Hubei Province, China, together with a further 150 cases in a later study. They concluded that, when Hegu was included in the treatment, changes were detected in the circulating immune indices. They suggested that this may be why some sufferers feel an improvement in their general wellbeing. This meridian is often used as an interim measure for toothache or for pain relief after extraction.

The Large Intestine meridian is very useful for treating sinusitis. LI 20 used in conjunction with other local points, particularly Yintang, and combined with LI 11 Quchi and perhaps St 36 Zusanli, will help with stubbornly stagnated and infected sinuses.

The Large Intestine meridian is used in cases of Blood Heat, often manifesting as skin conditions such as herpes zoster. It is usually combined with Lung and Spleen points for this type of problem. It has a strong homeostatic effect and can also be used for food allergies and forms of allergic arthritis. LI 11 Quchi and St 36 have a strong systemic effect.

> The chief signs of a problem within the Large Intestine meridian are pain along the course of the channel, particularly toothache, sore throat, swollen and painful gums, running nose and epistaxis.

Gall Bladder

The Gall Bladder meridian is positioned on the lateral aspect of the body, neither truly Yin nor Yang; it is sometimes called 'half Yin–half Yang'. There is a very large concentration of Gall Bladder points on the side of the head, making this an ideal meridian for treating lateral headache and other problems in this area. As it is connected to the Liver meridian, the Gall Bladder meridian is also used in the more complex treatment of migraine. It can also be used to treat pathology of the Liver itself, and Gall Bladder points, particularly on the leg, are used in cases of digestive failure. GB 34 is recommended in cases of persistent vomiting, used in conjunction with Stomach points.

It is evident that this meridian will be ideal for the treatment of any kind of lateral pain or what is often described as flank pain. Indeed, the meridian runs over or close to a number of major joints, temporomandibular, neck, shoulder, hip, knee and ankle, all of which are often treated with Gall Bladder points. These joints are all frequently damaged by Bi syndrome. The laterality of the Gall Bladder channel makes it an obvious choice for conditions such as hemiplegia where the paralysis is one-sided. The proximity of the upper channel to the ear means that this meridian is useful in conditions such as tinnitus and some forms of deafness. It is also indicated for pain caused by inflammation of the ear. There is a link with the inner ear and thus balance problems such as vertigo can also be treated.

> The chief signs of problems within the Gall Bladder meridian are lateral pain of any kind, but particularly that concentrating on the hip and lateral aspect of the lower limb.
>   Points on this channel are also often used to treat lateral headaches and ear problems.

Small Intestine

Along with the Urinary Bladder, the Small Intestine channel is considered to lie very superficially. This makes it vulnerable to pathogenic invasion, particularly Wind and Cold. This channel does not have a great influence on the general body Qi balance and is used mainly for painful disorders along the course of the channel. Although one might expect an effect on the digestive process, particularly on fluid organization, there are other meridians that influence this more directly, and this meridian appears to exert little influence over the actual small intestine.

The meridian starts from the ulnar side of the nailbed of the little finger and runs up the ulnar side of the forearm. It then runs posterolaterally, crossing at the posterior aspect of the shoulder, zig-zagging over the scapula to the anterolateral side of the neck. Here it gives off a deep branch running to the Heart and then to the Small Intestine. The main channel continues up the face, ending at the ear.

The channel is used mainly for disorders of the head, neck, ear, eye and throat, but because of the link with the Heart it can be incorporated into treatment formulae for mental problems.

The most interesting point on this meridian is SI 3 Houxi. This is a commonly used distal point for scapular or posterior shoulder pain. This is a Shu Stream point and also one of the confluent points, allowing access to the extraordinary meridians, in this case the Du meridian. It can be used alone to treat a disease within the Du meridian or in combination with UB 62 Shenmai. The most practical use of this is in dealing with acute low back pain. Houxi is also said to have a mild sedative effect.

Another use of SI 3 Houxi is in muscle spasm. Combined with Liv 3 Taichong and used bilaterally, it can be quite effective in reducing severe muscle spasm and can lead to a clinical decrease in contracture of the major muscles. It seems to be best to insert the two Small Intestine points first.

The Xi Cleft point SI 6 Yanglao is used for painful shoulder, back, neck, head and torticollis. It is also thought to be useful for hiccups.

From a physiotherapist's point of view, the Small Intestine channel is of most use for superficial channel pain; SI 3 Houxi is frequently used as a distal point for this, but the collection of points in the scapular area is very good for local scapular pain. Some are quite likely to correspond with familiar trigger points.

Pearce (2000) suggested that SI 12 Bingfeng may be indicated in the treatment of fibromyalgia, partly because of its positional relationship to one of the diagnostic tender points and partly because of its properties as a reunion point, linking the Small Intestine meridian with the Gall Bladder, Sanjiao and Large Intestine meridians.

> The chief signs of problems within the Small Intestine meridian are pain along the lateral side of the arm and in the scapular area. Pain in the neck and a stiff neck may also be associated.

Spleen

The Spleen meridian runs up the medial surface of the lower limb and enters the abdomen, passing through the Spleen to the Stomach. It ends externally at Sp 21 Dabao on the chest wall in the mid-axillary line, 6 cun below the axilla, level with the free end of the 11th rib. It has an internal branch to the root of the tongue. The branch from the Stomach flows upward through the diaphragm and links to the Heart meridian.

The Spleen has a strong centralizing, supporting and stabilizing influence on the body, and the dynamic energy in the Spleen meridian is used to raise structures that require support, being applied to patients with prolapse or Spleen Qi sinking. This can include haemorrhoids, varicose veins, prolapsed uterus, rectum or bladder, and protuberant, sagging abdominal wall.

As the Spleen is one of the two primary organs of digestion, points on this meridian are used in digestive disorders, frequently in combination with Stomach points. The key words associated with Spleen activity are transformation and transportation, both referring to digestion and subsequent utilization of foodstuffs. The Spleen is sometimes compared to the Kidney in importance for its function in maintaining general health. Certainly, tonifying Spleen points is regarded as essential in the weakened or debilitated patient.

The function of the Zang organ has a lot to do with fluid control throughout the body; the Spleen itself is damaged by excess Damp, and the meridian is often used to combat an invasion of external Damp or to clear the stasis resulting. In practical terms, Spleen points are always used for oedema in the lower limbs (Sanjiao points are more appropriate in the upper limb).

Spleen points have an effect on the Heat in the Blood, with Sp 6 Sanyinjiao and Sp 10 Xuehai being the most effective. These two are often included where there are itchy skin problems associated with the Blood Heat.

> The chief signs of problems within the Spleen meridian are weakness in the muscles of the leg, a cold feeling along the channel with possible swelling, and chronic urogenital problems such as vaginal discharge.

Stomach

According to TCM theory, the Stomach and Spleen are referred to collectively as the 'Root of Post-Heaven Qi'. They both need to be tonified in order to improve the assimilation of Nutritional Qi. The Stomach meridian also has an important role to play in the smooth flow of Qi and is responsible for transporting the food Qi to all the tissues, most particularly the limbs. The associated tissue of the Stomach channel is contractile tissue or muscle bulk, leading to the use of Stomach points to treat muscle-wasting disease. The Stomach has a high fluid requirement in order to function.

This is the third major Yang channel, running the whole length of the body and available for use with all types of pain on the anterior aspect of the body. It is used for musculoskeletal pain, particularly anterior hip or knee pain, and the distal point St 44 Neiting is often used to control general pain in the lower limb.

The meridian has an effect on the whole energetic balance of the body and use of St 36 Zusanli can enhance the general energy. It is used to treat problems of digestion and assimilation of food. It is used for frail debilitated patients recuperating after a long illness, or those simply in need of a Qi boost. Points along the channel are useful for gastrointestinal pain and irregularities of the bowel. St 25 Tiantu is a useful regulatory point, often used for acute intestinal pain.

The points may be used for local problems, in particular: points 1–8 for facial disorders; points 21, 25 and 29 for abdominal disorders; and points 36, 40, 41 and 44 for lower limb problems.

Previous research on rats, and more recently on humans, suggested that the stimulation of St 36 Zusanli together with LI 4 Hegu induces a 'rebalancing of cell-mediated immunity' (Petti et al 1998). In this experiment, T lymphocytes, known to be directly involved with the immune response, increased by 77% 30 minutes after treatment. In the same study, 60% of patients demonstrated an increase in the number of white blood cells 24 hours after treatment. The control group demonstrated no such effects. Further work is under way to examine these changes.

One of the most interesting points along the Stomach meridian is St 38 Tiaokou. This point is used to treat shoulder conditions, most especially chronic frozen shoulder where there is severe lack of mobility. This is the lower He Sea point of the Large Intestine and may therefore be used to treat problems along that meridian. It should be stimulated strongly while the patient attempts to mobilize the shoulder. The best position to do this in is side-lying while the affected limb is suspended in a Guthrie Smith suspension frame.

St 40 Fenglong is worthy of note. This is the Luo connecting point with the Spleen channel, but also eliminates Phlegm, and is frequently used for chest conditions, particularly asthma. Some texts translate the name as 'rich and prosperous', implying that it can be used to deal with the accumulation of Damp resulting either from rich foods or from being rich enough to eat unwisely and too well!

> The chief signs of problems within the Stomach channel are pain along the course of the channel, cold legs and feet, pain in the head and paralysis in the face.

Pericardium

This Yin channel begins lateral to the nipple in the fourth intercostal space and runs down the anteromedial aspect of the arm to the tip of the middle finger. It is paired with the Sanjiao channel. Another branch arises from

Pe 8 Laogong, in the centre of the palm, and terminates on the radial aspect of the tip of the ring finger, connecting with the Sanjiao channel. There is an internal connection to the Pericardium, descending through the diaphragm to the abdomen, linking the upper, middle and lower Jiaos. The Pericardium Luo channel extends from Pe 6 Neiguan to the Heart.

In basic acupuncture the Pericardium channel is somewhat overlooked. Pe 6 Neiguan is acknowledged for the treatment of travel sickness and nausea in pregnancy. This is mainly because of the enormous amount of research that has been published on this single point, which is also the only acupuncture point widely known to the general public because of the commercially available sea sickness acupressure remedy. It is used by some therapists as a point for calming and relaxing a patient. The combination of Pe 6 Neiguan and Pe 7 Daling is also widely used to treat carpal tunnel syndrome.

Consideration of the Pericardium as an individual organ is an idea peculiar to TCM. As the perceived function is to protect the Heart, wrapping around it to prevent damage from the exogenous Pathogens, the Pericardium serves as a primary and less powerful vehicle for treatment of the Heart and, more particularly, the Heart Shen or spirit. There are three main categories for the use of the Pericardium channel:

- ☯ treatment of mental and emotional disorders
- ☯ treatment of conditions affecting the heart and lungs
- ☯ treatment of gastrointestinal disorders.

Mental and emotional disorders

Disturbed Shen may manifest simply as insomnia or, more seriously, as excessive dreaming, hysteria, mania or insanity. Pathogens destined to enter the Heart will attack the Pericardium first. The Pericardium influences the mental and emotional state in several ways. Phlegm is produced as a result of stagnation of Body fluids brought on by pathogenic activity, i.e. Heat or fright. This phlegm obstructs the functioning of the Heart, and leads to poor memory, restlessness, agitation and ultimately mania. The key action of Pe 5 Jianshi is to transform Phlegm in the upper Jiao, predominantly in the Heart.

The Heart also rules the Blood and blood vessels, and regulates the flow of Blood. If Blood and Qi are in harmony, the Shen is nourished and calm. When this harmony is impaired, it may manifest as insomnia, forgetfulness, excessive dreaming or, more seriously, as hysteria, irrational behaviour or delirium. Pe 4 Ximen is the Xi Cleft point and affects emotional disorders by assisting regulation of Blood and Qi, and resolving stasis.

Heat is a dangerous Pathogen for the Heart, and the acupoint Pe 7 Daling can be used to eliminate it, working through the connection to the coupled Liver channel.

Conditions affecting the heart and lungs

Acute neck, back and left arm pain are generally ascribed to Blood stasis in the Heart and chest, but pain and pressure in the Heart and chest may also be due to stagnation of Liver Qi. Hence the two points Pe 6 and Pe 4 may be used to treat this.

Pe 6 Neiguan is the Luo connecting point. It links directly with the Heart and can therefore be used for physical manifestations of Heart disorders, such as palpitations and irregular beat.

Pe 5 Jianshi is the main point for transforming Phlegm, and this point will affect stagnation of Qi and Phlegm collecting in the chest. High fever can also produce Phlegm as it condenses the Body fluid in this area.

Studies inducing arrhythmia in rabbits involved applying electroacupuncture to Neiguan and measuring ventricular fibrillation. The researchers concluded that this treatment was as effective as lidocaine (lignocaine) in correcting ventricular arrhythmia and preventing ventricular fibrillation, but the quality of the work was not great.

Treatment of gastrointestinal disorders

The Pericardium channel can be used to counteract stagnation of Liver Qi as it has a connection to the Liver channel. This type of stagnation includes nausea and vomiting. The stagnation of Liver Qi transforms to Heat, which invades the Stomach causing rebellious Qi to ascend.

Neiguan is the most influential point because it is the Luo connecting point with the Sanjiao channel. The many links of the Pericardium channel throughout the three Jiaos mean that is has a strong influence over the movement of Qi. Pirog (1996) has described it as the Stomach meridian of the upper limb.

A recent double-blind randomized controlled study found that using acupressure wrist bands over Neiguan significantly reduced nausea and vomiting in 47 subjects before, during and after operation (Harmon et al 2000).

> The chief signs of problems within the Pericardium channel are pain along the course of the channel, particularly at the wrist, and stiffness of the elbow or the neck.

Heart

The inner links of the Heart are as important as the primary course with regard to the way the meridian is used. It originates in the Heart, spreads over the surrounding tissues, passes through the Lung and runs down the inner surface of the arm. However, the Heart meridian has branches connecting it to the Small Intestine, the oesophagus, the cheek, the root of the tongue and the eye.

The connection to the eye is considered to be the link to the brain, enabling theoretical control of the mind. Interestingly, early Chinese literature, before AD 652, does not cite Heart channel points for treating the mind. The particular connection with the root of the tongue, and therefore the effect on speech problems, arises from Ht 5 Tongli. This point can be used for stammering or loss of voice, particularly that associated with hysteria.

The Heart meridian can be used to treat pain in the heart and chest (although the Pericardium channel is often used in preference) and for heart symptoms, such as palpitations. It is used to calm the spirit or Shen, and Heart points are used in insomnia, stress or anxiety; the most important point in this regard is Ht 7 Shenmen. The Heart meridian is also sometimes used for eye or facial problems, mostly those relating to excessive reddening.

> The chief signs of problems within the Heart meridian are pain on the inner aspect of the arm, mimicking angina, and pain in the eyes.

Sanjiao

This is a fascinating meridian that is somewhat underused, perhaps because the whole concept of the three Jiaos or Body spaces is so alien to the Western mind. In fact, if the points are used unilaterally, there is probably little effect on physiology, but when bilateral treatment is undertaken the whole Jin Ye circulation is susceptible to change. The variety of names given to the channel perhaps expresses the general confusion.

The primary channel starts at the ulnar corner of the ring fingernail and runs up the posterior aspect of the forearm. It then passes over the shoulder and lateral side of the neck and terminates at the lateral canthus of the eye. A branch runs from the supraclavicular fossa down through the chest to where it connects with the Pericardium channel.

The functions of the Zang Fu organ relate mostly to water circulation. The Sanjiao Qi regulates the movement of fluids between the Spleen, Kidney, Stomach, Large Intestine, Small Intestine and Urinary Bladder. As the Sanjiao is hard to visualize as an individual organ, it is useful to imagine it merely as a series of functions that are brought into being the moment the umbilical cord is cut. (See Figure 2.5 for a diagram of Jin Ye circulation.)

The acupuncture points on this meridian are used to facilitate the movement of Qi through the three Jiaos, using the appropriate points for conditions in which movement of fluid is required to facilitate this flow. The Sanjiao is concerned with the physiological function of all the Yang organs within the body. The most effective points for balancing this are SJ 5 Waiguan and SJ 6 Zhigou. SJ 5 Waiguan is frequently included in the treatment of oedema, particularly in the upper body, along with Ren 9 Shuifen and Sp 9 Yinlingquan.

The points on the meridian are also useful for local pain, being appropriate for hand and wrist problems, and also for the face and ear. The last three points on the channel – Yifeng, Ermen and Sizhukong – are all useful for both the ear and facial paralysis. The Shu Stream point, SJ 3 Zhongzhu, is useful when there is an acute or hot ear problem and may be effective in treating tinnitus where the cause is Liver Heat or Wind. SJ 5 Waiguan is often used as a distal point for shoulder or arm pain, particularly when it is difficult to establish whether the pain is predominantly anterior or posterior. The posterior eye of the shoulder lies on the Sanjiao channel and this point, SJ 14 Jianliao, is commonly used for all types of shoulder pain. It is associated with an inability to elevate the arm at the shoulder.

There is an interesting link with Western theory with regard to SJ 16 Tianyou. This point often corresponds with a trigger point in levator scapulae, and direct pressure is put on this point when mobilizing C2. If this nerve root is affected, the symptoms exhibited by the patient – reduced mobility, hemispherical headache with eye pain and tinnitus – are similar symptoms to those mentioned in the literature as being alleviated by Tianyou.

> The chief signs of problems within the Sanjiao meridian are pain along the course of the channel, deafness and pain in the ear.

Lung

This is a straightforward Yin meridian running down the inner surface of the arm. It originates in the middle Jiao near the stomach, descends to the Large Intestine and then reverses, ascending through the diaphragm, through the upper Jiao and the Lungs, up towards the throat, and then down laterally to where it emerges at Zhongfu, the first point. After running upwards for a short distance, the meridian runs down the anterolateral aspect of the arm, through the cubital fossa and down to the lateral aspect of the thumb.

Probably the most commonly used point on this meridian is Lu 7 Lieque. Among other actions, this point has an opening effect on the Ren channel. It is indicated particularly for sore throat. As it is linked through the Ren Mai, this point can be incorporated in prescriptions for urinary symptoms.

Lu 7 Lieque is used with LI 4 to transfer energy from the more abundant Large Intestine meridian to the less active Lung meridian. The Lung meridian is said to control the lower respiratory tract, whereas the Large Intestine meridian is said to control the upper respiratory tract. The progress of energy from one to the other gives the Lung point Lu 7 a strong expectorant effect. Lu 7 is most associated with Wind dispersal. As it also draws energy from the interior to exterior, it can be used without fear of driving invading Pathogens deeper. (Lu 5 Chize is a bit more risky.)

Lu 9 Taiyuan can be used in more chronic situations. It is an influential point for the pulse but, as an Earth point, it has some value in the treatment of Lung conditions with copious Phlegm. As the Source point, it is often combined with St 36 Zusanli and Sp 3 Taibai in cases of chronic cough.

Lu 11 Shaoshang can be needled and bled for the relief of severe sore throat, although this not recommended as part of normal patient care. Lu 10 Yuji is a useful point for physiotherapists because, although it is a little tender to needle, it is an excellent treatment for 'physiotherapist's thumb'.

> The chief signs of problems within the Lung channel are a tight, obstructed feeling in the chest, fever, and pain along the course of the channel.

References

Auteroche B, Gervais G, Auteroche M et al 1986 Acupuncture and Moxibustion. Edinburgh: Churchill Livingstone.

Ballegaard S, Karpatschoff B, Holck JA et al 1995 Acupuncture in angina pectoris: do psychosocial and neurophysiological factors relate to the effect? Acupuncture & Electrotherapeutics Research 20: 101–116.

Cho ZH, Lee SH, Hong IK et al 1999 Further evidence for the correlation between acupuncture stimulation and cortical activation. Proceedings of a workshop at New Directions in the Scientific Exploration of

Acupuncture, Society for Acupuncture Research, University of California, 22 May 1999, pp 1–8.

Darras JC, Vernejoul P, Albarede P 1992 Nuclear medicine and acupuncture: a study on the migration of radioactive tracers after injection at acupoints. American Journal of Acupuncture 20: 245–256.

Harmon D, Ryan M, Kelly A, Bowen M 2000 Acupressure and prevention of nausea and vomiting during and after spinal anaesthesia for caesarian section. British Journal of Anaesthesia 84: 463–467.

Jayasuriya A 1967 Clinical acupuncture. Kalubowila, Sri Lanka: Medicina Alternativa International.

Low R 2001 Acupuncture: techniques for successful point selection. Oxford: Butterworth-Heinemann.

Lundeberg T, Hurtig T, Lundeberg S, Thomas M 1988 Long term results of acupuncture in chronic head and neck pain. Pain Clinic 2: 15–31.

MacPherson H, Blackwell R 1994 Rheumatoid arthritis and Chinese Medicine – a review. European Journal of Oriental Medicine 1: 17–29.

Mann F 1992 Re-inventing acupuncture: a new concept of Ancient Medicine, 1st edn. Oxford: Butterworth-Heinemann.

NIH Consensus Development Panel on Acupuncture 1998 Acupuncture. Journal of the American Medical Association 280: 1518–1524.

Pearce L 2000 Fibromyalgia – a clinical overview. Journal of the Acupuncture Association of Physiotherapists October: 34–40.

Petti F, Bangrazi A, Liguori A et al 1998 Effects of acupuncture on immune response related to opioid-like peptides. Journal of Traditional Chinese Medicine 18: 55–63.

Pirog JE 1996 The practical application of meridian style acupuncture, 1st edn. Berkeley, CA: Pacific View Press.

Wu MT, Hsieh JC, Xiong J et al 1999 Central nervous pathway for acupuncture stimulation: localisation of processing with functional MR imaging of the brain – preliminary experience. Radiology 212: 133–141.

Further reading

Auteroche B, Gervais G, Auteroche M et al 1992 Acupuncture and Moxibustion, a guide to clinical practice. Edinburgh: Churchill Livingstone.

Superficial acupuncture – just under the skin

KEY CONCEPTS

- Acupuncture can also be used with shallow subdermal needling.
- Japanese acupuncture is associated with superficial techniques and a need for greater sensitivity in palpation.
- In neuropathic pain associated with muscle shortening, the release of the shortening by intramuscular stimulation may provide relief.
- Musculotendinous acupuncture, with origins in massage therapy, is the ancient precursor of trigger point acupuncture.
- Trigger point acupuncture, or dry needling, is a modern medical technique based on the work of Travell & Simons.
- Segmental acupuncture can also address visceral symptoms, supporting the use of Back Shu points.
- A combination of these techniques can produce good results.

Superficial layers

It is possible to obtain good acupuncture results from a relatively superficial insertion; indeed, some Japanese acupuncture – Hinaishin or intradermal needling – is characterized by this (Birch & Ida 1998). This type of acupuncture depends greatly on the operator's palpatory skills and the ability to sense differences in energy and trophic changes in the skin surface. The needles utilize acupuncture points that generally correspond with those in Traditional Chinese Medicine (TCM), but wide variation may be encountered according to the energies palpated on the skin surface. Japanese acupuncture is essentially a superficial technique, but is very complex and subtle in application. Only a brief summary will be given here of the main variations on the technique.

Contact needling

No attempt is made to insert the needle. The tip is just rested on the skin surface and the needle is rotated in this position. This type of needling is used on frail, fatigued patients or those showing psychosomatic symptoms or depression. It is also useful with children or patients afraid of needle insertion. Sometimes the needle does just enter the tissues, less than 1 mm, and this can be used for patients who are showing signs of a deficiency condition such as low back pain caused by osteoporosis.

Insertion

The needle is often inserted but not retained. This is a similar technique to tonification in TCM. It is used with deficiency or for particularly sensitive patients.

The needles may be retained for varying lengths of time according to the condition being treated. The supporting points may only be pricked, but the needle is left longer in the point considered to be most influential. The decision on which points are less important depends on the sensitivity of the practitioner to the presence or absence of Qi and the diagnosis.

Intradermal needling

Intradermal needles are commonly used in Japan but less often in the UK, except for auriculotherapy. The needles resemble small thumbtacks with a sharp pin only 2 mm long. There is a broad base, which prevents the needle from being inadvertently pushed further into the tissues, and the whole needle is covered with a small piece of sticky tape, which prevents it from being dislodged. The Chinese type of needle is slightly different from the Japanese, being generally heavier and thicker, but the use is similar.

These needles are used primarily to increase and extend the effect of a treatment. The most influential point, or the point that is situated directly over the most intense pain, is selected and the needle retained until the next treatment. It could be suggested that this is counterproductive as the patient will be encouraged to focus on the pain rather than develop further coping strategies, but this technique is widely and successfully used clinically throughout Japan.

Intradermal needles are not generally recommended in the UK because of the danger of the site becoming infected. They are seen more commonly in ear acupuncture for smoking cessation, even though the danger of infection is rather worse because of the relatively poor blood supply to the cartilage. Leaving needles in the ear is not recommended by the Acupuncture Association of Chartered Physiotherapists and non-penetrative ear seeds are preferred (AACP 1997).

This type of needling has been used in the treatment of chronic respiratory disease and an interesting study has been published in which intradermal needles were used, particularly at Ren 17 Shanzhong, in the treatment of disabling breathlessness in patients with terminal lung cancer (Davis et al 2001). An additional advantage to using this type of needle in research is that removing the point can make a form of placebo needle; the patient remains unaware of the difference because it is masked by the sticky tape.

Moxa

Moxibustion, or burning a form of dried *Artemesia vulgaris* close to the skin, is also widely used and often utilized in place of invasive needling. It is added to extend the effect of treatment and, as in the UK, frequently given to patients to continue the treatment on specific points at home. The small adhesive Ibuki moxa is favoured over moxa rolls for home use.

Japanese direct moxibustion is a little different, however, with two broad categories of treatment: that which is intended to scar and that which is not. The scarring technique is rarely used.

Non-scarring, or indirect, moxibustion involves the use of very tiny amounts of moxa, often only rice grain-sized, placed very accurately on the required points and lit using an incense stick. This technique requires considerable practice and manual dexterity. The dose, as described by Denmei & Brown (2003), is three sesame seed-sized cones on each point for children or very depleted patients, with a standard dose of five half-rice grain-sized cones on each point. Other moxa techniques are also used extensively. The Japanese are less concerned with the effect of moxa on 'Hot' conditions, and tend to use moxa in most situations, unlike TCM practitioners.

Sensitivity to Qi

The ability to feel and facilitate the arrival of Qi is probably the most important aspect of Japanese acupuncture treatment. (Most TCM practitioners would also consider it vital to the success of any treatment.) The 'DeQi' sensations felt by the patient are an indicator that something is happening, but the acupuncturist should also experience some sensation when Qi is encountered. There are many descriptions of this – probably as many as there are practitioners – because the sensation is so subjective, but commonly used phrases are: 'tissue grip on the needle', 'a pleasant sensation', 'a desire to take a deep breath', 'a relaxation', 'increased saliva in the mouth', 'some tingling or warmth in the hand contacting the patient'.

Use of these sensations as a guide sometimes leads the Japanese practitioner to appear to be needling some way off the recorded location of an acupuncture point. While irritating to the purists, it is possible that there is a slight variation in the course of meridians – after all, most body structures exhibit variability between one patient and the next, or even from one side to the other. Perhaps following the Qi sensation leads the acupuncturist to be more accurate in point location, not less. At any rate it is a fascinating study; for more information on how points are located and used within this tradition, Brown's translation of Denmei's book is recommended (Denmei & Brown 2003).

Some of the most interesting modern techniques, particularly trigger point acupuncture, discussed below, show close links with the known patterns of nerve root distribution. These can be detected by palpation of temperature or trophic changes in the skin surface. The following technique, musculotendinous acupuncture, is from a very old TCM theory with very modern applications.

Musculotendinous acupuncture

When considering relatively superficial acupuncture techniques, use of the musculotendinous (MT) meridians, sometimes referred to as the muscle sinew channels, or the Jing Jin, must be included. These are topographical areas of the body that correspond to a defined area of influence belonging to any of the 12 paired meridians.

TCM theory considers them to be the first line of defence against invading pathogenic factors. As the MT meridians are located superficially, just under the skin, they are in close contact with the environment; this is well illustrated in major acupuncture textbooks (e.g. Deadman et al 1998).

Simple use of these areas can treat most musculoskeletal pain. Many sports therapists using acupuncture rely on the mapping of these areas to treat acute problems such as soft tissue injuries. The TCM theories and classification of symptom patterns associated with each Pathogen will be discussed in this chapter, but a glance at the location of these areas will serve to confirm the opinion of those who see segmental distribution as the clearest reason for the choice of acupuncture points.

Illustrations of selected MT meridians can be seen in Figures 6.1 & 6.2.

Figure 6.1   Urinary Bladder musculotendinous meridian. (Reprinted from *A Manual of Acupuncture*, by Peter Deadman and Mazin Al-Khafaji, with Kevin Baker, with kind permission of Journal of Chinese Medicine Publications.)

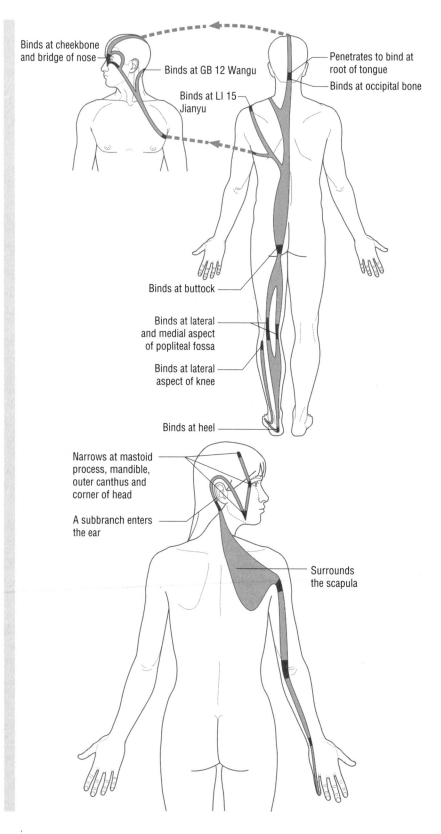

Binds at cheekbone and bridge of nose

Binds at GB 12 Wangu

Binds at LI 15 Jianyu

Penetrates to bind at root of tongue

Binds at occipital bone

Binds at buttock

Binds at lateral and medial aspect of popliteal fossa

Binds at lateral aspect of knee

Binds at heel

Figure 6.2   Small Intestine musculotendinous meridian. (Reprinted from *A Manual of Acupuncture*, by Peter Deadman and Mazin Al-Khafaji, with Kevin Baker, with kind permission of Journal of Chinese Medicine Publications.)

Narrows at mastoid process, mandible, outer canthus and corner of head

A subbranch enters the ear

Surrounds the scapula

It is thought that use of the MT meridians originated as an aid to massage, as this form of therapy requires manipulation of wider expanses of muscle tissue than the narrow line of a meridian. The MT meridians do not have points as such, and do not connect with the Zang Fu organs. They form a network under the skin and are influenced by use of the points on the associated meridians, usually the Jing Well (Tsing) or end points or the Jing River points (see Ch. 5). The Jing River points have the ability to 'overflow' the riverbanks into the surrounding tissues if the Qi is stimulated. They tend to narrow as they run over joints, corresponding to ligaments and tendons rather than muscles at these points.

The functions of these meridians is said to be to bind the bones and permit the movement of the joints, thus equating them with the perceived function of muscles and tendons in modern Western medicine.

Energy in these meridians flows centripetally and is particularly active in the Yang meridians by day and in the Yin meridians by night. The order of flow is generally given as:

UB→GB→St→ SI→SJ→LI→ Pe→Kid→Ht

The Yang meridians of the leg unite at St 3 Juliao on the face, and those of the arm unite at GB 13 Benshen. The Yin meridians of the leg unite at Ren 3 Zhongji, and those of the arm unite at GB 22 Yuanye.

None of these points is commonly used in basic pain relief acupuncture and careful checking is needed to ensure safe needle insertion. They are called into action only when there is widespread involvement of the superficial muscle tissues, as in general muscular atrophy after serious traumatic injury.

In order to understand the use of the MT meridians it is necessary to examine the relative depths of the TCM structures. The MT meridian is just below the skin surface, with the main meridian flowing beneath it. The Luo points on the main meridian connect it. Even deeper below the main meridian, the extraordinary vessels or extra meridians can be found. These are thought to lie just above the periosteum, but they are closed vessels and not part of the Jing Luo circulation of Qi and Blood.

From Figure 6.3 it can be seen that the MT meridian is the first barrier to an invading Pathogen and may indeed prevent it from reaching the

Figure 6.3 Section through tissues.

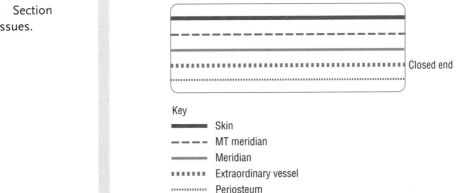

Key

━━━━ Skin

- - - - MT meridian

──── Meridian

▪▪▪▪▪▪ Extraordinary vessel

··········· Periosteum

main meridian. Ah Shi points, mentioned in Chapter 5, will occur in the superficial tissues or MT meridian in the acute stages of pathogenic invasion. These are said to be due to the Wei Qi or Defensive Qi attacking the Pathogen and creating local Heat. This situation is described as the MT meridian being 'full' while the main meridian is 'empty'.

Treatment of this situation takes the form of shallow needling of the Ah Shi points in order to deactivate or 'drain' them. Needling the Yuan Source point or Tonification point, or the strongest distal point, should then reinforce the main meridian. Moxa can be used on the meridian points, usually after Ah Shi points have been drained. This kind of treatment, attempting to balance the energies between the two types of meridian, is appropriate for acute injuries such as a sprained ankle, muscle strains or haematoma, and needs to be combined with immediate active movement of the affected area.

However, the Pathogen may still penetrate to a deeper level if the Wei Qi is not strong enough to expel it, resulting in a chronic situation. This leaves the MT meridian comparatively 'empty' because the Wei Qi is exhausted and the main meridian is now active and relatively 'full'. There will still be Ah Shi points but they will now lie deeper, at the level of the main meridian, and they will be much less easy to elicit with palpation. The area may be numb rather than actively painful. Old traumatic injuries, scars or burnt-out rheumatic disease often produce this type of situation in the tissues. An attempt is still required to balance the energies, but this is now done by adding energy to the MT meridian by the use of moxa and tonification needling techniques, applying these to the Ah Shi points, where palpable. The main meridian now requires draining, again done by strongly stimulating a major distal point. The condition may seem to require extensive drainage to the main meridian if it is very well established, and this may be easier to do by using mild stimulation on several distal points, thus spreading the load.

The pain may have different causes, although old trauma is a common reason for this type of musculoskeletal pain. If stasis of Blood is suspected, Luo connecting points can usefully be added. Shu Stream points may be added if Damp is the main Pathogen, and Ying Spring points used if there is a need to expel Heat. The group Luo points might be a useful addition in cases of stagnation in the MT meridian (Table 6.1).

Thus far, use of the MT meridians is fairly simple and the acute form of sports injury generally responds well. A further refinement to the use of MT meridians is the identified type of pathogenic invasion. The Eight

Table 6.1 Commonly used Luo points

Luo–MT meridian connections	Group Luo points
Lu 7 Lieque	Sp 6 Sanyinjiao (connects Yin meridians of the leg)
Pe 6 Neiguan	GB 39 Xuanzhong (connects Yang meridians of the leg)
SJ 5 Waiguan	Pe 5 Jianshi (connects Yin meridians of the arm)
UB 58 Feiyang	SJ 8 Sanyangluo (connects Yang meridians of the arm)

Principles can be applied to differentiation. The symptoms of the Pathogens follow the pattern established in Chapter 2, dividing into six main categories as in Table 6.2. This is essentially a pragmatic list which recognizes that Pathogens do not usually occur singly and describes the type of symptom picture seen with a combination of invasive factors.

Table 6.2 Pathogenic factors affecting the MT meridians (Rodger-Withers 1999)

Pathogen	Symptoms	Area affected
Wind	Cold surface Pores open, sweating may occur Pain with no fixed site Twitching Muscle spasm Itching Tremor	Upper part of the body
Wind and Cold	Pores closed No sweating Skin is pale Sharp pain Relieved by warmth Slowing and stagnation of Qi Wind may also cause cramping	Any part of the body
Wind Heat	Aching, dull pain Dry, warm surface Pores open Sweating may occur Muscle function affected, leading to muscle atrophy Skin may be rosy, becoming pale as Wei Qi is consumed	Upper part of the body Groin
Wind Damp	Obstructs circulation of Yang Qi Difficult to treat Numbness Heavy sensation	Lower part of the body
Wind–Cold–Damp	A combination of Pathogens with Damp usually the most prevalent, but presenting with a combination of symptoms Cold surface	Lower part of the body

Continues

Table 6.2 cont'd

Pathogen	Symptoms	Area affected
	Pale skin Numbness Muscle cramps Muscle spasm Stiffness	

Wind–Heat–Damp	The Heat disperses Wei Qi
	Dampness dries and turns
	    into Phlegm
	Muscle weakness
	Laxness of ligaments
	Muscle atrophy
	Heaviness
	Numbness
	Swelling and tension in
	    the tissues
		Upper part of the body
		Groin

While this may seem rather complicated, the most important point to bear in mind is that the presence of raised muscle tone indicates the prevalent underlying Pathogen is Cold in nature. It will be appropriate to use a form of heat in the treatment of this condition. However, if the muscles appear to be slightly soft or flaccid, the main underlying Pathogen is Heat and the further application of heat will be damaging, only adding to the internal state of excess energy.

This may also manifest by a relatively 'full' state in the MT meridian superimposed on an underlying deficiency, so care must be taken to assess all the other presenting symptoms. As with all acupuncture, patients exhibit widely differing combinations of symptoms, and care must be taken with the initial diagnosis and the prevalent Pathogen identified in terms of the Eight Principles (see Ch. 1).

In addition to the preceding differentiation, the MT meridians display symptoms related to the course of the named meridian involved. On the whole these tend to correspond to problems of pain or cramping in the major muscle areas along the course, but there are one or two variations worth noting (Table 6.3).

All of the symptoms shown in Table 6.3 require treatment as described at the beginning of this section, depending on the perceived depth of the pathogenic invasion and the characteristic pains of Hot or Cold, according to the Eight Principles.

Trigger point acupuncture

Trigger point acupuncture is a modern variation on a TCM technique – the use of Ah Shi points. The needling used is very shallow and brief in duration, 30 seconds being the recommended time for each insertion.

This acupuncture method is easier to use with a working knowledge of segmental innervation, but some of the pain referral patterns are counterintuitive. The technique is based on the work on trigger points done by

Table 6.3 Characteristics of MT meridians

MT meridian	Characteristic symptoms	Comments
Urinary Bladder	Pain, swelling and strain of leg structures including little toe, heel, popliteal region Spasm and tension at nape of neck Inability to raise shoulder Pain and strain in axilla; pain and strain in supraclavicular area	There is an MT strap running from the thoracic area, through the axilla, across the clavicular area and joining with the main meridian just under the eye
Gall Bladder	Muscle cramp from the fourth toe up to the knee Stiff knee Muscle spasm and cramping of vastus lateralis Cramping type of pain in sacral area radiating to lateral costal area Ribs said to 'belong to the Gall Bladder' Muscle spasm in supraclavicular fossa and lateral aspect of neck Muscle disturbances in the eye	Branch linking across to the sacrum and across to the breast area, otherwise follows meridian
Stomach	Muscle problems following the course of the meridian, starting at the middle toe and involving some or all of the anterior tibial muscles and quadriceps Swelling in anterior inguinal region Spasm in abdominal muscles Deviation of the mouth Problems with opening or closing the eye Opening (Hot), closing (Cold)	Runs very close to the course of the meridian
Small Intestine	Strained little finger Pain along medial aspect of forearm and elbow Pain on posterior aspect of axilla and across scapula Some connected neck pain Tension in the neck leading to swelling and muscle atrophy Tinnitus, ear pain Eye problems	Runs very close to the meridian Broad area over scapula

Continues

Table 6.3   cont'd

MT meridian	Characteristic symptoms	Comments
Sanjiao	Any muscle strain or cramp along the course of the meridian Curling of the tongue	Runs very close to the course of the meridian A branch separates at the angle of the mandible and runs to the root of the tongue
Large Intestine	Muscle cramps along the course of the meridian Inability to raise shoulder Restricted range of neck rotation	Branch to the thoracic spine attaching T1–7 Branch crosses over the top of the head to the opposite mandible
Pericardium	Local muscle problems, cramps and strains along the course of the meridian Chest pain Distressed breathing Sensation in diaphragm	Runs very close to the course of the meridian Spreads over anterior chest wall with an internal branch to the diaphragm
Kidney	Foot cramps Associated with some forms of back pain Associated with some types of epilepsy	Runs very close to the course of the meridian; wide spread on inner surface of thigh Branch ascends on inner surface of spine
Heart	Internal tension, feeling of discomfort, around and below the heart Pain and muscle cramping along the course of the meridian	Runs very close to the course of the meridian Spreads over the anterior costal area and a branch runs down to the umbilicus
Lung	Muscle cramps along the course of the channel Some association with lung disease, involving tightness of lateral costal area and haemoptysis	Runs very close to the course of the meridian and spreads over the anterior chest wall with an internal branch to the diaphragm

Continues

Table 6.3   cont'd

MT meridian	Characteristic symptoms	Comments
Liver	Muscle problems associated with great toe, medial aspect of calf and knee, and medial aspect of thigh Dysfunction of genitalia; clear demarcation between symptoms of Heat and Cold	Runs very close to the course of the meridian
Spleen	Muscle problems associated with great toe, medial aspect of ankle and leg Twisting pain in genital region Umbilical pain spreading to the lateral costal region or to internal aspect of spine	Runs very close to the course of the meridian Branches internally from genitals first to umbilicus, then to internal surface of spine

Travell & Simons (1983) and later extended by Baldry (1989). It is often called 'dry needling' in order to imply that, although a quasi-medical technique, nothing is injected into or taken out of the patient. The needles used are, in fact, normal solid acupuncture needles.

Travell & Simons discovered that there are trigger points present in all muscles that give rise to referred pain in clear repeatable patterns when pressure is exerted. Injecting saline solution into the muscles and thus producing a painful response enabled the mapping of most of these areas of referred pain.

The use of trigger points resembles that of Ah Shi points in some respects, but there are clear differences between the two techniques, as shown in Box 6.1.

Box 6.1   Ah Shi points and trigger points

Ah Shi points	Trigger points
Very painful on pressure	Very painful on pressure
Very few in number	Many to be found
Not usually palpable as bands	Palpable band in muscle tissue
No referred pain pattern	Characteristic referred pain pattern
DeQi obtained	No DeQi
Needle to normal depth for tissue	Shallow subdermal needling
20-minute treatment time, accompanied by other acupuncture needles	30-second insertion with optional repeat of a further 30 seconds
No repeat in same day	Immediate repeat if unsuccessful
Normal acupuncture response from patient	Patient exhausted if many trigger points treated
No pattern to location	Each muscle has clearly mapped major trigger points
Unlikely to be found at next treatment	Frequently need several treatments to deactivate
Customarily used in normal acupuncture protocols	Can be used alongside normal body acupuncture

Characteristics of trigger points

The structures that are likely to contain trigger points include muscles, tendons, joint capsules, ligaments, the periosteum and the skin. Trigger points are most often found and used in muscle tissue. Each muscle has its own characteristic specific pattern of pain referral from the trigger points contained within it (Fig. 6.4).

Exerting pressure on, or inserting a needle into, any active trigger point may sometimes reproduce the spontaneous pattern of pain complained of by a patient. Neural hyperactivity causes both latent and active trigger points to be exquisitely tender. As a result of this, when such a point is palpated the patient flinches in a manner that is out of proportion to the amount of pressure exerted on it. This is the so-called 'jump and shout' sign. Active trigger points are responsible for the referral of pain, either locally or at some distant site, or both. Active trigger points are sometimes associated with autonomic disturbances in the zone of pain referral. A local twitch may be observed when a palpable band in a superficially placed muscle is smartly 'plucked'.

Trigger points can be described as latent or active depending on the degree to which they are activated. When there is an active trigger point in a muscle, this often causes it to become shortened and somewhat weakened. The aim of treatment is to deactivate the point and decrease or abolish both the local tenderness and the referred pain in the characteristic area.

Uses of trigger point acupuncture

Trigger point acupuncture is used for persistent muscle pain, particularly when the muscles are tight and spastic. It may be of use in long-standing chronic conditions such as muscle spasticity after stroke (Case study 6.1). It will not cure the basic problem of paralysis but may make mobilization of the tissues easier and remove a source of pain. Head and neck pain responds well; patients with pain problems that correspond to the patterns of pain referral for trigger points are frequently referred for physiotherapy. Headache often has its roots within hotspots in the neck and shoulder

Figure 6.4 Trigger points and radiating pain referral pattern in the infraspinatus muscle. (Redrawn with kind permission from Baldry 1989.)

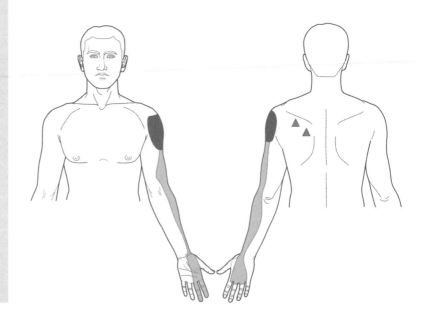

CASE HISTORY

Case study 6.1 Stroke

52-year-old woman. Stroke 25 years ago, caused by contraceptive pill. Permanent left-sided paralysis and increased tone causing marked spinal rotation to the opposite side. Awkward high-stepping gait, using a stick. High muscle tone in both arm and leg, but coping well with disability. Main presenting problem: chronic left-sided pain. Unhappy about visible deformity. Sleeping poorly.

Impression
TCM sequelae of stroke; long-standing problem considered unlikely to be amenable to acupuncture treatment. However, left-sided symptoms fall directly into Gall Bladder MT area. Treat with a mixture of body acupuncture and MT meridian techniques.

Treatment 1

- GB 26 Daimai, GB 43 Xiaxi, GB 34 Yanglingquan, left only
- Liv 3 Taichong, SI 3, Small Intestine, bilaterally.

Treatment 2

- Slight decrease in pain, lasted for only 24 hours. Slept better
- Repeated points.

Treatment 3

- Same result
- GB 34, GB 43 and Liv 3, left only
- Added local superficial trigger points in left lateral costal area
- 30 seconds, superficial insertion. Approximately 15 points neutralized
- Patient exhausted.

Treatment 4

- Pain greatly improved.
- Decrease in muscle tone in costal muscles
- Repeated treatment.

This patient had a further three treatments with very good results. While the Gall Bladder remained the meridian most affected, neutralizing the trigger points was very effective. The patient was able to sleep better, walk more easily, and seemed to be more upright. The pain she had sought help with was almost gone.

muscles. These hotspots can be caused by poor working postures (Case study 6.2). Treatment of repetitive strain injury can also incorporate trigger point deactivation.

Trigger point acupuncture is used successfully for postoperative pain, the most painful points often being at either end of the scar. Certainly surgery anywhere in the body may involve damage to muscle tissue with resulting trigger points. Fibromyalgia responds well, but because it is often widespread protracted treatment may be needed; there are usually many trigger points that can be found on palpation. My personal experience is that neutralization of about 15 points at any one treatment is as much as most patients can tolerate.

Commercially available wall charts showing trigger point patterns can be useful in the clinic.

CASE HISTORY

Case study 6.2
'Restless legs'

Middle-aged man suffering from 'restless legs'. No real problems during his relatively sedentary working day, but unable to sit still in the evenings. Unable to watch a whole television programme; had to get up and walk around to stop his legs from twitching. Disturbed sleep; had to get up and walk about every 2–3 hours. Not really painful.

Impression
TCM stagnation, treated by trigger point acupuncture.

Acupuncture treatment
Superficial needle into gluteus maximus trigger point, 3 cun below the iliac crest (injection point). Palpable band at that level. Distal points, GB 34 and UB 60. Short stimulus, 30 seconds for trigger point in first treatment, but little response. For subsequent treatments, trigger point needle manipulated strongly with deeper insertion. Local DeQi response; needles left for 20 minutes.
After six treatments, twice weekly, the problem resolved.

Intramuscular stimulation

This technique does not really belong in the superficial category, but it is so closely linked with trigger point acupuncture that it is described here. Chronic musculoskeletal pain is defined as pain that persists in the absence of repeated injury or inflammation and is due to some functional disorder of the nervous system. It can be treated in many ways. The use of myofascial trigger points is described by Gunn (1989) and offered as an alternative to trigger point or dry needling.

The theory behind this type of treatment claims that each myofascial trigger point consists of a sensory component (sensitive locus) and a motor component (motor locus). Needle stimulation at the sensitive locus produces both a local muscle twitch response and referred pain. The sensitive loci are probably sensitized nociceptors, widely distributed through the muscle but concentrated in the endplate zone. The active loci are now thought to be dysfunctional endplates, as the spontaneous electrical activity they generate is the same as recorded endplate noise (Hong 2002). The referred pain zoning and the local muscle twitch are both mediated via spinal cord mechanisms. The pathogenesis of the myofascial trigger points themselves seems to be associated with the disturbance of nerve endings and the resulting abnormal contractile mechanism at the dysfunctional endplates. It is not clear which occurs first. Several forms of physiotherapy are used to treat these trigger points and the consequent muscle shortening: stretch and spray, electrotherapy, laser therapy, heat and acupuncture.

Clearly, these points could also be associated with some of the Travell & Simons' trigger points, but the needle treatment is usually relatively deep and much longer in duration. It is also quite painful for the patient.

The primary goal is to desensitize supersensitive structures and thus restore normal motion and function. This is effected by inserting the needle into the muscle at a site where muscle spasm is palpated. The needle is inserted directly into the tight tissue zone and the resulting muscle grasp confirms the correct siting. The patient is likely to experience a strong cramping sensation; at this point the needle should gently be pushed further in. If the spasm is not felt, this technique is not likely to be successful. This treatment can be applied at several loci, one after the other.

The technique as taught by Gunn requires the use of a single heavy-gauge needle of between 1 and 3 inches, the longer needle being used where there is a thick layer of muscle. To make penetration easier and avoid finger contact with the needle, an insertion tube is always used. As many as eight needles may be inserted at one time, but it must be borne in mind that this is quite a painful process for the patient so fewer needles would be advisable for a tense or less robust person.

There are few specific contraindications to this technique; the most important ones are early pregnancy, patient on anticoagulants or local infection. Otherwise contraindications and precaution are as with any other form of acupuncture. Electrostimulation is sometimes applied when there are at least two needles; Gunn (1989) recommends a frequency of between 30 and 100 Hz, producing a muscle contraction but allowing for a relaxation in the tissues between each stimulation and avoiding tetany.

While this is accepted as a relatively painful treatment, the argument runs that one painful needle is worth several less painful ones in treatment effect. There is no research to back this view, but patients are generally quite accepting of the intramuscular stimulation (IMS) technique because they can feel a change almost immediately. It is clear that the mechanism of action in the superficial trigger points, the deeper Ah Shi points and the still deeper IMS sites must be different, but they do all seem to have a beneficial clinical effect. Some research specifies the depth to which the needle must penetrate; this is helpful in identifying which of the techniques is in use.

Six Chiaos

Working from the outside to the inside using the six channel syndromes or the six Chiaos can be a useful way of organizing the symptomatology. It is really a way of describing the characteristics of the body defence system, layer by layer, and is credited to Zhang Zhong Jing (AD 158–166). The channels are considered as pairs, with the pairing following a clearly layered pattern starting with the most superficial (Table 6.4). One of the maxims of TCM is that treatment should never drive a Pathogen deeper into the tissue, but always attempt to move it to a more superficial level or expel it. Given the damage that pathogenic invasion can cause, this is a logical treatment aim.

Table 6.4 Arrangement of Chiaos

Layer		Channel pairing	
Yang	Tai Yang (Great)	Small Intestine	Urinary Bladder
	Shao Yang (Lesser)	Sanjiao	Gall Bladder
	Yang Ming (Light)	Large Intestine	Stomach
Yin	Tai Yin (Great)	Lung	Spleen
	Jue Yin (Diminishing)	Pericardium	Liver
	Shao Yin (Lesser)	Heart	Kidney

In some texts, the channels are named in terms of the Chiao to which they belong, for example Hand Taiyin = Lung. Each pairing of channels displays characteristic symptoms indicating the depth at which one should work.

In the three Yang stages the Wei Qi is generally relatively strong and the symptoms tend to Excess or Heat, treatment being focused on their elimination. In the Yin stages treatment is not so straightforward as the defences have been breached; the situation has become both more chronic and diffuse, with the symptoms frequently being those of Cold.

The Tai Yang channels, translating as Greater Yang, are the Urinary Bladder and Small Intestine, and are the most superficial. Symptoms that indicate problems in this area include:

- headaches
- neck pain
- stiffness of the lower back
- fever, chill, palpable cold on the surface of the body
- body ache
- absence of sweating
- floating pulse.

Shao Yang, or Lesser Yang, is formed from the Sanjiao and Gall Bladder channels and is regarded as a hinge or transitional layer between the two other Yang Chiaos.

Typical symptoms usually involve the two organs and may include:

- fever with shivering
- pain over the heart
- bitter taste in the mouth.

Yang Ming or Sunlight Yang is formed from the Large Intestine and Stomach channels. Typical symptoms usually involve:

- fever
- aversion to heat
- perspiration
- thirst
- anxiety
- pain in the affected organs, stomach and large bowel with intolerance of pressure and constipation
- deep forceful pulse
- paralysis.

The Yang Ming is particularly associated with the treatment of any type of paralysis; the Stomach meridian and the Chong Mai are envisaged as supporting the integrity of the lumbar spine and the abdominal and inguinal muscles by nourishing them. Paralysis is seen as a lack of nourishment in the legs, with the Stomach meridian failing to supply the muscles with Blood and Qi.

Tai Yin, or Greater Yin, is formed from the Lung and Spleen channels. Typical symptoms are caused by the penetration of Cold and Damp to this deeper layer:

- abdominal distension
- diarrhoea
- indigestion
- slow, weak pulse.

Jue Yin, or Diminishing Yin, is formed from the Pericardium and Liver channels. It is regarded as the transition between Yang and Yin energy, and produces a complex symptomatic picture. Typical symptoms usually involve:

- sensation of alternating hot and cold when the Heat is of Yang origin and relatively acute and the Cold is of Yin origin and rather more chronic
- Yang Heat causes painful diarrhoea
- Heat in the upper part of the body and Cold below
- pain in the heart
- vomiting; hungry but unable to eat.

Shao Yin, or Lesser Yin, refers to the Heart and Kidney channels. This is the deepest level housing the Yang fire of the Heart and the Yin energy of the Kidney. Symptoms can be profoundly damaging and, again, manifest as a complex mixture according to whether Yang or Yin predominates.

Yang deficiency:

- diarrhoea
- vomiting
- cold limbs
- extreme fatigue
- thin, soft pulses.

Yin deficiency:

- pain in the chest, and throat and heart area
- restlessness
- thin, soft pulses.

While not included in all diagnostic frameworks, use of the six Chiaos enables the therapist to estimate the relative severity of the patient's symptoms. Use of the six Chiaos is closely related to the use of the Eight Principles (see Ch. 1) and also links easily to Five Element acupuncture. It is useful to be able to track the progress of a Pathogen as it moves deeper into or out of the tissue layers.

Use of Huatuojiaji points

The Huatuojiaji points, or Hua Tuo's paravertebral points, are included in this section because they are generally used in a segmental fashion, often in conjunction with trigger points. They are listed as extra points in most acupuncture atlases, but are believed by some teachers to be a secondary branch of the Urinary Bladder channel.

These points are located 0.5 cun from the midline of the spine or the Du channel, and are identified in pairs on a level with the lower border of the spinous process of each vertebra in the spinal column. They require relatively shallow needling, and are much safer than the Back Shu points found alongside because there are no major organs situated directly underneath; they are perhaps safer than the points on the Du channels because there is no chance of penetrating to the spinal cord.

The Huatuojiaji points are selected either because they are situated at the appropriate segmental level or because they can be associated with the desired Back Shu points and thus the Zang Fu organs. They can be used in TCM to regulate Yin and Yang, which is why they are always inserted in balanced pairs to refresh the mind and send down rebellious Qi. They are generally used in pairs in Western applications too, and often as a pair above and a pair below the perceived segmental innervation.

A list of spinal innervations and associated muscles is given in Tables 6.5 and 6.6. This can serve as a reminder whether using MT meridians or trigger points with the Huatuojiaji points.

Table 6.5 Segmental innervation of muscles: upper limb

Muscle	Spinal innervation						
Trapezius	C3	C4					
Levator scapulae		C4	C5				
Rhomboid major and minor		C4	C5	C6			
Latissimus dorsi				C6	C7	C8	
Pectoralis major				C6	C7	C8	T1
Serratus anterior			C5	C6	C7	C8	
Pectoralis minor						C8	T1
Deltoid		C4	C5	C6	C7		
Coracobrachialis			C5	C6	C7	C8	
Biceps brachii			C5	C6			
Teres major			C5	C6			
Triceps brachii				C6	C7	C8	
Supraspinatus		C4	C5	C6			
Infraspinatus		C4	C5	C6			
Teres minor		C4	C5	C6	C7		
Brachialis			C5	C6			
Brachioradialis			C5	C6			
Pronator teres			C5	C6	C7		
Pronator quadratus				C6	C7	C8	T1
Palmaris longus				C6	C7	C8	T1
Supinator			C5	C6	C7		
Extensor carpi radialis brevis			C5	C6	C7	C8	
Extensor carpi			C5	C6	C7	C8	
Extensor carpi ulnaris				C6	C7	C8	
Extensor digitorum				C6	C7	C8	
Extensor indicis				C6	C7	C8	T1
Extensor digiti minimi				C6	C7	C8	T1
Extensor pollicis longus				C6	C7	C8	T1
Extensor pollicis brevis				C6	C7	C8	
Flexor carpi ulnaris					C7	C8	T1
Flexor carpi radialis				C6	C7	C8	
Flexor pollicis brevis				C6	C7	C8	T1
Flexor digiti minimi brevis				C6	C7	C8	T1

Continues

Table 6.5 cont'd

Muscle	Spinal innervation			
Abductor pollicis	C6	C7	C8	T1
Flexor digitorum sublimis	C6	C7	C8	T1
Flexor digitorum profundus		C7	C8	T1
Flexor pollicis longus	C6	C7	C8	T1
Lumbricales	C6	C7	C8	T1
Abductor brevis	C6	C7	C8	T1
Abductor digiti minimi	C6	C7	C8	T1
Dorsal and palmar interossei			C8	T1
Opponens pollicis	C6	C7	C8	T1
Opponens digiti minimi		C7	C8	T1
Adductor pollicis			C8	T1

Table 6.6 Segmental innervation of muscles: lower limb

Muscle	Spinal innervation					
Pectineus	L2	L3	L4			
Tensor fascia lata			L4	L5	S1	
Adductor brevis	L2	L3	L4	L5		
Rectus femoris	L2	L3	L4	L5		
Vastus lateralis	L2	L3	L4	L5		
Vastus medialis	L2	L3	L4	L5		
Vastus intermedius	L2	L3	L4	L5		
Sartorius	L2	L3	L4			
Adductor longus	L2	L3	L4			
Adductor magnus	L2	L3	L4	L5		
Gluteus maximus			L4	L5	S1	S2 S3
Semimembranosus			L4	L5	S1	S2 S3
Semitendinosus				L5	S1	
Biceps femoris			L4	L5	S1	S2 S3
Gluteus medius			L4	L5	S1	S2
Gracilis	L2	L3	L4	L5		
Gluteus minimus			L4	L5	S1	
Quadratus femoris			L4	L5	S1	
Piriformis					S1	S2 S3
Gastrocnemius			L4	L5	S1	S2 S3
Soleus			L4	L5	S1	S2 S3
Flexor hallucis longus			L4	L5	S1	S2 S3
Flexor digitorum longus			L4	L5	S1	S2
Peroneus longus			L4	L5	S1	S2
Peroneus brevis			L4	L5	S1	S2
Tibialis posterior			L4	L5	S1	S2
Tibialis anterior			L4	L5	S1	S2
Extensor digitorum longus			L4	L5	S1	S2
Extensor hallucis longus			L4	L5	S1	S2
Flexor hallucis brevis				L5	S1	
Flexor digitorum brevis				L5	S1	
Plantar and dorsal interossei					S1	S2
Extensor digitorum brevis			L4	L5	S1	S2

Advanced segmental acupuncture

The link between the individual segments and the internal organs is also worth noting. Table 6.7 shows the segmental innervation of the internal organs.

In traditional Chinese acupuncture the Back Shu points are used to treat the organs. Their correspondence with the segmental dermatome distribution is close if not exact, although UB 14 Pericardium and UB 22 Sanjiao do not fit easily into the segmental concept.

A segmental disturbance can maintain other segmental symptoms. A good example of this is the pain from angina pectoris, perhaps leading to shoulder and chest pain, and active trigger points with the local muscles.

A patient with stomach problems may display segmental disturbances in the segment C3–5 and/or T5–9. Any point in the dermatome, myotome, viscerotome or sclerotome could be used to treat this. Some points correspond with traditional acupuncture points; others may not.

Research

Recent work has indicated that the original ideas about the correlation between trigger points and acupuncture points may have been rather optimistic. The value given by Melzack et al (1977) was 71%, but Birch (2003) reviewed the original study and made an attempt to reidentify the acupuncture points. He found that the correlation was more likely to be 40%, as many points really corresponded only with Ah Shi points, not points customarily associated with acupuncture treatment.

Table 6.7   Segmental innervation of the internal organs (after Bekkring & van Bussel 1998)

Organ	C3	C4	C5	T1	T2	T3	T4	T5	T6	T7	T8	T9	T10	T11	T12	L1	L2	S2	S3	S4
Heart	C3	C4	C5	T1	T2	T3	T4	T5												
Lungs	C3	C4	C5	T1	T2	T3	T4	T5	T6	T7										
Spleen	C3	C4	C5						T6	T7	T8	T9								
Stomach	C3	C4	C5					T5	T6	T7	T8	T9	T10							
Duodenum	C3	C4	C5					T5	T6	T7	T8	T9	T10	T11						
Pancreas	C3	C4	C5					T5	T6	T7	T8	T9	T10	T11						
Liver and Gall Bladder	C3	C4	C5					T5	T6	T7	T8	T9								
Proximal colon	C3	C4	C5						T6	T7	T8	T9	T10	T11	T12	L1				
Distal colon															T12	L1	L2			
Kidney	C3	C4	C5										T10	T11	T12	L1				
Urinary Bladder														T11	T12	L1	L2	S2	S3	S4
Uterus														T11	T12	L1	L2	S2	S3	S4

References

Acupuncture Association of Chartered Physiotherapists 1997 Guidelines for safe practice. Mere, UK: AACP.

Baldry PE 1989 Acupuncture, trigger points and musculoskeletal pain. Edinburgh: Churchill Livingstone.

Bekkring R, van Bussel R 1998 Segmental acupuncture. In: Filshie J, White AR, eds. Medical acupuncture, pp 105–135. Edinburgh: Churchill Livingstone.

Birch S 2003 Trigger point–acupuncture point correlations revisited. Journal of Alternative and Complementary Medicine 9: 91–103.

Birch S, Ida J 1998 Japanese acupuncture: a clinical guide. Brookline, MA: Paradigm.

Davis CL, Lewith GT, Broomfield J, Prescott P 2001 A pilot project to assess the methodological issues involved in evaluating acupuncture as a treatment for disabling breathlessness. Journal of Alternative and Complementary Medicine 7: 633–639.

Deadman P, Al-Khafaji M, Baker K 1998 A manual of acupuncture, 1st edn. Hove: Journal of Chinese Medicine Publications.

Denmei S, Brown S 2003 Finding effective acupuncture points. Seattle: Eastland Press.

Gunn C 1989 Treating myofascial pain. Seattle: University of Washington.

Hong CZ 2002 New trends in myofascial pain syndrome. Zhonghua Yi Xue Za Zhi 65: 501–512.

Melzack R, Stillwell DM, Fox EJ 1977 Trigger points and acupuncture points for pain: correlations and implications. Pain 3: 3–23.

Rodger-Withers S 1999 Understanding acute disharmonies of the channel sinews. American Journal of Acupuncture 27: 141–149.

Travell JG, Simons DG 1983 Myofascial pain and dysfunction. The trigger point manual. Baltimore: Williams & Wilkins.

Acupuncture microsystems (mini onions)

- ☙ Microsystems enable treatment of the whole body from one small region.
- ☙ Ear acupuncture (auriculotherapy) is the most commonly used system.
- ☙ It is a reflex system using organ–cutaneous and cutaneous–organ reflexes.
- ☙ It is important to detect tender ear points before using body points.
- ☙ Among other systems are the scalp, the hand, the navel, the nose and any long bone.
- ☙ These areas are often associated with particularly uncomfortable acupuncture points.
- ☙ There is some research to support the existence of the microsystems.

Introduction

Microsystems for diagnosing and treating medical problems have existed almost as long as medicine itself. These systems, which define correspondences with physiological, psychological and even cosmological phenomena, have been observed in many parts of the world from ancient times to the present. Perhaps the first example of this is palmistry, in which the history, current state and future situation of the enquirer can, supposedly, be read from the line on the palm.

The tongue and the radial pulse can also be considered as microsystems, but they are restricted to a diagnostic role. With the microsystems used in acupuncture treatment there is an implicit understanding that, not only can the history and present be read, but also the future can be altered in some way.

Ear acupuncture

Ear acupuncture is probably the best-known microsystem in acupuncture. It was first recognized as a reflex system by Paul Nogier in the 1950s. There are two distinct classifications of points: those according to Nogier and those according to Traditional Chinese Medicine (TCM).

The Chinese had recognized that some channels passed around or through the ear, and had described all the Yang meridians as having some connection, but they had not fully appreciated the reflexes involved. Nogier, on the other hand, spent many years studying the ear and slowly built up his concept of the 'man in the ear', in which he described a human fetus in an upside-down position with the head in the region of the ear lobe and the limbs towards the top of the ear. His ideas were imported into China in the mid 1950s, and barefoot doctors were trained in auricular therapy techniques, using the map of points illustrated, and enabling the treatment of a wide range of problems.

Nogier postulated that if there is a change in a body system due to pathology then a corresponding change can be shown in the ear, on the appropriate region. In the case of pain, the areas where pain is felt in the body have been shown to have a high correlation with tenderness in the points on the ear that correspond with the sites. Oleson et al (1980) provided the statistical evidence for these defined regions with a 74% accuracy rate in defining the musculoskeletal pains of 40 patients. This applies to many kinds of pathology, not just pain (Nogier & Nogier 1985). The area occupied on the ear surface is proportional to that in the cortex, so the upper limb, particularly the hand, and the face seem to be well represented.

The standardization of nomenclature for ear acupuncture points has been slow. The two main schools, that of Nogier and the TCM point locations, have now been joined by the work of Frank & Soliman (2000, 2001), who have built on the original Nogier extended work that described three basic phases: mesodermal, ectodermal and endodermal. The theory underlying this division is that the ear is composed of three different kinds of tissue in the developing embryo, and each of these types is involved in different somatotropic responses relating to the ear. Further, the different phases are associated with acute, intermediate and chronic pain conditions. A recent acupuncture atlas (Hecker et al 2000) gives all the points with little or no explanation, leading to much confusion among students.

Auricular therapy is defined as a physical reflex therapy that detects somatic level disturbances on the auricle. There are precise zones of representation of organs, although these are not thought of as fixed points as they tend to have fluctuating boundaries, depending as they do on the metabolism of the organ. The right ear is said to represent the left hemisphere of the brain, while the left ear represents the right hemisphere. Thus, actual treatment will be on the same side as the problem.

Nogier discovered that there was a change in the amplitude of the human pulse as monitored at the wrist when tactile stimulation of the ear occurred. This was evidence of a sympathetic reflex affecting peripheral blood vessel activity. He referred to this as the auricular cardiac reflex (ACR). The changes detected are in waveform or amplitude, not actually in pulse rate. This is an involuntary arterial reflex, also known as the vascular autonomic signal (VAS), and is found as a vascular–cutaneous reflex in response to other stimuli. This response to any form of tactile stimulus may explain the soothing effect of rubbing the ears – in both small children and dogs!

Acupuncture technique in the ear is slightly different to that for any other body surface. Short, fine needles are preferable, and these are inserted carefully without piercing the cartilage of the ear. The reason for this care is that the cartilage has a very poor blood supply, so that any infection is very difficult to eliminate. This has led to the recommended use of alcohol swabs to clean the surface before needle insertion. Originally auriculotherapy was recommended for the treatment of nicotine or alcohol addiction; subdermal needles like tiny tacks were left in situ from one treatment to the next, and covered by a small piece of plaster. This is discouraged nowadays because the risk of infection is too great.

The Chinese ear charts differ quite radically from those produced by Nogier, leading to considerable confusion among acupuncturists. There are many points on the TCM ear, located by way of a grid system and requiring a fine location skill. Chinese texts recommend the use of the points according to TCM principles (e.g. the Kidney point to treat bones), but as this appears to be a true reflex system this use is not supported scientifically.

More important is the nerve supply to each part of the structure. The ear has an abundant innervation, being supplied by the sensory fibres of the trigeminal, facial and vagus nerves. The endings of these nerves are closely interwoven and can influence many distant body areas. Bourdiol (1982) gives an explanation based on embryology, emphasizing the fact that these nerves travel only a short distance to the reticular formation of the brainstem.

There are several ways of classifying the points. Oleson & Kroening (1983) suggested nomenclature that depends on whether the points are located on raised, depressed or hidden areas in the ear. Otherwise, the Chinese or Nogier maps are commonly used.

The mechanism of acupuncture effect appears to be the same as that in the rest of the body. Ear acupuncture has been shown to affect the endorphin concentration and to be reversed by naloxone (Simmons & Oleson 1993). This study investigated changes in dental pain threshold after electroacupuncture stimulation to the ear, and showed that true electroacupuncture produced a significant rise in the pain threshold whereas a placebo treatment, using inappropriate ear points, did not.

All areas of the ear surface are utilized, with some points being located on raised areas, some in the depressions, some in hidden areas under folds of tissue, and still others on the posterior surface of the ear.

When the two maps – Nogier (Fig. 7.1) and TCM (Fig. 7.2) – are compared, it can be seen that some regions are similar but there are many

Figure 7.1
Representation of the 'inverted fetus' in the ear. (Redrawn with kind permission from Hopwood et al 1997.)

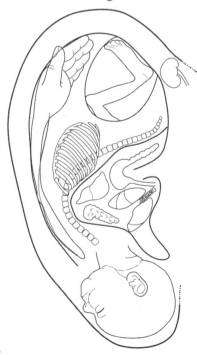

Figure 7.2 Chinese map of ear points.

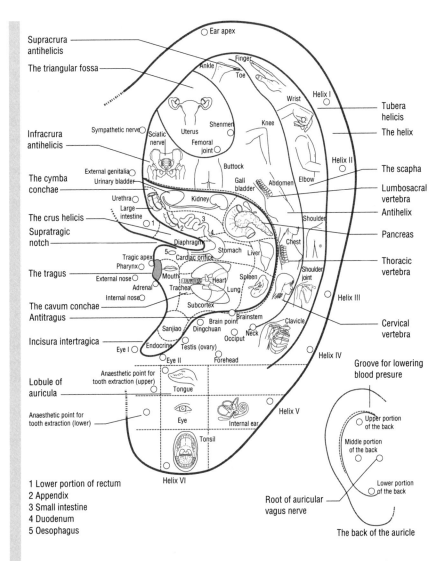

1 Lower portion of rectum
2 Appendix
3 Small intestine
4 Duodenum
5 Oesophagus

single points that do not seem to tally. In physiotherapy practice the most commonly used auricular point is Shenmen, which is common to both – a sedative point located in the navicular fossa. As might be deduced from the name, this point has similar applications to Ht 7 Shenmen, being used to calm anxious patients, often before further acupuncture is undertaken. The musculoskeletal zones are also frequently used, perhaps because they are easily located.

These points are used in conjunction with body acupuncture in many protocols for musculoskeletal acupuncture. They offer an alternative when points are inaccessible, either because of medical problems, plaster, etc., or simply because of the difficulty of positioning or undressing the patient.

Points derived from the Chinese system of ear acupuncture are used regularly in drug addiction withdrawal programmes. The National Acupuncture Detoxification Association (NADA) protocol uses five points – Shenmen, Liver, Lung, Sympathetic and Kidney – and is supported by some research (Smith & Khan 1988). This combination of points can produce profound relaxation in quite distressed patients, so it has an application beyond that of drug withdrawal, in my opinion. It would be interesting to set up a research protocol using it for anxiety.

Recent advances in ear acupuncture have advocated the use of three phases, or differing maps of point location, according to whether the problem is perceived as acute, intermediate or chronic (Frank & Soliman 2000). These locations are based on the Nogier theories rather than those of the Chinese, and echo the territories according to embryological origin: mesoderm, endoderm and ectoderm. The Chinese territories tend to correlate with those in the acute or mesodermal phase. To treat patients using this system, some ability with pulse diagnosis is required in order to monitor treatment events, checking the vascular autonomic signal (VAS). Also, a specially designed electrical instrument that works as both a point finder and a therapeutic tool will be helpful.

Technique

The indications of pathology are similar to those elsewhere in the body. Among these are: changes in the appearance of the skin, redness or small skin lesions, changes in tenderness or sensitivity of the skin, and changes in the electrical resistance of the skin. The usual way of detecting these tender points is to use manual pressure via the blunt end of an acupuncture needle or a blunt spring-loaded instrument. Care must be taken to maintain an even pressure. The location of tender spots indicates both the area of the body in trouble and the point in the ear to insert the needle.

Electrical point finders are often recommended for use in the ear. Where the points are very close together, distinguishing between one and the next might be a critical factor in treatment. While theoretically a good idea, these point finders are difficult to use in practice because it is easy to produce a false impedance reading if the pressure on the skin is too great or the patient is sweating. It is also possible to burn a low resistance pathway through the dermis if the current is too high, also producing a false point.

Treatment is usually most effective with the least possible number of needles. The needles are usually left in for 10–20 minutes (normal treatment time) and, as explained above, it is not recommended that they be left between treatments. Slight bleeding may occur after removal of the needles; use an alcohol swab to clear this. If a longer effect is required, patients can be asked to stimulate the point themselves. Sterilized mustard seeds or small ionic beads (Magraine) may be left securely stuck to the ear with small plaster patches. This makes it possible for the patient to apply acupressure between treatments, whenever the presenting problem recurs.

If body acupuncture is to be combined with the use of ear points, the points on the ear must be located first as the delicate organ–cutaneous reflex can be altered by body needling and the ear points will be harder to locate.

Research

Oleson et al (1980) did the original work supporting this theory. In a blinded trial, they found that body pathology in patients could be detected with 74% accuracy by testing for tenderness in the ear and measuring changes in the electrical resistance of the skin. The result was highly statistically significant, and anecdotal evidence from the same trial indicated that old pathology that the patients themselves had forgotten about was also detected.

A more recent study has taken this apparent correlation further. Given that the pathology of a particular organ appears to give rise to changes in the electrical impedance of the skin on the ear over the corresponding point, the researchers tested the validity of this reflex in patients undergoing surgery (Szopinski et al 2003). Forty-five patients, admitted for surgery for cholecystectomy, appendicectomy, partial gastrectomy, or dilatation and curettage after miscarriage, were tested. The initial value of skin resistance was estimated at the auricular organ projection area (OPA) on five occasions: before premedication, after medication, under general anaesthesia, after skin incision and after surgery. On each occasion, two healthy OPAs were measured on each patient as a control. The examiners performed all measurements without knowledge of the corresponding points.

The measuring equipment, a prototype organ electrodermal diagnostic device (OED) measuring impedance, took two values at each point, adjusting for anomalies such as sweat on the skin, to give a ratio. The rectification ratios at OPAs related to a diseased organ before premedication were approximately three times higher than readings from the control points. Premedication, medication and incision did not influence the results, but direct surgical manipulation of the diseased organs resulted in a rapid increase in the rectification ratios observed in the corresponding skin areas ($P < 0.001$). In addition, rectification ratios were significantly different for all conditions compared with control values ($P < 0.001$). It is suggested that, as the damage to the organ produced by surgical intervention produced such immediate changes in the electrical parameters, this type of OED could be used with confidence to detect pathology in patients unable to communicate, such as small children or unconscious patients.

A recent small controlled study (Kuruvilla 2003) has indicated that ear acupuncture may have an effect in obesity, although the National Institutes of Health report in 1998 concluded that there was no supportive evidence for this or for smoking cessation (NIH Consensus Development Panel on Acupuncture 1998). The points used were mouth, stomach, small intestine, the endocrine point and Shenmen. Both groups were given a calorie-controlled diet and an exercise programme. Interestingly, the entire acupuncture group described a decrease in appetite, although not necessarily a decrease in weight.

Ear acupuncture is a useful addition to the needling skills of a physiotherapist. It seems to have a reasonable evidence base and lends itself to use on nervous or debilitated patients (Case study 7.1). As it can also be utilized in patients when, for some reason, access to the normal body points is not possible – in cases of pain after major surgery, during childbirth or extensive application of plaster fixation – ear acupuncture can be very versatile.

A good atlas for locating ear points is the *Color Atlas of Acupuncture* (Hecker et al 2000) and there are two excellent texts (See Further reading list for Oleson 1996 and Rubach 2001).

CASE HISTORY

Case study 7.1

Elderly woman, aged 73 years, wife of a patient with multiple sclerosis visited in the community. Her husband required constant care, unable to walk more than a few steps, problems with transfer, registered blind. Wife very stressed, suffering from osteoporosis, with severe low back pain. Unwilling to undress but agreed to be treated while husband was having physiotherapy.

Treatment
Seated in an armchair, feet supported. Checked painful points in the ear.
Ear acupuncture: Shenmen, lumbar spine, Kidney point.
Body acupuncture: SI 3 Houxi, UB 62 Shenmai, Kid 3 Taixi.
Needles left for 20–30 minutes.

Response
Immediate pain relief, lasting for approximately 5–6 days each time. Patient usually fell asleep while being treated. Claimed to feel refreshed and cheerful after each treatment.

Comment
This patient was treated regularly whenever her husband was visited. The pain relief was maintained over several months and she was comfortable with the nature of treatment as she was not required to take off anything other than her tights. The ear points were an important element; pain relief was not so good when they were omitted.

The hand as a microsystem

Much of the basic work on microsystem acupuncture originates with Ralph Alan Dale and was published in various professional journals between 1974 and 1999. One of the more accessible is that of the hand.

There are, in fact, many classifications of hand acupuncture. One of the better known is Korean hand acupuncture, devised in Korea in the early 1970s and often credited to Dr Woo Tae Yoo. There is another type, also from Korea, called Su Jok.

The hand is regarded as representing the whole body, with the back of the hand corresponding to the back of the body and the palmar surface to the front (Fig. 7.3). The centre line passes down the centre of the middle finger and the right or left side of the hand is treated according to the site of the problem in the body. Vertebral or visceral problems can be treated on both hands. Stimulation is by very tiny needles, moxa or electroacupuncture. Diagnosis is made using a mixture of Five Element theory and pulse reading.

There are many points fitted into this small space; Yoo has identified the equivalent of all the 361 orthodox body points. He also claims to have discovered points that do not have a direct relationship with those on the regular meridians. I am not aware of any good-quality research, but it must be said that this system is widely used in Korea and anecdotal evidence from Western practitioners is usually very enthusiastic.

Less ambitious, but more likely to be incorporated into normal treatment, are the Baxie, so-called extra points on the hand, found in TCM theory. The usual combination contains LI 4 Hegu and SJ 3 Zhongzhu, with

Figure 7.3 The hand as a microsystem (Korean system). (Redrawn with kind permission of Dr Ralph Alan Dale 1990, 1999.)

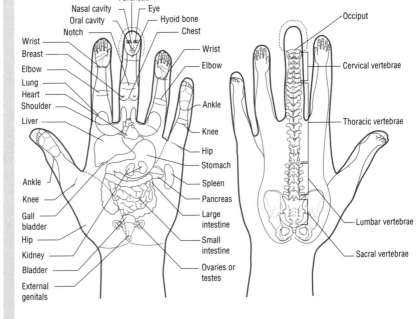

two intervening points corresponding in site to SJ 3, but between the second and third and the third and fourth fingers. These are not strictly speaking a microsystem in themselves, as they do not represent the whole body; however, if so many powerful points are truly clustered in this area, perhaps there is a connection.

The connection may be clearer between the Korean hand points on the back of the hand and the other well-known pair of extra points, Yatongdian, situated in the spaces between the proximal ends of the second and third and the third and fourth metacarpals, exactly where the lumbosacral area is on the Korean hand acupuncture map. These two points can be rather painful for the patient, but are used with some clinical success for severe low back pain.

Philtrum

The area just below the nose and above the upper lip is also said to be a microsystem. Fu Qiang first proposed this in 1971. There are nine points on a line corresponding to the Du channel. This is a remarkably sensitive area, commonly used to restore consciousness (Du 26 Renzhong). The points are in reverse order, with that relating to the head and face situated just above the line of the lip. This set of points is most associated with the three Jiaos and could logically be used together with the three Jiao type of tongue diagnosis.

Navel

The navel is sometimes considered as a microsystem, but not in the same sense as the other areas described in this chapter. The basic difference is that the navel itself is a forbidden point for acupuncture needling. Moxa can be used, but needles are never inserted. There are records of abdominal palpation dating from the Ming dynasty in China, but the practice seems to have been adopted far more enthusiastically by the Japanese acupuncturists. The ancient TCM views expressed in the Nanjing considered the navel as the centre of heaven, ruled by earth; according to the Five Elements its organs are the Spleen and Stomach.

The front Mu points, described briefly in Chapter 5, are acupuncture points located on the abdomen and are related directly to specific meridians. These points can serve for diagnosis as well as treatment, tenderness on palpation being an indication of a problem within the corresponding organ. They are normally considered to be linked in a Yin–Yang pairing with a corresponding Back Shu point. The Front Mu points do not really correspond with those used in navel or Hara diagnosis.

The abdomen is the cavity where the Qi force of the Zang Fu organs is sited. Those using abdominal diagnosis claim that palpation of the abdominal wall is a good guide to the imbalances among the Zang Fu organs and can be used prophylactically to predict future problems. This form of diagnosis is widely used in Japanese acupuncture, where it is known as Hara diagnosis.

The navel is the scar on the abdomen that marks where the umbilical cord was attached in fetal life. In most adults it is marked by a depression, in a minority by a protuberance. It is located at the level of the interspace of the third and fourth lumbar vertebrae, and lies about halfway between the infrasternal notch and the symphysis pubis.

One of the final roles of the umbilical cord is to deliver antibodies to the child at the time of birth. At delivery, after umbilical pulsation has ceased, these antibodies are released, a process that takes about 1 minute. These antibodies are critical to the establishment of immune function in the newborn child and help to activate the thymus gland, the major gland responsible for production of immune antibodies. The time of severance is believed to be critical: too early and the child will lack the necessary antibody stimulation, or too late when some of the mother's antibodies may have crossed the barrier setting up confusion in the T-cell response or immune reactions to 'foreign' substances, which may continue throughout life in the form of autoimmune disease. Thus the importance of the navel in TCM is echoed in Western medicine.

The condition and shape of the navel in a mature adult is said to indicate quite clearly the energetic balance of the organs beneath and adjacent to it.

This system of diagnosis and treatment is described in detail in Japanese acupuncture textbooks (e.g. Matsumoto & Birch 1988) and also by Gardner-Abbate (1996). Only a brief description will be attempted here.

The diagram of the areas of the abdomen with the Zang Fu–Five Element correspondences (Fig. 7.4) indicates the soft tissues that might give some information on the Liver, Lung and Kidney, whereas the zone for the Spleen and Stomach lies around the centre of the navel. On visual examination, a healthy navel should look symmetrical with a clear circular shape and firm surrounding tissue. A normal navel will be observed to have a slight depression above. The most important sign to look for is the symmetry of the surrounding circle of tissue. If there is an imbalance, the navel will appear to be 'looking' in one direction or another. This appearance is caused by the flattening or softening of the navel border and can be confirmed by palpation.

A navel with a collapsed border on the upper side (i.e. 'looking up') indicates a deficiency of the Spleen; looking to the left indicates a Liver Blood deficiency, to the right Lung Qi Xu, and looking down Kidney Qi Xu.

Figure 7.4 Abdominal map based on the Nanjing. (Redrawn from Gardner-Abbate 1997.)

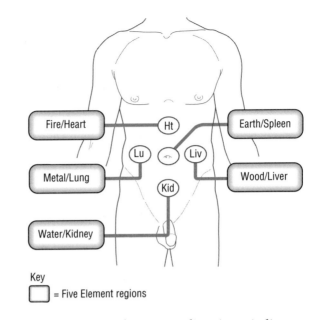

Fire/Heart — Ht

Earth/Spleen

Lu — Liv

Metal/Lung

Wood/Liver

Kid

Water/Kidney

Key
☐ = Five Element regions

Weakness or softness in the surrounding tissue indicates a poor constitution and capacity for healing; treatment should be according to the zone. If there is palpable oedema around the area, again the location is critical. A slight puffiness below the navel is said to indicate Kidney Yang deficiency. The navel itself is said to belong to the Spleen and the vitality of the patient can be assessed by the visibility of a slight pulse within the navel.

A lot of information can be drawn from the shape and size of the navel. If it is protuberant or particularly wide, there is obviously some disturbance of the surrounding connective tissue and this is held to indicate weak immunity. If the area around it is particularly hard on palpation, this may indicate rigidity in the muscles and an underlying Excess condition. Finally, there should be no pain or discomfort associated with navel palpation. When the response to an investigative touch is guarding, this indicates a Kidney deficiency.

Traditional Chinese acupuncture does not, as previously stated, advocate needling of the navel, although moxa is used quite frequently, usually through another medium such as salt or ginger, but sometimes indirectly using a moxa roll. The aims of treatment are to reinvigorate the Spleen and Kidney energies. Cupping is also used occasionally. Japanese acupuncture does advocate needling in the area around the navel, but this is not recommended if the tissues are hard and tight. There is a technique using eight needles inserted superficially at the compass points around the navel as a tonifying treatment for Lung, Spleen and Kidney.

This is probably not a technique that will be used frequently by physiotherapists without additional training in the subtleties of Japanese diagnosis and acupuncture, but it is worth observing the configuration of the navel when treating chronic pain problems. An indication of major Zang Fu imbalance can assist with the choice of valuable supplementary points.

Long bones

One of the strangest ideas on microsystems is that credited to Zhang Yin Qing. This system, called 'embryo containing the information of the whole organism', was first published in 1980. Zhang first discovered a microsystem on the second metacarpal bone, locating it along the dorsoradial aspect. He related 11 separate points along the length of the bone to specific body areas (Fig. 7.5). Later he postulated that the same system could be found in all the long bones of the body, although he separated 'leg' and 'foot', making 12 separate points along the shaft of the bones. He claimed that this was related to embryological development.

Research

This microsystem has been tested on postoperative wound pain following abdominal surgery in a randomized controlled clinical trial (Wang 1992). In this study 100 patients were randomized to two groups, one treated with acupuncture to the second metacarpal at appropriate levels (i.e. 'Liver' for biliary tract surgery and 'Stomach' for gastric surgery). The needles were manipulated to ensure DeQi and retained for 30–40 minutes. The control group received intramuscular injections of pethidine and promethazine. The patient group was balanced for sex, and ages ranged between 30 and 76 years. All patients were treated within 8–10 hours of operation.

The published results are interesting in that the two treatment groups showed no significant difference ($P > 0.05$). However, the advantages of the acupuncture were clear: the wound pain was relieved very rapidly, in 2–5 minutes. The technique was simple and involved none of the side-effects associated with the drugs.

No outrageous claims are made in this study, but it looks as though this microsystem may offer an alternative to drug control for postoperative wound pain.

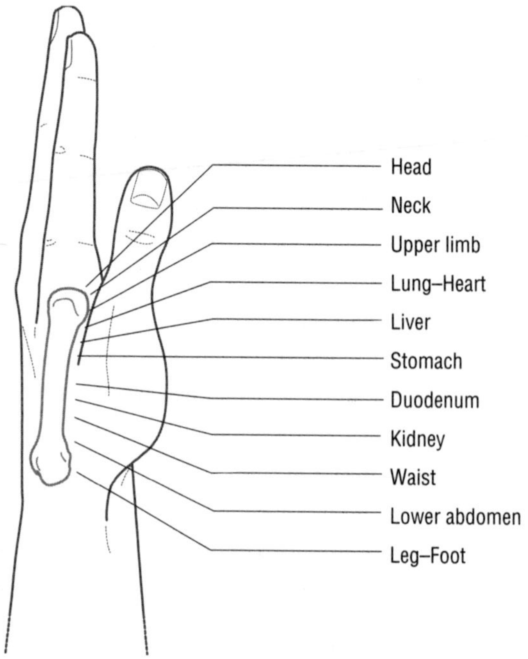

Figure 7.5 Second metacarpal bone microsystem.

Head
Neck
Upper limb
Lung–Heart
Liver
Stomach
Duodenum
Kidney
Waist
Lower abdomen
Leg–Foot

Scalp acupuncture

This is a relatively modern acupuncture technique credited to Chiao Shun Fa and introduced into China in 1971. Chiao claimed to have tried all the points on himself with the aid of a mirror! A full description of this technique can be found in his published text (Jiao 1997). There are links to traditional body acupuncture, auriculotherapy and the neuroanatomy of the brain. The Chinese research base is substantial, but of rather poor quality.

Two relatively recent Western papers indicate that acupuncture, when used with electrical stimulation, may enhance cerebral circulation (Ingvar & Gadea Ciria 1975, Yuan et al 1998). It is used for neurological conditions, most commonly for motor or sensory deficit in stroke, but also for Parkinson's disease, chronic muscle spasm, deafness, balance problems and speech problems. The application in stroke treatment, where the needles are inserted along the lines of the motor or sensory cortices, has some sort of logic to it: the establishment of a supplementary or peripheral circulation to the damaged areas of the cortex might theoretically prevent further cell death in the very early stages after stroke.

Technique

The hair needs to be moved out of the way; shaving is recommended if regular treatment is to be undertaken. The skin is sterilized with a solution of 2.5% iodine and 75% alcohol. The Chinese technique utilizes longer, finer needles of 40–70 mm inserted subdermally along the motor or sensory lines. Western practitioners use several short needles inserted obliquely at strategic intervals along the line. An electrostimulation current is applied to the needles, at a frequency of 200–300 Hz for 20–40 minutes.

Patients may feel a tingling, a sensation of pins and needles, or warmth locally; sometimes there is a distended sensation in the distal area affected by the treatment. Treatment may be contralateral, ipsilateral, or both, and can be combined with body acupuncture. Far from being uncomfortable, scalp acupuncture is very relaxing and patients tend to go to sleep while being treated.

Research evidence

Scalp acupuncture has been used in several trials of acupuncture for stroke with varying success, but never in the West as the only acupuncture modality. Two small controlled trials by Naeser et al (1992, 1994) showed a significant result overall for acupuncture, including scalp acupuncture, over the control. However, the most recent use of scalp acupuncture as part of an acupuncture 'package' in a major randomized controlled trial showed no significant differences between treatment and control groups (Hopwood 2003). However, anecdotal evidence from China seems to indicate that this technique is used widely for many neurological problems, perhaps with some success (Jiao 1997).

Liver 3

Finally, it is necessary to include a word or two about Liv 3 Taichong. This is not strictly a microsystem, but seems to have found its way into modern acupuncture literature as a universal treatment (Campbell 2003, Mann 1992). Both of these authors regard this as an area rather than a specific acupoint, describing it as a roughly rectangular area about 2.5 cm wide and 0.6 cm long, situated between the first and second metatarsal bones.

Taichong is recognized as a powerful point in TCM theory, but these two Western practitioners have used it extensively to treat conditions such as chronic urticaria, solar dermatitis, menopausal hot flushes, bronchial asthma, hay fever asthma, digestive disturbances, headache and migraine.

The purist TCM practitioner will naturally claim that these conditions may frequently have an element of Heat as Pathogen, and that this Liv 3 area is a good way to expel this as the location covers both Liv 2 Xingjian and Liv 3 Taichong, Ying Spring and Shu Stream points respectively.

Further research is probably necessary to see whether isolated treatment at Liv 3, with its segmental supply mainly from L5, is as good as a carefully constructed TCM prescription.

Summary

Acupuncturists have always been fascinated by these subsystems, and most will use at least one subsystem on occasion. There are quite possibly many more microsystems than we currently describe. The microacupuncture system may be used to treat the macroenergetics (Qi) and the viscera (Zang Fu), and also local symptoms relating to the musculoskeletal system.

Dale (1999, p 220) has summarized this beautifully in a quote taken from a Hindu sutra:

In the heaven of Indra there is said to be a network of pearls so arranged that if you look at one you see all the others reflected in it. In the same way, each object in the world is not merely itself but involves every other object, and in fact is in every other object.

References

Bourdiol RJ (ed.) 1982 Elements of auriculotherapy. Sainte-Ruffine: Maisonnerve.

Campbell A 2003 Acupuncture in practice; beyond points and meridians, 1st edn. Oxford: Butterworth-Heinemann.

Dale RA 1990 The holograms of hand micro-acupuncture: a study in systems of correspondence. American Journal of Acupuncture 19: 141–162.

Dale RA 1999 The systems, holograms and theory of micro-acupuncture. American Journal of Acupuncture 27: 207–242.

Frank BL, Soliman NE 2000 Atlas of auricular therapy and auricular medicine. Richardson.

Frank B, Soliman N 2001 Zero point: a critical assessment through advanced auricular therapy. Journal of the Acupuncture Association of Chartered Physiotherapists, February: 61–65.

Gardner-Abbate S 1996 Holding the tiger's tail. Santa Fe, New Mexico: Southwest Acupuncture College Press.

Gardner-Abbate S 1997 A brief guide to the use of the navel microsystem for diagnosis and root treatment according to classical Chinese and Japanese traditions. American Journal of Acupuncture 25: 115–131.

Hecker H-U, Steveling A, Peuker E et al 2000 Color atlas of acupuncture. Stuttgart: Thieme.

Hopwood V 2003 An investigation into the effects of acupuncture on stroke recovery. PhD thesis, Southampton University.

Ingvar D, Gadea Ciria M 1975 Assessment of severe damage to the brain by multiregional measurements of cerebral blood flow. Ciba Foundation Symposium 34: 97–120.

Jiao S 1997 Scalp acupuncture and clinical cases. Beijing: Foreign Languages Press.

Kuruvilla AC 2003 Acupuncture and obesity. Medical Acupuncture 14: 32–33.

Mann F 1992 Re-inventing acupuncture: a new concept of Ancient Medicine, 1st edn. Oxford: Butterworth-Heinemann.

Matsumoto K, Birch S 1988 Hara diagnosis: reflections on the sea. Brookline, MA: Paradigm Publications.

Naeser MA, Alexander M, Stiassny-Eder D et al 1992 Real versus sham acupuncture in the treatment of paralysis in acute stroke patients: a CT scan lesion site study. Journal of Neurological Rehabilitation 6: 163–173.

Naeser MA, Alexander M, Stiassny-Eder D et al 1994 Acupuncture in the treatment of paralysis in chronic and acute stroke patients. Improvement correlated with specific CT scan lesion sites. Acupuncture & Electrotherapeutics Research International Journal 19: 227–249.

NIH Consensus Development Panel on Acupuncture 1998 Acupuncture. Journal of the American Medical Association 280: 1518–1524.

Nogier PMF, Nogier R 1985 The man in the ear. Sainte-Ruffine: Maisonneuve.

Oleson TD, Kroening RJ 1983 A new nomenclature for identifying Chinese and Nogier auricular acupuncture points. American Journal of Acupuncture 11: 325–344.

Oleson TD, Kroening RJ, Bresler DE 1980 An experimental evaluation of auricular diagnosis: the somatotopic mapping of musculoskeletal pain at ear acupuncture points. Pain 8: 217–229.

Simmons M, Oleson T 1993 Auricular electrical stimulation and dental pain threshold. Anesthesia Progress 40: 14–19.

Smith MO, Khan I 1988 An acupuncture programme for the treatment of drug addicted persons. Bulletin on Narcotics XL: 35–41.

Szopinski JZ, Lukasiewicz S, Lochner GP et al 2003 Influence of general anesthesia and surgical intervention on the parameters of auricular organ projection areas. Medical Acupuncture 14: 40–42.

Wang X 1992 Postoperative pain: clinical study on the use of the second metacarpal holographic points for wound pain following abdominal surgery. American Journal of Acupuncture 20: 119–121.

Yuan X, Hao X, Lai Z et al 1998 Effects of acupuncture at Fengchi point (GB 20) on cerebral blood flow. Journal of Traditional Chinese Medicine 18: 102–105.

Further reading

Oleson T 1996 Auriculotherapy manual: Chinese and Western systems of ear acupuncture. Los Angeles: Health Care Alternatives.

Rubach A 2001 Principles of ear acupuncture: microsystem of the auricle. Stuttgart: Thieme.

Acknowledgement

I am indebted to Ralph Alan Dale for his original work on microacupuncture and his permission to use the hand holograms in Figure 7.3.

Pulling it all together – working in code

- Traditional Chinese Medicine is a truly holistic discipline.
- The many diagnostic prompts will guide the practitioner to an understanding of patterns or syndromes.
- It helps to be able to see the Zang Fu pattern.
- Use of this syndrome recognition is essentially safe.
- Knotty or complex problems can be solved in this way because the TCM 'code' is extremely subtle in the hands of an experienced practitioner.
- The most common syndromes are given for reference.
- There is some correspondence with Western disease categories, but this can sometimes be misleading.
- Treatment is often long term and may progress through several identified syndromes before the best outcome is achieved.

Introduction to syndromes

The classification and identification of syndromes involves the use of all the diagnostic tools of Chinese Medicine. All the aspects mentioned in previous chapters must play their part and will help to build a composite picture of what is wrong with the patient. The final combination of symptoms is what defines the syndrome. Very few patients fit the picture completely, but most will display a collection of identifiable symptoms, the majority of which can be classified into a syndrome pattern.

Mastery of this art is based on gaining a thorough understanding of the basics and then applying those basics in a rigorously consistent and logical manner. True acupuncture masters appear to be quite intuitive in their ability to sense the imbalances, but when questioned closely the procedural steps can be explained quite simply. The steps are simply accomplished more quickly with greater experience of working in this way.

Skill in TCM is primarily the ability to see the patterns. A secondary, but perhaps no less important skill, is the ability to sense how chronic the problem is and how deep the causes of the symptoms are. It is not uncommon to encounter, as in orthodox Western medicine, an acute pattern superimposed on a chronic deterioration. Often, in complex diseases, the slow penetration of a Pathogen to a deep level of body functioning has produced changes along the way, and teasing out the twists and turns in this process can be fascinating. This gradual and painstaking process is ultimately very beneficial to the patient, who may achieve a complete cure rather than temporary relief.

It is worth noting that the initial diagnosis is really only a working hypothesis. The response to the first treatments will clarify and vindicate the line of reasoning, or cause the therapist to rethink carefully. If the patient fails to respond over a period of time or actually gets worse, the tentative diagnosis is clearly wrong. However, any changes that have occurred should point to the new direction needed for the treatment plan. This regular self-audit for the therapist is built into the therapeutic encounter and serves as a real protection for the patient. Faulty lines of reasoning will not be pursued for more than a couple of sessions.

One of the simplest methods of determining a syndrome is to list the symptoms one by one and then allot each one to a group within the Eight Principle categories. A simple list of two columns will work well for the novice to TCM (Box 8.1), or a slightly more complex Eight Principles list (Box 8.2) will allow for greater differentiation and analysis (see Ch. 1, Box 1.1).

The table in Box 8.2 allows an initial sorting of the different types of symptom, although in any complex situation it is always difficult to decide which are really important and which are only minor or, indeed, just the logical result of a major imbalance. When they are all written down and categorized, it is at least possible to make value judgements.

A Five Element diagram (Fig. 8.1) is a useful tool, particularly if this type of TCM theory is well understood. Even if full Five Element theory is not being followed, the division of symptoms in this way is helpful and can lead to a better Zang Fu differentiation. Listing the observed symptoms

Box 8.1   Simple sorting of symptoms

Excess (Shi)	Deficiency (Xu)

Box 8.2   Sorting according to the Eight Principles

Eight Principle symptom categories	
External	Internal
Yang	Yin
Hot	Cold
Excess	Deficiency

Figure 8.1 Five Element diagram.

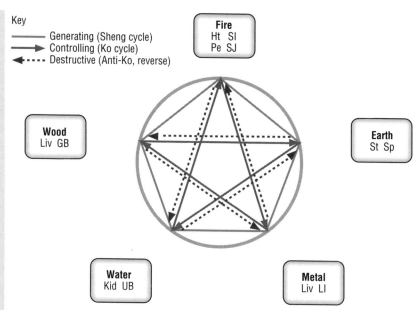

Key
- —— Generating (Sheng cycle)
- ——▶ Controlling (Ko cycle)
- ◀···· Destructive (Anti-Ko, reverse)

Fire
Ht SI
Pe SJ

Wood
Liv GB

Earth
St Sp

Water
Kid UB

Metal
Liv LI

close to the associated element allows the therapist to distinguish the possible classification of the majority of symptoms. Where the picture is confusing, application of Five Element dynamics may help to guide the treatment plan. There are some very good reference books in this field (Ross 1995, Seem 1987).

The following syndromes are given in the order of the Zang Fu organs as the Qi circulates in the body. The Zang Fu functions are described in detail in Chapter 3, so only a brief summary is given here to explain the symptoms. The points given in each section are only suggestions; if the treatment aims are followed each time, there may well be others that would be suitable. Those selected are perhaps the most obvious, given the TCM interpretation of their indications. While not dealt with directly in this chapter, the innervation of the acupuncture points might also be relevant to their selection.

At the end, two important general syndromes, Collapse of Yin and Collapse of Yang, are included, because these require a fairly urgent and global treatment if they are recognized. The widely identified Bi syndrome has been discussed in Chapter 2.

The Front Mu and Back Shu points are frequently offered in the points lists. These points would not be used at the same time, partly for practical reasons, as positioning the patient can be difficult. The Mu points tend to have a more general Yin effect and the Back Shu points more Yang, and the Shu points are also perhaps more specific to the Zang Fu organ in question.

In each section a list of symptoms is given to help differentiate between Excess and Deficiency. The syndrome symptoms are those that general TCM theory ascribes to each condition and an approximate Western diagnosis is also included. It will be apparent that the same Western diagnosis can apply to several syndromes; this highlights the sophistication of the original TCM diagnoses. When in doubt, the final decision as to the exact syndrome should be guided by whether there is Excess or Deficiency present. It is always best not to depend too closely on the Western diagnosis, although it may be helpful to have a familiar starting place.

Many physiotherapists will feel that some of the following conditions and situations are beyond the scope of their professional practice. However, some of them are seen very frequently in Western society and may arise as complications to an otherwise simple pain problem. Some form of intermediate TCM training is necessary to gain a clearer understanding of the diagnostic prompts and the 'code'.

A simple rule is that, if the therapist feels unsure, the patient should be referred to an experienced TCM practitioner, after consulting with the responsible medical practitioner. Certainly some situations, included here for interest, are medical emergencies and should be dealt with as such. Acupuncture has its limitations!

Patterns of Lung disharmony

Functions of the Lung:

- ☯ respiration, intake of Qi
- ☯ governs Wei Qi
- ☯ controls the skin, pores and body hair
- ☯ controls perspiration
- ☯ to disperse and descend Qi
- ☯ regulates water circulation.

The Lung has a clear connection to the Kidney, being reliant on Kidney energies for efficient function, so symptoms involving problems with the water circulation may necessitate treatment of Kidney points.

There is a convention when treating the Lung that moxa is not used, as excess Heat or Dryness is damaging to that organ.

In all syndromes the problem may be one of Excess or Deficiency, and the symptoms for the Lung can be identified as in Box 8.3.

Syndromes
Invasion of Lungs by Cold

Western diagnoses: common cold, acute or chronic bronchitis, bronchial asthma.

Symptoms: chills, fever, slight headache, aching muscles, lack of perspiration, thin cough, stuffy or runny nose, superficial wheeze, dislike of cold.

Box 8.3 Simple differentiation of Lung symptoms

Excess (Shi)	Deficiency (Xu)
Pain in upper back, chest, shoulder	Pain and coldness in upper back and shoulder
Head cold with a stuffy nose	Shortness of breath
Wheezing respiration, hoarse voice	Pallor, flushed cheeks
Heaviness in the chest	Loose bowel movements
Frequent urination, small amount	Chills
Cough	Sensitive to cold
Nasal discharge	Wet, runny nose

Tongue: thin white coating.

Pulse: floating, light.

Treatment

Expel the Cold and Wind, improve Lung function:

GB 20 Jianjing	expels Wind
UB 10 Tianzhu	dispels Wind
LI 4 Hegu	tonifies the Wei Qi
UB 13 Feishu	Back Shu point for the Lung
UB 12 Fengmen	use with UB 13 for Lung and Qi
Lu 7 Lieque	circulates Lung Qi, disperses Wind
St 36 Zusanli	tonifies generally.

Explanation

This is an external invasion of Wind or Cold, or both. The Cold constricts the tiny vessels and obstructs the free flow of Wei Qi. Thus the Lung becomes congested and blocked. Lung Qi flows upwards, causing coughs and sneezing and producing excess fluid in the Lung. The fever is due to the accumulation of Wei Qi close to the surface.

Invasion of Lungs by Wind Heat

Western diagnoses: common cold, acute or chronic bronchitis, pneumonia, pulmonary inflammation.

Symptoms: fever, chills, swelling and soreness of the throat, hoarse cough, thick yellowish phlegm, asthma, headache, possible nose-bleed, thirst, sweating, constipation, dark scanty urine.

Tongue: red with thin yellow coat.

Pulse: fast.

Treatment

Expel the Wind, disperse the Heat:

Du 14 Dazhui	disperses excess Heat
SJ 5 Weiguan	disperses excess Heat
GB 20 Fengchi	expels Wind
UB 10 Tianzhu	expels Wind
LI 4 Hegu	expels Wind and Heat
Lu 5 Chize	sedation point
LI 11 Quchi	used with LI 4 for stronger effect
Pe 6 Neiguan	regulates Qi
Lu 11 Shaoshang	bleed to relieve Heat.

While the common cold may frequently be encountered in patients, it is probably not the problem that brought them to seek treatment. Family, friends and colleagues are more likely to derive general benefit from the treatments described above. However, therapists working in specialist clinics with patients who are frail or elderly, or those who can ill afford another chest infection, may find the points useful. Certainly, patients who have an underlying chest problem will benefit from this.

Explanation

The Wind causes congestion in the Lung and thus reverses Qi flow with coughing and sneezing. The Heat produces the fever and the thicker yellowish phlegm.

Phlegm Damp obstructs the Lungs

Western diagnoses: chronic bronchitis, bronchial asthma, bronchiectasis.

Symptoms: shortness of breath, cough, asthma with copious phlegm, wheezing, rattling sounds in the throat or chest. Sometimes there is tenderness in the side and a full sensation in the chest. The breathing discomfort increases when the patient lies down. The full sensation within the chest may indicate involvement of the Heart.

Tongue: thick, white, greasy coating (Cold); thick, yellow, greasy coating (Heat).

Pulse: slippery.

Treatment

Improve Lung and Spleen function. Disperse Excess:

St 40 Fenglong	transforms Phlegm
St 36 Zusanli	regulates Spleen and Stomach
UB 20 Pishu	Back Shu point for the Spleen
UB 13 Feishu	Back Shu point for the Lung
UB 12 Fengmen	use with UB 13 for Lung and Qi
LI 11 Quchi	eliminates excess Heat if necessary.

Explanation

Caused originally by Heat, the Phlegm obstructs the Lung Qi, thus producing poor Lung function, stagnation and further Heat. (Anecdotal evidence suggests that prolonged acupressure (15–20 minutes) to the infrascapular fossa may relieve asthmatic symptoms.)

Deficient Lung Yin

Western diagnoses: pulmonary tuberculosis, chronic pharyngitis, chronic bronchitis, bronchiectasis.

Symptoms: dry unproductive cough, occasional blood in sputum, dry mouth, flushed cheeks, night sweats, low voice, afternoon fever. Poor general health, thin appearance. Five palm sweating (sweating on soles and palms and also chest).

Tongue: slightly red with dry coating.

Pulse: thin and rapid.

Treatment

Tonify Lungs and Kidney Yin:

Lu 5 Chize	use for dry cough
Lu 7 Lieque	affects Lung Qi, also treats cough
UB 17 Geshu	Back Shu point for the diaphragm
UB 13 Feishu	Back Shu point for the Lungs
Kid 3 Taixi	Kidney source point
Kid 7 Fuliu	tonifies Kidney
Sp 6 Sanyinjiao	tonifies Yin energies
Pe 6 Neiguan	regulates Qi.

Explanation

This syndrome may occur as a result of a poor constitution, ageing or chronic disease. Long-term Heat in the Lungs may have consumed Yin. The link with Kidney deficiency is very marked and the condition may arise from original Kidney problems.

Deficient Lung Qi

Western diagnoses: emphysema, chronic bronchitis, allergies affecting the lungs, pulmonary tuberculosis.

Symptoms: affects the voice, low voice, no desire to talk, weak respiration, weak cough, shortness of breath, spontaneous sweating, weakness and general lassitude, low resistance to cold.

Tongue: pale, thin white coating.

Pulse: weak.

Treatment

Tonify Lung and Spleen Qi:

Lu 7 Lieque	used for throat infection and cough (could be used with LI 4 Hegu in allergic asthma)
LI 4 Hegu	used to strengthen Wei Qi
St 36 Zusanli	regulates Stomach and Spleen Qi
UB 13 Feishu	Back Shu point for the Lungs
UB 20 Pishu	Back Shu point for the Spleen
Ren 17 Shanzhong	regulates Qi in the upper Jiao
Liv 13 Zhangmen	Front Mu point for the Spleen.

Explanation

A combination of both Lung Yin and Qi deficiency is often seen in clinical practice. Recurrent coughing tends to weaken the Spleen as well.

Patterns of Large Intestine disharmony

Functions of the Large Intestine:

- governs transportation and transformation of turbid waste
- absorbs fluid

- Large Intestine Qi descends
- connected functionally to the Lung; influence on Wei Qi, facial and sinus problems.

Symptoms of Large Intestine disharmony can be differentiated as in Box 8.4.

Syndromes
Insufficient fluid in the Large Intestine

Western diagnosis: constipation.

Symptoms: constipation, difficulties defaecating, dry mouth and throat.

Tongue: red, dry.

Pulse: thin.

Treatment
Tonify both Qi and Yin of the Large Intestine:

Ren 6 Qihai	tonifies lower Yin
Sp 6 Sanyinjiao	tonifies Yin generally
St 36 Zusanli	tonifies Qi
LI 4 Hegu	regulates Qi of the Large Intestine
UB 25 Dachangshu	Back Shu point of the Large Intestine
St 25 Tianshu	Mu point of the Large Intestine.

Explanation
The Large Intestine loses nourishment, resulting in abdominal distension and constipation. This often occurs as a result of Heat in the Lung.

Stagnation of Blood and Heat in the Large Intestine

Western diagnosis: corresponds to an intestinal abscess or appendicitis.

Symptoms: a severe fixed pain in the lower abdomen that increases with pressure, accompanied by either constipation or mild diarrhoea. There may be fever or vomiting.

NB: It is not advisable to treat this syndrome with acupuncture. The opinion of a medical specialist should be sought. Emergency surgery may be necessary.

Damp Heat in the Large Intestine

Western diagnoses: acute colitis, acute dysentery.

Symptoms: abdominal pain, urgency in defaecation, blood or pus in the stool, fever.

Box 8.4 Simple differentiation of Large Intestine symptoms

Excess (Shi)	Deficiency (Xu)
Warmth	Cold
Swelling along the course of the channel	Shivering
Distended abdomen	Bowel noises
Dizziness	Unable to get warm
Constipation	Diarrhoea
Strong urine	

Tongue: red with greasy yellow coating.

Pulse: slippery and rapid.

Treatment
Clear Heat and Damp:

St 36 Zusanli	reduces Heat and resolves Damp
GB 34 Yanglingquan	clears Damp and Heat
St 25 Tianshu	clears Heat from the Large Intestine
St 44 Neiting	pulls Heat down
LI 4 Hegu	clears Heat from the system
LI 11 Quchi	He Sea point, clears Heat
St 37 Shangjuxu	(sometimes used, lower He Sea point of Large Intestine).

Explanation
This syndrome is often due to overeating sweet, fatty or spicy foods. It results from an accumulation of Damp in the body. This transforms quickly into Heat after consumption of further very hot peppery foods or excess alcohol.

Deficient Qi in the Large Intestine

Western diagnoses: often compared to viral infection or possibly a parasitic invasion.

Symptoms: chronic diarrhoea, moderate, persistent abdominal discomfort made better by pressure, tired, cold limbs, constipation, bowel noises. Linked with Spleen deficiencies.

Tongue: pale with white coating.

Pulse: weak.

Treatment
Increase Qi in the Large Intestine:

LI 4 Hegu	tonifies Qi
St 25 Tianshu	Front Mu point for Large Intestine
UB 25 Dachangshu	Back Shu point, Large Intestine
Ren 12 Zhongwan	tonifies the middle Jiao
Liv 13 Zhangmen	Front Mu point for the Spleen.

Explanation
The separation of clear and turbid substances in the Large Intestine does not happen efficiently. This is most often caused by Damp disturbing the functions of the Large Intestine.

Cold Damp in the Large Intestine

Western diagnoses: chronic diarrhoea or chronic indigestion.

Symptoms: abdominal pain, watery diarrhoea, bowel noises, cold feet and hands, clear copious urine, clouded spirit, general feeling of malaise.

Tongue: moist with pale white coating.

Pulse: deep and slow.

Treatment
The aim is to warm and tonify the lower Jiao:

Ren 12 Zhongwan	Front Mu point of the Stomach
Ren 4 Guanyuan	tonifies the lower Jiao
St 25 Tianshu	Large Intestine Front Mu point
St 36 Zusanli	tonifies the Stomach and Spleen
UB 23 Shenshu	Back Shu point for the Kidney.

Moxa could be applied at all these points.

Explanation
This is a chronic effect of Damp obstructing the flow of Qi. If the Damp moves upwards, this may affect the spirit, producing a feeling of cotton wool or fog in the head.

Patterns of Stomach disharmony

Functions of the Stomach:

- governs nourishment
- controls digestion
- controls downward movement of Qi
- susceptible to dryness
- source of Post-Heaven Qi together with Spleen.

Symptoms of Stomach disharmony can be differentiated as shown in Box 8.5.

Syndromes
Stagnation of Stomach Qi

Western diagnoses: gallstones, anorexia.

Symptoms: distended and painful epigastric area, sour taste in the mouth, belching, nausea and vomiting, anorexia.

Tongue: thick, greasy, yellowish coating.

Pulses: wiry.

Box 8.5 Simple differentiation of Stomach symptoms

Excess (Shi)	Deficiency (Xu)
Hot abdominal area	Cold in the abdominal area
Overactive digestive system	Abdomen swollen and full
Hunger and thirst	Gastritis
Dark yellow urine	Loss of appetite
Halitosis	Diarrhoea
Swollen gums	Nausea
Dry red lips	Shivering
Leg cramps	Weakness in legs

Treatment

Tonify the Stomach, treat the stagnation:

St 36 Zusanli	tonifies Stomach and Spleen
Ren 12 Zhongwan	Front Mu point for the Stomach
Ren 10 Xiawan	clears stagnation in the middle Jiao
Pe 6 Neiguan	clears middle Jiao
St 44 Neiting	clears excess Heat, pulls down Qi
Liv 3 Taichong	moves stagnation
Liv 14 Qimen	moves stagnation
UB 20 Pishu	Back Shu point for the Spleen
UB 21 Weishu	Back Shu point for the Stomach.

Moxa could be used with these points.

Explanation

This syndrome is often caused by Damp Heat affecting the Spleen, so care should be taken when applying moxa; more heat may be damaging.

Western diagnoses: gastric ulcer, virus infection.

Symptoms: pain in the epigastrium, improved by warmth and by pressure and eating; diarrhoea.

Tongue: pale, moist white coating.

Pulse: deep, moderate or weak.

Treatment

Tonify and warm the middle Jiao:

Ren 6 Qihai	tonifies Yang
Ren 12 Zhongwan	Front Mu point for the Stomach
St 36 Zusanli	tonifies Stomach and Spleen
UB 21 Weishu	Back Shu point for the Stomach
UB 20 Pishu	Back Shu point for the Spleen
Liv 13 Zhangmen	Front Mu point for the Spleen.

Explanation

Closely linked with a diet containing too much raw and cold food. Also affects the Spleen.

Western diagnoses: ulcers, gastritis, diabetes, hyperthyroidism.

Symptoms: dryness of the mouth, constipation, excessive thirst and appetite, halitosis, swollen and painful gums, burning sensation in the epigastrium, preference for cold drinks, bleeding gums.

Tongue: red with thick yellow coating; may be ulcerated.

Pulse: rapid and full.

Stomach invaded by Cold (Spleen Yang Xu)

Stomach Fire blazing

Treatment
Clear Stomach Fire, remove Excess:

St 44 Neiting	clears Stomach Heat
St 45 Lidui	disperses Stomach Heat and Excess
UB 21 Weishu	Back Shu point of the Stomach.

Explanation
This syndrome is due to overeating greasy, fried, spicy foods and drinking too much alcohol. These produce an accumulation of Heat in the Stomach and intestines. This tends to travel upwards, affecting the head and upper body.

Stomach Yin Xu

Western diagnosis: anorexia.

Symptoms: hunger but inability to eat or poor appetite, dry mouth and lips, dry vomit, belching, constipation.

Tongue: red, peeling, no coating.

Pulse: fine and rapid.

Treatment
Tonify Stomach Yin:

St 44 Neiting	Water point
Ren 12 Zhongwan	Front Mu point for the Stomach
Pe 6 Neiguan	tonifies Stomach Yin
St 25 Tianshu	clears intestines, relieves constipation.

Explanation
This is a pattern often seen in elderly patients where Stomach Yin has been consumed by poor dietary habits over a long period.

Stomach Blood stasis

Western diagnosis: gastric ulcer.

Symptoms: stabbing pain in the epigastrium, abdominal distension and pain made worse by pressure, dark stools, blood in the stools.

Tongue: dark red, some dots, thin yellow coating.

Pulse: wiry and choppy.

Treatment
Clear stagnation:

Sp 6 Sanyinjiao	clears obstruction
Sp 10 Xuehai	Sea of Blood
LI 11 Quchi	harmonizes Blood
UB 17 Geshu	master point for Blood.

Explanation

This syndrome is caused primarily by a long-term stagnation of Qi and Blood in the Stomach. There is often severe pain. Medical help should be sought for this type of patient.

Patterns of Spleen disharmony

Functions of the Spleen:

- governs transportation and transformation of food
- transforms food into Blood
- controls Blood, keeps it in the blood vessels
- controls bulk of muscles and flesh
- maintains the position of internal organs
- includes the functions of the pancreas
- controls taste, connected with saliva
- opens to the mouth and lips
- controls upward movement of Qi
- regulates Water circulation.

The Spleen is particularly liable to the effects of excessive thinking, brooding or obsessing over a problem. Long-term studying or attempting to memorize material is also damaging. This type of activity tends to weaken the Spleen Qi.

The Spleen is also susceptible to the effects of 'comfort eating' when large quantities of sweet, highly processed foods are eaten. This, of course, is quite likely to be happening during long periods of intensive study.

As for all syndromes, the problem may be one of Excess or Deficiency, and the symptoms for the Spleen can be identified as in Box 8.6.

Syndromes
Deficient Spleen Qi

Western diagnoses: chronic dysentery, gastric or duodenal ulcers, anaemia, hepatitis, nervous dyspepsia.

Symptoms: abdominal pain and distension relieved by pressure, poor appetite, lassitude, anaemia, blood in the stools, prolapse of the rectum or uterus, uterine bleeding, chronic haemorrhage, anorexia; sometimes patients describe a bearing down or sagging sensation in the abdomen; chronic catarrh.

Box 8.6 Simple differentiation of Spleen symptoms

Excess (Shi)	Deficiency (Xu)
Abdominal pain	Tight, distended abdomen
Irregular appetite	Craving for sweet food
Stickiness in the mouth	Flatulence
Red lips	Pale lips
Constipation	Nausea
Congested chest	Mild oedema
Fatigue	Failing memory
	Heavy feeling in legs
	Chronic diarrhoea

Tongue: pale, thin white coating.

Pulse: empty.

Treatment
Tonify Spleen Qi:

Sp 3 Taibai	Source point for the Spleen
Sp 2 Dadu	tonification point
UB 20 Pishu	Back Shu point for the Spleen
UB 21 Weishu	Back Shu point for the Stomach
St 36 Zusanli	regulates Stomach and Spleen Qi
Liv 13 Zhangmen	Front Mu point for the Spleen
Ren 12 Zhongwan	strengthens and regulates Qi.

Moxa can be used on all points.

Explanation
This set of symptoms may be due to all the dietary sins that normally affect the Spleen, but Spleen Qi Xu is a common diagnostic finding in Western patients and is a frequent complication of other syndromes. As this syndrome can occur together with other common syndromes, such as Liver invading the Spleen, Spleen and Kidney Qi Xu, Stomach Heat and Qi Xu and Spleen Blood Xu, it is rarely seen in isolation.

Deficient Spleen Yang

Western diagnoses: gastric or duodenal ulcers, gastritis, enteritis, hepatitis, nephritis, dysentery.

Symptoms: cold limbs, abdominal pain and distension, relieved by heat or pressure. There is often undigested food in the loose stools, diarrhoea, anaemia, poor appetite. Difficulty with urination, leucorrhoea, oedema.

Tongue: swollen, moist and pale.

Pulse: slow, weak.

Treatment
Tonify the Spleen, particularly the Yang energy:

Sp 3 Taibai	Source point for the Spleen
Sp 2 Dadu	tonification point
UB 20 Pishu	Back Shu point for the Spleen
St 36 Zusanli	regulates Stomach and Spleen Qi
Liv 13 Zhangmen	Front Mu point for the Spleen
Ren 4 Guanyuan	tonification of Yang.

Moxa should be used.

Explanation
This could be caused by general Spleen Qi deficiency consuming the Yin.

Spleen Qi sinking

Western diagnoses: uterine or rectal prolapse.

Symptoms: abdominal distension and pain, poor appetite, prolapse of the uterus or rectum, chronic diarrhoea, urinary incontinence.

Tongue: enlarged, pale.

Pulse: soggy.

Treatment
Raise the Qi and tonify Spleen:

Du 20 Baihui	to raise Qi
Liv 13 Zhangmen	Front Mu point for the Spleen
Ren 12 Zhongwan	to strengthen and regulate Qi
UB 20 Pishu	Back Shu point for the Spleen.

Note: Some authorities suggest that the use of points on the lower limbs is counterproductive.
Moxa can be used.

Explanation
The Spleen Qi may not be able to restrain or hold in place the abdominal contents. This could be due to prolonged standing or excessive fatigue during the birth process.

Spleen unable to govern the Blood

Western diagnoses: haemorrhoids, bleeding disorders.

Symptoms: arises from Spleen Qi Xu. Blood in the stools, excessive menstrual flow, uterine bleeding, subcutaneous haemorrhages, petechiae or blood spots under the skin.

Tongue: pale.

Pulse: fine.

Treatment
Tonify Spleen, tonify Blood:

UB 20 Pishu	Back Shu point of the Spleen
St 36 Zusanli	regulates Stomach and Spleen
Sp 6 Sanyinjiao	tonifies Yin (Blood) and Spleen
Sp 10 Xuehai	Sea of Blood, nourishes Qi, clears Heat
UB 17 Geshu	regulates and tonifies Blood
UB 43 Gaohuangshu	point used for anaemia.

Explanation
The Spleen Qi does not have sufficient strength to hold the Blood within the walls of the vessels. This may sometimes be seen in obese patients with clear symptoms of Phlegm or Damp.

External Damp invades the Spleen

Western diagnoses: viral or bacterial infection.

Symptoms: acute onset, low fever, loss of appetite, loss of taste, nausea. There is a sensation of fullness or heaviness in either the chest or the head. Watery stools.

Treatment
Resolve the Dampness and tonify the Spleen:

St 40 Fenglong	transforms dampness
St 36 Zusanli	regulates Stomach and Spleen Qi
Ren 12 Zhongwan	Front Mu point for the Stomach
UB 20 Pishu	Back Shu point for the Spleen
LI 4 Hegu	tonifies Qi, treats muzzy head
Liv 13 Zhangmen	Front Mu point for the Spleen.

Explanation
External Damp can invade the Spleen, causing damage. The inability of the Spleen to transport and transform liquids results in further accumulation of Dampness. This may also have its origin in a poor constitution. Take care that this does not develop into chronic fatigue syndrome.

Damp Heat in the Spleen

Western diagnoses: acute hepatic infection, cholecystitis, cirrhosis of the liver, jaundice, acute gastritis.

Symptoms: jaundice, loss of appetite, fullness and discomfort in the epigastrium and abdomen, nausea and vomiting, loose stools, sensation of extra weight.

Tongue: red body with greasy yellow coating.

Pulse: rapid and slippery.

Treatment
Disperse Heat, resolve Damp and tonify Spleen:

GB 34 Yanglingquan	cools Damp Heat generally
Sp 9 Yinlingquan	transforms Damp
St 40 Fenglong	clears Damp
St 36 Zusanli	regulates Stomach and Spleen Qi
UB 20 Pishu	Back Shu point for the Spleen
Liv 13 Zhangmen	Front Mu point for the Spleen.

Explanation
Damp Heat may invade externally and lodge in the Spleen and Stomach. There it hinders digestion and blocks the normal secretion of bile. The bile is forced out of the Gall Bladder and turns the skin yellow.

Turbid mucus invades the head

Western diagnoses: hypertension, Menière's disease.

Symptoms: extreme dizziness and nausea, 'cotton wool' in the head, excessive mucus and sinus blockage, general symptoms of Damp.

Tongue: very cheesy-looking white or yellow coating.

Pulse: slippery or wiry.

Treatment
Resolve Phlegm, tonify Spleen:

St 40 Fenglong	transforms Damp
Sp 2 Dadu	tonifies Spleen
Sp 3 Taibai	resolves Phlegm
St 36 Zusanli	regulates Spleen and Stomach Qi
GB 20 Fengchi	disperses Wind, clears head
Du 20 Baihui	clears dizziness.

Explanation
This syndrome is sometimes secondary to Spleen Qi Xu. The Dampness accumulates in the Lungs and upper Jiao, where it manifests as Phlegm.

Liver invading the Spleen

Western diagnoses: long-term emotional problems, overwork and exhaustion.
   This is usually listed under Liver syndromes, but is included here because it is relatively common in Western society and may manifest with a majority of Spleen symptoms. Essentially due to Liver stagnation.

Symptoms: irritability, abdominal distension and slight pain; loose stools more common than constipation but the picture may be mixed, flatulence, tiredness.

Tongue: pale.

Pulse: weak on the right and wiry on the left.

Treatment
Tonify the Spleen and harmonize the Liver:

Liv 14 Qimen	promotes smooth flow of Liver Qi
Liv 13 Zhangmen	harmonizes Liver and Spleen
GB 34 Yanglingquan	promotes smooth flow of Liver Qi
Liv 3 Taichong	soothes and cools Liver
Sp 6 Sanyinjiao	tonifies Spleen, regulates Liver
St 36 Zusanli	tonifies Spleen
Ren 6 Qihai	calms abdominal pain.

Explanation
Linked to Spleen Qi Xu.

Patterns of Heart disharmony

Functions of the Heart:

- ☯ governs the circulation of Blood (blood vessels and pulse)
- ☯ stores the mind and spirit (Shen)
- ☯ governs speech
- ☯ opens to the tongue
- ☯ manifests in the face.

The Heart is usually unaffected by external climatic Pathogens, although external Heat may be damaging. The Pericardium stands as protection for the Heart and is likely to be affected first. However, the Heart is very susceptible to the emotions – the internal Pathogens. Imbalances may manifest as speech problems. Symptoms of Heart disharmony can be differentiated as in Box 8.7.

Syndromes
Deficient Heart Blood

Western diagnoses: tachycardia, arrhythmia, anaemia, hypertension, hyperthyroidism, depressive neurosis, extreme malnutrition.

Symptoms: palpitations, forgetfulness, dream-disturbed sleep, difficulty getting to sleep, easily startled, general inability to concentrate, feeling of unease, lethargy, dizziness, dull pale 'spiritless' face.

Tongue: pale.

Pulse: choppy.

Treatment
Tonify Heart Yin and Blood. Support Kidney Yin:

Ht 7 Shenmen	Source point for the Heart
Sp 6 Sanyinjiao	tonifies Yin Qi generally
Sp 10 Xuehai	harmonizes and cools Blood
Sp 9 Yinlingquan	fluid problems
UB 17 Geshu	Back Shu point for Blood
UB 43 Gaohuangshu	poor memory
Ren 14 Juque	Front Mu point for the Heart
Ren 6 Qihai	Source point for Yin energy.

Box 8.7 Simple differentiation of Heart symptoms

Excess (Shi)	Deficiency (Xu)
Anxiety	Inability to speak
Vivid, scary dreams	Restless sleep
Nervousness	Loss of memory
Oppressive pressure in the chest	Palpitations
Hot sweats	Cold sweats
Tongue feels numb and heavy	Cold feeling in the chest
Dark urine	Nocturnal emission

Heart Yin Xu

Explanation

This syndrome is usually caused by a poor constitution, ageing, debilitating chronic disease or blood loss.

Western diagnoses: tachycardia, arrhythmia, anaemia, hypertension, hyperthyroidism, depressive neurosis, overexhaustion, 'running on empty'.

Symptoms: agitated manner, palpitations, forgetfulness, insomnia, dream-disturbed sleep, wakes easily, restlessness, patient often very uncomfortable lying flat, night sweats, sweaty chest, palms and soles (five palm sweat), thirst, afternoon fever, flushed cheeks.

Tongue: red, peeled.

Pulse: floating empty.

Treatment

Tonify Heart Yin and Kidney Yin:

Pe 6 Neiguan	calms the Heart, tonifies Heart Yin
Ren 14 Juque	Front Mu point for the Heart
Ht 3 Shaohai	calms the spirit
Kid 3 Taixi	Kidney Source point, tonifies Yin
Kid 7 Fuliu	tonifies Kidney
GB 25 Jingmen	Front Mu point for Kidney.

Explanation

Often emotional in origin. Because of damage by the internal emotions, Heart Blood and Yin may be reduced. This means that the Heart Shen or spirit is not nourished and becomes restless.

Heart Qi Xu

Western diagnoses: cardiac insufficiency, general heart disease, arrhythmia, neurosis.

Symptoms: lethargy, palpitations, shortness of breath aggravated by exertion, spontaneous sweating, feeling of pressure in the chest.

Tongue: pale, enlarged.

Pulse: thin, weak, interrupted.

Treatment

Tonify Heart Qi:

UB 15 Xinshu	Back Shu point for the Heart
Ren 14 Juque	Front Mu point for the Heart
Ht 7 Shenmen	calms Heart
Ht 9 Shaochong	tonifies Heart and Blood
LI 4 Hegu	controls pain, tonifies Wei Qi
Lu 7 Lieque	use with Ren 17 for feeling of pressure
St 36 Zusanli	regulates Qi and Blood.

Explanation

This syndrome may have many causes, including poor constitution, over-work, stress, worry, chronic disease, or just old age.

Heart Yang Xu

Western diagnoses: angina pectoris, cardiac insufficiency, coronary arterio-sclerosis, general bodily weakness, nervous disorders.

Symptoms: lethargy, shortness of breath made worse by exertion, profuse sweating, cold limbs, aversion to cold, blueness of the lips, mental confusion.

Tongue: pale, moist.

Pulse: slow, thin, weak.

Treatment

Tonify Heart and Kidney Yang:

UB 15 Xinshu	Back Shu point for the Heart
Ht 7 Shenmen	Heart Source point, calms the Heart
Du 4 Mingmen	tonifies Kidney Yang
Kid 3 Taixi	tonifies Kidney Yin and Kidney Yang.

Explanation

Excess effort exhausts the Heart Qi and, eventually, Heart Yang.

Stagnant Heart Blood

Western diagnoses: angina pectoris, coronary artery disease, pericarditis.

Symptoms: stabbing pain in the precordial or substernal region, pain sometimes in the left shoulder or forearm, lassitude, shortness of breath, blueness of lips and nails.

Tongue: purple.

Pulse: deep, hesitant, irregular rhythm.

Treatment

Move Blood stagnation:

Ht 7 Shenmen	calms the spirit, moves stagnation
Pe 6 Neiguan	calms the spirit, regulates Qi
UB 17 Geshu	influential point for circulation
UB 15 Xinshu	Back Shu point for the Heart
Ren 17 Shanzhong	treats stagnation and Phlegm
LI 11 Quchi	harmonizes Blood and Ying Qi.

Explanation

Often due to long-lasting Liver Qi stagnation, which, itself, is a result of anger or stress or of debility in chronic disease. As the Liver can no longer ensure the smooth flow of Qi through the Heart, the condition can only get worse.

Phlegm misting the orifices of the Heart

Western diagnoses: mental illness, epilepsy.

Symptoms: coma, drooling, muttering to oneself, sudden blackouts, rattling sound in the throat, stupor, inability to talk, vomiting.

Tongue: greasy white coating.

Pulse: slow, slippery.

Treatment
Resolve Phlegm. Tonify Heart Qi and Spleen Qi:

UB 15 Xinshu	Back Shu point for the Heart
UB 44 Shentang	calms Heart and spirit
UB 43 Gaohuang	treats weakness
Ht 7 Shenmen	calms the spirit
Ht 9 Shaochong	bled to clear Heart and open orifices
Sp 2 Dadu	tonification point, resolves Phlegm
St 36 Zusanli	regulates Spleen and Stomach
St 40 Fenglong	transforms Phlegm and Damp.

Explanation
Usually caused by Damp within the Spleen, in addition to Liver stagnation. This results in an upward movement of Damp and Phlegm. The Spleen problems may be caused by poor or unsuitable nutrition, whereas the Liver is damaged by the pathogenic emotions of anger and frustration. A common manifestation in frustrated career overachievers.

Flaring up of Heart Fire

Western diagnoses: neurosis, bladder infection.

Symptoms: ulceration, pain and swelling of the mouth and tongue, bitter taste in the mouth, thirst, insomnia and restlessness, strong, dark yellow urine with a burning pain on urination.

Tongue: red with ulceration at the tip.

Pulse: full and rapid.

Treatment
Cool Fire, tonify Heart and Kidney Yin:

Ht 7 Shenmen	calms the spirit
Ht 9 Shaochong	bled to clear Heat
Pe 6 Neiguan	calms the Heart, regulates Qi
Pe 8 Laogong	cools Heart and disperses Heat
LI 4 Hegu	controls pain, tonifies Wei Qi
Kid 3 Taixi	tonifies Kidney Yin and Kidney Yang
Kid 7 Fuliu	tonifies Kidney
Sp 6 Sanyinjiao	general Yin tonification
GB 14 Yangbai	disperses Wind as a result of Fire.

Explanation
Very similar causes to the preceding syndrome.

Patterns of Small Intestine disharmony

Functions of the Small Intestine:

☯ responsible for digestion and nutrient absorption
☯ affects quality of Blood
☯ linked with the Heart
☯ separates Body fluids, connection with Bladder:
—clear becomes Body fluid
—turbid becomes waste.

The Small Intestine syndromes are usually linked with problems involving either the Spleen or the Yang energy of the Kidney. This means that the type or temperature of food eaten can affect the Small Intestine. Symptom differentiation as Excess or Deficiency is shown in Box 8.8.

Syndromes
Heart Fire spreads to the Small Intestine

Western diagnosis: urinary tract infection.

Symptoms: burning pain in the urethra, hot dark-yellow urine, frequent urination, haematuria, lower abdomen feels sore, sore throat, sores in the mouth, flushed face, insomnia, irritability.

Tongue: red with yellow coating.

Pulse: rapid and slippery.

Treatment
Drain Heat of Small Intestine and Stomach:

SI 8 Xiaohai	sedation point for Small Intestine
St 44 Neiting	drains Heat from the upper body
Sp 6 Sanyinjiao	expels Damp Heat from the lower Jiao
Sp 9 Yinlingquan	expels Damp Heat from the lower Jiao
SI 2 Qiangu	Water point.

Explanation
It is often difficult to decide which way round this originates. The original cause is usually extreme emotional damage, transferred from the Heart but affecting both organs with excess Heat. *Medical help will be necessary as a quick resolution is important.*

Box 8.8 Simple differentiation of Small Intestine symptoms

Excess (Shi)	Deficiency (Xu)
Congestion in the abdomen	Pain bearing down in the abdomen
Pain in temples	Swelling, formation of nodules
Pain at the side of the neck	Tinnitus
Painful joints in the upper limb	One-sided headache
Flaccidity of muscles	Ear pain
Reddish urine	

Stagnant Qi in the Small Intestine

Western diagnosis: hernia.

NB: This syndrome is sometimes referred to as Cold stagnation of the Liver meridian.

Symptoms: pain in the hypogastrium and groin area, low back pain, hernia.

Tongue: white coating.

Pulse: deep and wiry or tight.

Treatment
Move the stagnation, disperse Cold:

Ren 4 Guanyuan	disperses Cold from the lower Jiao
Ren 6 Qihai	benefits Qi and Yang
Liv 3 Taichong	moves the Qi in the channel
Liv 5 Ligou	clears the channel
Liv 8 Ququan	Water point, tonifies the Liver
Sp 6 Sanyinjiao	benefits the Liver.

Explanation
Very closely linked to Liver Qi stagnation.

Obstruction of Qi in the Small Intestine

Western diagnoses: bowel obstruction, food poisoning.

Symptoms: constipation, intense pain in the abdomen relieved by flatulence and increased by pressure, vomiting.

Tongue: yellow, greasy coating.

Pulse: wiry and full.

Treatment
Remove obstruction:

SI 3 Houxi	tonifies the Small Intestine
St 36 Zusanli	clears Heat
St 44 Neiting	clears Heat
St 25 Tianshu	used for stagnation in the bowels
St 39 Tiaokou	lower He Sea point of Small Intestine
Ren 12 Zhongwan	tonifies middle Jiao
Ren 6 Qihai	controls Qi.

NB: This condition may be serious enough to require surgery, so great care should be taken when considering acupuncture treatment. *It would be advisable to seek a medical opinion before proceeding.*

Small Intestine Deficient and Cold

Western diagnoses: gastric or duodenal ulcers, nervous dyspepsia, chronic dysentery.
Sometimes classified as Spleen Qi Xu.

Symptoms: general discomfort in the lower abdomen, borborygmi (rumbling in the gut), watery stools.

Tongue: pale with thin white coating.

Pulse: empty.

Treatment
Tonify Small Intestine and Spleen:

St 25 Tianshu	strengthens lower Jiao
St 28 Shuidao	clears the lower Jiao
St 39 Tiaokou	lower He Sea point of Small Intestine
St 36 Zusanli	tonifies the Spleen
UB 20 Pishu	Back Shu point for the Spleen.

Explanation
This may be caused by overeating raw or chilled foods, or a chronic disease process.

Patterns of Urinary Bladder disharmony

Functions of the Urinary Bladder:

- ☯ receives, stores and transforms fluids prior to excretion
- ☯ Urinary Bladder Qi should descend
- ☯ imbalance is said to be connected to long-standing jealousy or grudges.

There are only a few identifiable Urinary Bladder syndromes, most involving some form of Heat invasion. The Bladder is also affected by Fear, like the Kidneys. This is thought to be the possible cause of nocturnal enuresis in children. Symptoms can be differentiated as shown in Box 8.9.

Syndromes
Damp Heat pours down into the Bladder

Western diagnosis: urinary tract infection.

Symptoms: frequent, urgent, and painful urination; fever, thirst, dry mouth; low backache; cloudy urine.

Tongue: red, greasy yellow coating.

Pulse: rapid, wiry or slippery.

Box 8.9 Simple differentiation of Urinary Bladder symptoms

Excess (Shi)	Deficiency (Xu)
Headache	Nose bleeds
Olfactory problems	Frequent urination
Pain along the channel, particularly spine	Excessive urination
Congestion in the abdomen	Pain in the lower back
Insufficient urine	Nocturnal enuresis
Cloudy urine	

Treatment

Dispel Damp, clear Heat:

Liv 8 Ququan	dispels Damp Heat
St 40 Fenglong	dispels Damp
Sp 9 Yinlingquan	dispels Damp
Sp 6 Sanyinjiao	tonifies Yin
UB 28 Pangguangshu	Back Shu point for the Bladder
Ren 3 Zhongji	Front Mu point for the Bladder
UB 32 Ciliao	useful point for Bladder problems
UB 23 Shenshu	Back Shu point for the Kidneys.

Explanation

This pattern is due to invasion by exogenous Damp Heat. The Damp originally manifests in the Spleen and is aggravated by a heavy consumption of sugars. The Damp finds its way into the lower Jiao and the Bladder. It may also be associated with Liver stagnation.

Medical treatment is quicker and more effective than acupuncture for an acute Urinary Bladder infection.

Western diagnosis: kidney stones.

Symptoms: gritty feeling in urine, obstruction of urine, pain in groin or low back, blood in the urine.

Tongue: normal.

Pulse: rapid.

Treatment

Dispel Damp, clear Heat:

Liv 8 Ququan	dispels Damp Heat
St 40 Fenglong	dispels Damp
Sp 9 Yinlingquan	dispels Damp
Sp 6 Sanyinjiao	tonifies Yin
UB 28 Pangguangshu	Back Shu point for the Bladder
Ren 3 Zhongji	Front Mu point for the Bladder
UB 32 Ciliao	useful point for Bladder problems
UB 23 Shenshu	Back Shu point for the Kidneys
UB 65 Shugu	Bladder sedation point.

Explanation

As above. TCM texts describe ways of treating patients in order to expel kidney stones, but this is not recommended. *Medical help should be sought.*

Western diagnosis: urinary tract infection.

Symptoms: cloudy, offensive urine.

Tongue: red, greasy coating.

Pulse: soggy but rapid.

Damp Heat accumulates in the Bladder

Turbid Damp Heat obstructs the Bladder

Treatment
Dispel Damp, clear Heat:

Liv 8 Ququan	dispels Damp Heat
St 40 Fenglong	dispels Damp
Sp 9 Yinlingquan	dispels Damp
Sp 6 Sanyinjiao	tonifies Yin
UB 28 Pangguangshu	Back Shu point for the Bladder
Ren 3 Zhongji	Front Mu point for the Bladder
UB 32 Ciliao	useful point for Bladder problems
UB 23 Shenshu	Back Shu point for the Kidneys
UB 65 Shugu	Bladder sedation point.

Explanation
As with the two preceding syndromes, *medical help should be sought.* Acupuncture may help to prevent further problems.

Deficient Bladder Qi

Western diagnoses: bladder infection, kidney infection.

Symptoms: pale, abundant urination, incontinence, low backache, enuresis.

Tongue: pale, wet.

Pulse: slow, deep and weak.

Treatment
Tonify Bladder and Kidney Qi:

UB 28 Pangguangshu	Back Shu point for the Bladder
UB 23 Shenshu	Back Shu point for the Bladder
Ren 4 Guanyuan	strengthens Qi and Yang in the lower Jiao.

Explanation
This syndrome is very similar to Kidney Yang Xu and may be treated in the same way. Kidney energy is required to control the fluid within the Bladder.

Patterns of Kidney disharmony

Functions of the Kidney:

- responsible for reproduction, growth and development
- rules bones and marrow
- governs water metabolism
- foundation for Yin and Yang of all organs
- opens to the ears, responsible for hearing
- activates Spleen and Lung
- stores Jing.

The Kidney is an important organ and responsible for the basic constitution of the patient. The most common indication of a Kidney problem is the presence of low back pain as a symptom. Differentiation of symptoms as Excess or Deficiency is shown in Box 8.10.

As Kidney energy is so vitally important to all body processes it is considered quite wrong to deplete it in any way. The Kidney syndromes are all thought to be of Deficiency, and treatment is aimed at restoring the normal balance.

Further information on Kidney syndromes including 'Kidney Qi not firm' and 'Kidney fails to hold Qi', and the combined syndromes frequently found in the elderly, can be found in Chapter 12.

Syndromes
Kidney Jing Xu

Western diagnoses: impotence, frigidity, arthritis, prostate problems, asthma.

Symptoms: soreness and weakness in the lower back, weak knees, frequent urination, enuresis, incontinence, nocturnal emission, sexual dysfunction, infertility, shortness of breath, asthma, premature ageing and greying of hair, memory problems, poor teeth; there may be vertigo, tinnitus or deafness. If this occurs in children, there may be poor skeletal development and a weak constitution with mental dullness.

Tongue: pale (Yang Xu), slightly red (Yin Xu).

Pulse: thin.

Treatment
Tonify Kidney and Spleen:

Kid 3 Taixi	tonifies Kidney Yin and Yang
Kid 7 Fuliu	tonifies Kidney
UB 23 Shenshu	Back Shu point of the Kidney
UB 52 Zhishi	used in chronic Kidney problems
Du 3 Yaoyangguan	used for Cold and Damp in the Kidney.

Explanation
This can arise from a Lung problem. If there is a chronic cough and lung disease, the Kidney may fail to grasp the weakly descending Qi, thus not completing the Lung–Kidney Qi cycle. The patient having difficulty inhaling but no problem exhaling often identifies it.

Box 8.10 Simple differentiation of Kidney symptoms

Excess (Shi)	Deficiency (Xu)
No problems of Excess identified	Lumbago
False Heat symptoms common	Sciatica
	Lack of will
	Low sex drive
	Impotence
	Coldness in the lower limbs
	Premature senility, loss of hair
	Poor memory
	Mental dullness

Kidney Yang Xu

Western diagnoses: pulmonary heart disease, nephritis, chronic enteritis, often caused by long, chronic illness.

Symptoms: lassitude, apathy, low back pain, sensation of cold in the back and knees, chills, diarrhoea, poor appetite, oedema in the lower limbs, impotence, premature ejaculation, infertility in women.

Tongue: pale, swollen and moist.

Pulse: slow and weak.

Treatment
Tonify Kidney Yang:

Kid 3 Taixi	tonifies Kidney Yin and Yang
Kid 7 Fuliu	tonifies Kidney
UB 23 Shenshu	Back Shu point of the Kidney
UB 52 Zhishi	used in chronic Kidney problems
Ren 4 Guanyuan	nourishes Kidney
Ren 6 Qihai	used for increase of sexual energy
Du 4 Mingmen	builds up Yuan Qi
Du 3 Yaoyangguan	used for Cold and Damp in the Kidney
St 36 Zusanli	regulates Stomach and Spleen.

Moxa may be used.

Explanation
This deficiency could be caused by old age or general debility. It is also attributed to excessive sex and use of drugs. It is also often seen as part of the menopause.

Kidney Yin Xu

Western diagnoses: lumbago, hypertension, chronic ear problems, diabetes, chronic urogenital problems.

Symptoms: tinnitus, blurring of vision, dizziness, flushed cheeks, poor memory, hot palms and soles, night sweats, constipation, weakness of the legs, weak and sore back, nocturnal emission.

Tongue: red with little coating.

Pulse: thin and rapid.

Treatment
Tonify Kidney Yin:

Ren 6 Qihai	tonifies Kidney Qi
Ren 4 Guanyuan	preferred for men to tonify Kidney
Ren 3 Zhongji	used for women, affects uterus
Sp 6 Sanyinjiao	tonifies Yin Qi of Spleen Kidney and Liver
UB 23 Shenshu	Back Shu point of the Kidney
Kid 3 Taixi	tonifies Kidney Yin and Yang
Kid 7 Fuliu	tonifies Kidney.

Explanation
The causes of Kidney Yin deficiency are similar to those of the preceding syndromes, but in addition this syndrome may arise after heavy loss of blood, sometimes as the cycle becomes irregular at the onset of menopause.

Kidney Yin and Yang Xu

Symptoms: vertigo, dizziness, tinnitus, weak low back, cold limbs, alternating sensations of cold and heat; heat above, cold below.

Tongue: pale.

Pulse: deep, thready and weak.

Treatment
As for individual syndromes above.

Explanation
Simultaneous deficiency in Kidney Yin and Yang is not unusual as the two energies are very closely related. The practitioner needs to decide which to correct first, according to the symptom history.

Patterns of Pericardium disharmony

Functions of the Pericardium:

☯ protects the Heart
☯ circulates Kidney Yang Qi
☯ activates all the Yin channels.

For differentiation of Pericardium symptoms as Excess or Deficiency, see Box 8.11.

Syndromes

There are few frank Pericardium syndromes; instead, links with the Heart or the Kidneys should be investigated.

Heat invades the Pericardium

Western diagnoses: coma, nervous disorders, mental illness.

Symptoms: delirium, coma, convulsions, high fever, constipation, restlessness.

Tongue: deep red with dry tallow coating.

Pulse: wiry and rapid.

Box 8.11 Simple differentiation of Pericardium symptoms

Excess (Shi)	Deficiency (Xu)
Cardiac pain	Stiff neck
Light sleep	Loose stools
Frequent dreams	Low-grade fever
Heavy head	
Headache	
Stomach pain	
Impacted faeces	

Treatment
Clear the Heat:

St 36 Zusanli	clears Heat (pulls it down)
Pe 5 Jianshi	calms the spirit
Pe 6 Neiguan	calms the Heart, balances Yin and Yang
Ht 7 Shenmen	calms the Heart
Ren 14 Juque	clears excess Yang.

Phlegm obstructs the Pericardium

Western diagnoses: mental illness, nervous disorders.

Symptoms: impairment or loss of consciousness, diarrhoea, low-grade fever.

Tongue: red with white greasy coating or yellow greasy coating (Heat).

Pulse: slippery or soggy and rapid.

Treatment
Resolve Phlegm, clear the Pathogen causing the problem:

St 40 Fenglong	used for Damp throughout the body
St 36 Zusanli	transforms mucus, expels Heat
Pe 6 Neiguan	calms the spirit, tonifies upper Jiao Yin
UB 14 Jueyinshu	Back Shu point for Pericardium
UB 15 Xinshu	Back Shu point for Heart.

Patterns of Sanjiao disharmony

Functions of the Sanjiao:

- upper Jiao linked particularly with the functions of the Lung
- middle Jiao linked mainly with the Stomach
- lower Jiao linked with the functions of the Urinary Bladder, Kidneys and Intestines.

Sanjiao patterns are not usually described because the Sanjiao is not, strictly speaking, a single organ. As described in Chapter 3, the predominant function of the Sanjiao is the control of Water circulation throughout the body. This means that, for practical purposes, the syndromes affecting the major Zang Fu organs may occasionally be assisted by needling points on the Sanjiao meridian. This is applied most often when the circulation of Body fluids is affected.

Syndromes affecting the Spleen or Kidney will often manifest in symptoms localized in the various areas of the Sanjiao.

Patterns of Gall Bladder disharmony

Functions of the Gall Bladder:

- storage of bile
- closely linked to the functions of the Liver
- linked with courage and the ability to make decisions.

The Gall Bladder is very susceptible to the Pathogen Damp. It is sometimes affected when the function of the Spleen is impaired. Both organs can be damaged by the excessive consumption of rich and fatty foods. Symptoms of Gall Bladder disharmony are differentiated in Box 8.12.

The Gall Bladder is also affected by anger, like the Liver. The emotional Pathogens that affect the function of the Liver produce Heat, which will also unbalance the Gall Bladder.

Syndromes
Damp Heat in the Gall Bladder

Western diagnoses: cholecystitis, hepatitis.

Symptoms: hypochondriacal pain, feeling of distension in this area, jaundice, dark, scanty urine, fever, nausea, vomiting, thirst without desire to drink, bitter taste in the mouth.

Tongue: yellow, greasy coating.

Pulse: wiry, slippery.

Treatment
Clear Heat, dispel Damp:

GB 34 Yanglingquan	Gall Bladder He Sea point
GB 37 Guangming	cools the Liver
GB 39 Xuanzhong	cools the Gall Bladder
UB 18 Ganshu	Back Shu point for the Liver
UB 19 Danshu	Back Shu point for the Gall Bladder
Liv 3 Taichong	removes Heat from the Liver
St 36 Zusanli	reduces Heat and Damp.

Explanation
This syndrome also affects the Liver and is caused by invading Damp Heat or overeating hot, acrid, peppery, greasy foods, or drinking too much alcohol.

Gall Bladder Qi Xu

Western diagnoses: hypertension, eye problems.

Symptoms: vertigo, blurred vision, easily frightened, timidity, lack of courage, sighing.

Tongue: thin white coating.

Pulse: thin and wiry.

Box 8.12 Simple differentiation of Gall Bladder symptoms

Excess (Shi)	Deficiency (Xu)
Lateral headache	Vertigo
Muscular spasm	Weakness in the legs, difficulty standing
Tinnitus	Chills
Deafness	Insomnia
Limbs slightly cold	Indecisiveness
Heaviness in the head and stomach	Excessive sighing
Bitter taste in the mouth	Fearfulness

Treatment
Tonify the Gall Bladder:

GB 34 Yanglingquan	Gall Bladder He Sea point
GB 43 Xiaxi	used in deficiency conditions
UB 19 Danshu	Back Shu point for the Gall Bladder
GB 40 Qiuxu	Gall Bladder Source point
GB 24 Riyue	Front Mu point for the Gall Bladder.

Explanation
This syndrome is said by Maciocia (1989) to be a description of a personality type typified by timidity, lack of courage and a lack of initiative. It is usually caused by the effect of long-term stress on Liver Qi. Spleen Qi Xu, when present, will lead to excess Phlegm, which complicates matters. In addition, the Stomach may be affected by the blockage of Qi with resultant reverse flow.

Patterns of Liver disharmony

Functions of the Liver:

- stores Blood
- rules the smooth flow of Qi around the body
- governs muscles, tendons and ligaments
- responsible for secretion of bile
- important in menstrual flow
- influences emotional balance
- controls mental function of planning
- opens to the eyes
- condition seen in the nails.

Symptoms of Liver disharmony can be differentiated as shown in Box 8.13.

Syndromes
Stagnation of Liver Qi

Western diagnoses: mastitis, scrofula, menstrual problems, nervous disorders.

Symptoms: headache, pain in the hypochondrium and lower abdominal regions, swelling of the breast, belching, irrational anger, sighing, depression, sensation of a 'lump or plum-stone in the throat', menstrual pain or irregularity.

Tongue: reddish-purple.

Pulse: wiry.

Box 8.13 Simple differentiation of Liver symptoms

Excess (Shi)	Deficiency (Xu)
Excitability	Timidity
Insomnia	Vertigo
Compulsive energy	Pruritus
Red, watery eyes	Dry skin
Moodiness	Bad temper
Bitter taste in the mouth	Difficulty raising or lowering the head
Genital diseases	Depression
Excessive sex drive	Asthma

Treatment

Move Liver stagnation:

Liv 1 Dadun	Jing Well point, used for stagnation
Liv 3 Taichong	balances Liver and regulates the Blood
Ren 3 Zhongji	transformation of Qi
Liv 14 Qimen	Front Mu point for the Liver
UB 18 Ganshu	Back Shu point for the Liver
Liv 13 Zhangmen	Front Mu point for the Spleen
Ren 17 Shanzhong	controls Qi in the upper Jiao
Sp 6 Sanyinjiao	transforms Damp, benefits the Liver.

Explanation

Liver Qi stagnation is sometimes referred to as Liver depression. It is caused primarily by emotional stress, anger and frustration. The result is that the smooth flow of Qi is disrupted and tends to accumulate in parts of the body associated with the Liver.

Liver Fire rising

Western diagnoses: hypertension, migraine, acute conjunctivitis, otitis, labyrinthitis.

Symptoms: severe headache, dizziness, red face and eyes, sensation of pressure or distension in the head, bitter taste in the mouth, tinnitus, hearing difficulty, epistaxis, violent anger, insomnia, uterine bleeding, constipation, dark scanty urine.

Tongue: red edges, thin yellow coat.

Pulse: wiry and rapid.

Treatment

Disperse Fire, tonify Liver Yin:

GB 34 Yanglingquan	cools Damp Heat anywhere in the body
Liv 2 Xingjian	Fire point, disperses Fire in the Liver
Liv 3 Taichong	Liver Source point
Liv 14 Qimen	Front Mu point for the Liver
St 8 Touwei	intersection between Gall Bladder and Stomach meridians
Ren 4 Guanyuan	increases Yuan Qi.

Explanation

This syndrome is often due to emotional stress. It can be exacerbated by intense anger, described in TCM as apoplexy. The Heat present in the Liver flares up, affecting the parts of the head associated with the Liver.

Liver Yin Xu

Western diagnoses: hypertension, nervous disorders, chronic eye problems, menstrual problems.

Symptoms: depression, dizziness, afternoon fever, flushed cheeks, nervous tension, dry eyes, blurring of vision, warm palms and soles, headache, tinnitus, tremors in the muscles, fragile nails, disturbance of menstrual pattern, general irritability.

Tongue: red.

Pulse: thin, rapid.

Treatment
Tonify Liver and Kidney Yin:

Liv 2 Xingjian	Fire point, disperses Fire in the Liver
Liv 3 Taichong	Liver Source point
Sp 6 Sanyinjiao	tonifies Spleen, balances Liver and regulates Blood
Liv 13 Zhangmen	Front Mu point for the Spleen
Liv 8 Ququan	Water source point, tonifies Yin
Kid 3 Taixi	tonifies Kidney Yin and Yang
GB 25 Jingmen	Front Mu point for the Kidney
Kid 7 Fuliu	tonifies Kidney; Metal point.

Explanation
Yin becomes too weak to control Yang, resulting in symptoms of Heat in the upper part of the body and of Cold and Deficiency in the lower part. This is strongly associated with Kidney Yin Xu.

Liver Qi and Yang Xu

Western diagnoses: chronic fatigue syndrome, chronic hepatitis, cirrhosis of the liver, chronic gastritis, irregular bowel movements.

Symptoms: mood swings, poor digestion, problems in the eyes and tendons, muscle spasms, stifling sensation in the chest, bloating in the abdomen, constipation or loose stools, sadness, fear, difficulty making decisions, feeling of inner cold, severe heartburn, acid reflux.

Tongue: sticky white coating (if Cold predominates), red with yellow coating (if Heat predominates).

Pulse: wiry.

Treatment
Strengthen Liver Qi and tonify Kidney and Spleen:

Liv 3 Taichong	Liver Source point; balances Liver, moves Qi
UB 18 Ganshu	Back Shu point for the Liver
Kid 7 Fuliu	tonifies both Kidney and Liver
Sp 6 Sanyinjiao	tonifies Spleen, balances Liver and regulates Blood
GB 34 Yanglingquan	cools Damp Heat anywhere in the body
Liv 14 Qimen	Front Mu point for the Liver.

Explanation

Liver Qi Xu occurs first but is often followed by a combination of the two syndromes. This combination may occur in chronic fatigue syndrome or myalgic encephalopathy.

Stirring of Liver Wind

Western diagnoses: hypertension, stroke, epilepsy, trigeminal neuralgia.

Symptoms: vertigo, tremor, convulsion, spasms, stiff neck, facial paralysis, tinnitus, apoplexy, hemiplegia.

Tongue: red or dark purple with dry fur.

Pulse: wiry.

Treatment

Calm Liver, disperse Wind:

Liv 2 Xingjian	Fire point, disperses Fire in the Liver
Liv 3 Taichong	Liver Source point; balances Liver, moves Qi
GB 20 Fengchi	expels Wind
UB 18 Ganshu	Back Shu point for the Liver
LI 4 Hegu	expels Wind; used for face and neck
Du 20 Baihui	used to calm the Liver and expel Wind
Kid 3 Taixi	tonifies Kidney Yin and Yang
Kid 7 Fuliu	tonifies both Kidney and Liver
UB 23 Shenshu	Back Shu point for the Kidneys.

Explanation

There are three different syndromes associated with the stirring of Liver Wind. They can be caused by:

1. Internal Heat, caused by penetration of an exogenous Pathogen to the interior. This is characterized by serious febrile diseases in children (e.g. measles, meningitis).
2. Inability of the deficient Liver Yin to control the Liver Yang with subsequent internal Wind symptoms.
3. Deficiency of Liver Blood.

Treatment of all three syndromes aims to subdue the Liver Wind, which can be very dangerous. Otherwise, the Liver energies need controlling or tonifying according to whether the underlying symptoms exhibit Excess or Deficiency. The prevention of stroke depends on getting this balance correct.

Liver Blood Xu

Western diagnoses: hypertension, chronic eye problems, chronic menstrual problems, anaemia.

Symptoms: dizziness, blurring of vision, dryness of the eyes, seeing spots before the eyes, muscle spasms and tics, limb numbness, pale face, irregular and meagre menstrual flow.

Tongue: pale.

Pulse: thin and wiry.

Treatment

Tonify Liver Yin and tonify the Spleen:

Sp 6 Sanyinjiao	tonifies Spleen, balances Liver and regulates Blood
UB 23 Shenshu	Back Shu point for the Kidneys
UB 20 Pishu	Back Shu point for the Spleen
UB 18 Ganshu	Back Shu point for the Liver
UB 15 Xinshu	Back Shu point for the Heart
St 36 Zusanli	tonifies and regulates the Stomach and Spleen
Ren 4 Guanyuan	builds up the Kidney and Yuan Qi
Liv 14 Qimen	Front Mu point for the Liver.

Explanation

This syndrome may be caused by extreme or repeated blood loss, leading to a deficiency of stored Liver Blood. Poor constitution or Kidney Yin and Spleen Qi Xu will also contribute to the overall problem. There will be poor nourishment of the tissues and poor Liver function.

Western diagnoses: hypertension, migraine, nervous disorders.

Symptoms: anger, depression, throbbing unilateral headaches, visual problems, heart palpitations, dizziness, tinnitus.

Tongue: red body.

Pulse: wiry.

Treatment

Disperse Liver Yang, tonify Liver Yin:

Liv 2 Xingjian	disperses Liver Heat
GB 34 Yanglingquan	calms the Liver and Gall Bladder
UB 18 Ganshu	Back Shu point for the Liver
GB 20 Fengchi	used for headache, expels Wind
Sp 6 Sanyinjiao	tonifies Spleen, Liver and Kidney Yin
Kid 3 Taixi	tonifies Kidney Yin and Yang.

Explanation

The Liver loses control over the smooth flow of body Qi due to stress, anger or frustration, so the Qi accumulates and stagnates. As it is essentially Yang, it tends to rise.

Western diagnoses: infectious hepatitis, cholecystitis.

Symptoms: jaundice, bitter taste in the mouth, fullness and pain in the chest and hypochondrium, nausea, fever with thirst and dark urine, loss of appetite, vaginal discharge and itching, pain and swelling of the scrotum.

Tongue: red with yellow greasy coating.

Liver Yang rising

Liver–Gall Bladder invaded by Damp Heat

Pulse: wiry, slippery and rapid.

Treatment
Clear and disperse the Damp Heat:

GB 34 Yanglingquan	disperses Damp Heat
Liv 2 Xingjian	disperses Liver Heat
Sp 9 Yinlingquan	transforms Damp
UB 48 Yanggang	point used for jaundice
GB 24 Riyue	regulates Liver Qi, soothes Damp
St 36 Zusanli	regulates the Stomach and Spleen
UB 19 Danshu	Back Shu point for the Gall Bladder
UB 18 Ganshu	Back Shu point for the Liver
LI 11 Quchi	resolves Damp, clears Heat.

Explanation
The bitter taste in the mouth is said to be due to Heat forcing the bile out of the Gall Bladder. This syndrome is caused by a diet containing too many rich, greasy, spicy foods and alcohol. This tends to cause Heat in the Liver and Damp in the Spleen, which combine to become Liver–Gall Bladder Damp Heat.

NB: Although there are acupuncture points recommended for this condition, *medical help should be sought immediately*. Cholycystectomy may prove necessary and any type of hepatitis needs to be treated with great care.

As long as the situation is monitored, carefully reviewing all the usual laboratory test results, it has been shown in an interesting case study that this condition responds to a mixture of acupuncture and Chinese herbal medicine (Williams 1992).

Cold stagnation in the Liver channel

Western diagnoses: pelvic inflammatory disease, hernia.

Symptoms: pain in the lower abdomen, pain improved by warmth and made worse by cold, pain sometimes described as being on the sides of the body, swelling and painful distension in the scrotum.

Tongue: damp with white glossy coating.

Pulse: wiry, deep and slow.

Treatment
Move the stagnation, disperse Cold:

Liv 3 Taichong	move the Qi in the channel
Liv 5 Ligou	clears the channel
Liv 8 Ququan	Water point, tonifies the Liver
Sp 6 Sanyinjiao	benefits the Liver
Ren 4 Guanyuan	disperses Cold from the lower Jiao
Ren 6 Qihai	benefits Qi and Yang.

Box 8.14 Symptom list for Liver invading Spleen

Excess (Liver)	Deficiency (Spleen)
Constipation	Diarrhoea
Abdominal distension	Abdominal distension
Marked pain	Little pain
Tongue, red sides	Tongue, pale
Irritability	Tiredness

Explanation

This is an essentially painful condition. The Pathogen Cold is always associated with a deep, penetrating type of pain. Cold congeals or 'freezes' the flow of Qi and Blood.

Liver invades Spleen

Western diagnoses: stress due to overwork or emotional problems.

Symptoms: Possible combinations between the two lists in Box 8.14.

Tongue: pale with red sides.

Pulse: weak on the right, wiry on the left.

Treatment

Move stagnating Liver Qi and tonify Spleen Qi:

Liv 14 Qimen	smooth flow of Liver Qi
Liv 13 Zhangmen	harmonizes the Liver and Spleen
GB 34 Yanglingquan	promotes smooth flow of Liver Qi, calms pain
Liv 3 Taichong	promotes smooth flow of Liver Qi, calms pain
St 36 Zusanli	tonifies the Spleen
Sp 6 Sanyinjiao	tonifies the Spleen, regulates the Liver.

Explanation

This is a somewhat modern interpretation of TCM syndromes and described by Maciocia as a combined pattern. It implies that indigestion has occurred due to the secretion of large amounts of acidic digestive juice (produced by the Liver) in comparison to alkaline digestive juice (produced by the Spleen). The symptoms can present either as a deficiency, when the Spleen permits the 'invasion', or as an excess, when Liver symptoms predominate. Either way, it is linked to long-term emotional stresses, poor eating habits or overworking (Maciocia 1989).

Collapse of Yin and Yang

These two patterns tend to stand alone and they both require urgent treatment if recognized.

Collapse of Yang

Western diagnoses: total exhaustion, severe shock.

Symptoms: chills, cold clammy skin, cold extremities, cold sweat, feeble breathing, lack of spirit, exhaustion, desire for hot drinks.

Tongue: swollen, pale, wet.

Pulse: deep and weak.

Treatment
Rescue Yang, prevent further loss:

Ren 4 Guanyuan	tonifies Yang
Du 20 Baihui	tonifies Yang
Ren 8 Shenque	rescues Yang
St 36 Zusanli	raises Yang.

Explanation
Collapse of Yang is due to continuous, extreme vomiting or diarrhoea. Excessive bleeding or perspiration in the case of heat stroke can also cause it. The patient needs to be kept warm. If associated with shock, the feet should also be elevated. The specific Yang organs should be treated on their respective Fire points to guard against further collapse. *Medical help is advisable.*

Collapse of Yin

Western diagnoses: mental overwork, high stress, emotional collapse.

Symptoms: restless, insomniac, dull spirit, inability to focus or make decisions; often linked with the overuse of stimulants or tranquillizers.

Tongue: red, peeled, dry.

Pulse: floating, empty, rapid.

Treatment
Tonify Qi and Yin. Calm the spirit, disperse Fire:

Sp 6 Sanyinjiao	tonifies Yin
Kid 6 Xaohai	tonifies Yin
St 36 Zusanli	tonifies Qi and Blood
Yintang	for restlessness
Anmian	for insomnia
Ren 17 Shanzhong	Yin Xu with anxiety.

Explanation
Changes in lifestyle are required or this will become a chronic state, eventually leading to collapse of Yang as Yang rages out of control. Relaxation techniques should be taught. Some form of meditation or Qi Gong will also be helpful.

Using syndrome differentation

The preceding syndromes are very basic and, in reality, most patients tend to show more than one during the course of any lengthy disease. More complex diseases such as multiple sclerosis actually progress quite clearly from one syndrome to another. Blackwell & MacPherson (1993) described a staging for multiple sclerosis in terms of syndromes (Table 8.1). The first

Table 8.1 Staging of multiple sclerosis (after Blackwell & MacPherson 1993)

Stage	Description
1	Remission
2	Meridian problem Damp Heat in channels Support Spleen and Stomach
3	Internal Damp Spleen Qi Xu Liver Blood Xu
4	Kidney Yang Xu Kidney Yin Xu

stage, or remission, shows no symptoms and the aim of acupuncture treatment is to return patients to that situation.

Acupoints are selected as appropriate for each stage, but treatment of the superficial meridian symptoms continues throughout (Blackwell & MacPherson 1993).

No rigorous research has been done in the field of multiple sclerosis; achieving a homogeneous group of patients would be almost impossible, and any study would require very large numbers to power it adequately. However, anecdotal clinical findings seem to indicate that this type of treatment may be useful in delaying the progression of the disease. It is certainly worthwhile suggesting this type of treatment early in the course of the disease (Case study 8.1).

Evolving TCM

Physiotherapy is a profession closely associated with the treatment of neurological disease, but the TCM textbooks often do not give the information we require. The following is an exercise undertaken with a group of neurological physiotherapists, reasoning from basic TCM principles but applying these to physiotherapy as it is generally practised.

Acupuncture and Parkinson's disease

The following is a list of problems observed in a patient with Parkinson's disease; the most important TCM link is given in parentheses:

1. slow and limited movement (stagnation of Qi, Blood and Body fluids)
2. difficulty initiating movement (Kidney Yang Deficiency)
3. stooping posture (associated with Du channel and Kidney Qi)
4. tremor (Liver)
5. mask-like face, lack of expression (Heart)
6. drooling (Heart)
7. dull monotone in speech (Heart)
8. cold painful limbs (Blood stasis)
9. depression (Liver, Heart).

This is obviously a long and complicated list of symptoms, all of which combine to make up a picture that is not unlike the TCM idea of old age – a slow decline of supporting Kidney energy. It is not suggested that

CASE HISTORY

Case study 8.1

Young woman, aged 34, with an early diagnosis of multiple sclerosis. Had minor symptoms for 2 years. Sent by her general practitioner to the physiotherapy department for 'some exercises'.

Main problem
Lack of sensory perception in the extremities: 'a feeling that she was wearing rubber gloves on her hands and that she was walking through soft sand'. This tended to produce a slightly clumsy gait. Otherwise, few physical symptoms, slight double vision occasionally. Patient very anxious in view of her diagnosis.

Impression
Stage 2 Damp Heat in the channels, producing mainly channel symptoms.

Treatment
The aim was to clear channels, support the Stomach and Spleen.

Points:

- Baxie (extra points on the hand)
- Bafeng (extra points on the foot)
- St 36 Zusanli
- Sp 6 Sanyinjiao.

Treatment was given twice weekly for 3 weeks, then once a week for 3 weeks. Very gentle coordination exercises were given.

Outcome
Restoration of normal sensation in limbs. Some improvement in gait. Patient much more serene. Unfortunately, the patient moved out of the area and was not treated again.

Parkinson's disease can be cured by acupuncture, but it is reasonable to suppose that the known physiological effects may help with symptom control.

Using TCM reasoning, the following points could be used, but not all at once:

- St 36 Zusanli and Sp 6 Sanyinjiao – to assist with the formation and better circulation of Qi; used as a tonic and boost
- Kid 3 Taixi – stimulates both Kidney Yin and Yang
- Du 20 Baihui or moxa to Du 4 Mingmen – to access and support the energy in the Du meridian. Kid 3 Taixi could also be useful
- Liv 3 Taichong – for control of muscle tremor. (Use with SI 3 Houxi if spasm is also present)
- Ht 7 Shenmen – for mask, lack of emotion
- Ht 6 or 7 – for excess or uncontrolled saliva
- Heart points associated with speech problems (Ht 5 Tongli)
- Sp 10 Xuehai – for Blood stasis in lower limbs; SJ 6 Zhigou in the upper limb. Also moxa to UB 17 Geshu for general circulation. Ren 6 Qihai can be used to support body Qi

☯ All of the preceding points will have some effect on the mood of the patient because of the anticipated increase in serotonin levels. TCM suggests points such as Yintang to 'lift the spirits'.

It is important to remember that these patients are characterized by a slowing down of body processes and a general lack of energy. Acupuncture can be a draining type of therapy and should be used with caution. However, it can be seen that with a basic understanding of TCM a useful prescription can be drawn up for a patient manifesting with a clear neurological disease process.

Research

Published research in this field has been limited. The papers from China available in the West do not help the situation. Usually the rationale for the selection of points is not given. There are two reasons for this. First, it may be assumed that the readers are perfectly familiar with the TCM theories guiding point selection and that no explanation is needed. Second, the feeling that Western scientific institutions will neither understand nor accept the reasons given for the selection of points may compound the natural reticence of the researchers. There are some notable exceptions, however. For example, Aune et al (1998) investigated a well defined and described Bladder syndrome with promising results and a TCM-guided choice of points.

There has been little research in which TCM syndromes have been specifically identified and described. This is a great pity because this is the cutting clinical edge of acupuncture. Many hundreds of years of empirical experience are distilled into the description of the individual syndromes. The great variety and subtlety of both differentiation and subsequent choice of points for treatment makes it difficult to standardize treatments. Unfortunately, controlled clinical trials require this kind of precision in order for the results to be analysed and quantified with any confidence.

There is now a strong move in acupuncture circles to ensure that the TCM aspect of treatment is not neglected, but carefully reported, in future trials (MacPherson et al 2002). Birch (1997) has identified the main problems facing the researcher in traditionally based acupuncture, and has offered some solutions.

The current emphasis in scientific research is to specify and report on all aspects of the research protocols. This means that the underlying theories are made extremely clear and the treatments specified are repeatable (MacPherson et al 2002). The Standards for Reporting Interventions in Controlled Trials of Acupuncture (STRICTA) protocol published by MacPherson et al (2002) will assist in allowing full evaluation of the systems of syndrome differentiation. It is likely that only the simpler and more obvious syndromes will be examined, with those corresponding to a Western diagnosis being regarded as easier to tackle first.

A handful of interesting papers has been published, however, with regard to TCM-type treatments. Some researchers have looked at cardiac disease, particularly angina pectoris and coronary artery disease, finding that acupuncture appears to be beneficial (Bueno et al 2001, Richter et al 1991).

The proven effect of acupuncture on peristalsis and gastric motor function deserves better recognition, and the papers by Chang et al (2001a, b) are worth reading. Acupuncture has been shown to be effective in treating two patients with persistent hiccups (Schiff et al 2002).

Acupuncture with clear roots in syndrome differentiation has been used with success in cases of dysmenorrhoea (Griffiths 2000, Proctor et al 2002). Porzio et al (2002), who looked at the use of acupuncture to combat menopausal symptoms in women after tamoxifen was used to treat their cancer, investigated a similar application.

The use of acupuncture for morning sickness and nausea is based entirely in TCM theory, but has been almost adopted by Western practitioners, first because it is so simple, involving only a few points in addition to Pe 6 Neiguan, and second because it has been investigated so comprehensively by researchers. A recent trial (Smith et al 2002) showed acupuncture to be an effective treatment for women who experienced nausea and dry retching during early pregnancy.

The use of syndrome differentiation has seriously complicated the approach of researchers. In their paper on the diagnosis and treatment of low back pain by traditional Chinese medical acupuncturists, Sherman et al (2001) found that only two acupoints (UB 23 and UB 40) were common to all 150 treatments for chronic low back pain, although more than 85 different points were used. A diagnosis of Qi and Blood stagnation, or of Qi stagnation, was made for 85% of the patients, with a diagnosis of Kidney Deficiency (or one of the three subtypes) made for 33–51% of patients. As Sherman et al (2001) pointed out, selecting a single treatment that has wide applicability is certainly challenging.

More recently there has been an attempt to establish manualized research protocols (Schnyer & Allen 2001). This team has published what is, in effect, a textbook for the TCM acupuncture treatment of depressive illness, taking into consideration the various syndromes that may be constituted from the symptoms. Thus, a clear framework is established within which individualized treatment may be given. This is a truer pragmatic test for acupuncture than most, and is hopefully indicating a way forward for syndrome research.

Herbal medicine

Use of TCM syndrome patterns in acupuncture treatment can be very rewarding, but it is important to bear in mind that treatment suggestions given here do not address the herbal component. Acupuncture is only part of a full traditional treatment, and sometimes only a minor part. Physiotherapists are not currently involved in prescribing, although things are changing. It is unlikely that the prescription of Chinese herbs will be part of normal practice for some time to come, if ever. It is, however, worth noting that many proprietary brands of common herb combinations are available and, if advice is sought from a registered herbal practitioner, good advice could be given to the patient. The underlying principles of the syndromes need to be understood first in order to avoid recommending the wrong herbal combinations, and further training in TCM would be advisable.

References

Aune A, Alraek T, LiHua H, Baerheim A 1998 Acupuncture in the prophylaxis of recurrent lower urinary tract infection in adult women. Scandinavian Journal of Primary Health Care 16: 37–39.

Birch S 1997 Testing the claims of traditionally based acupuncture. Complementary Therapies in Medicine 5: 147–151.

Blackwell R, MacPherson H 1993 Multiple sclerosis. Staging and patient management. Journal of Chinese Medicine 42: 5–12.

Bueno EA, Mamtani R, Frishman WH 2001 Alternative approaches to the medical management of angina pectoris: acupuncture, electrical nerve stimulation, and spinal cord stimulation. Heart Disease 3: 215–216.

Chang CS, Ko CW, Wu CY, Chen GH 2001a Effect of electrical stimulation on acupuncture points in diabetic patients with gastric dysrhythmia: a pilot study. Digestion 64: 184–190.

Chang X, Yan J, Yi S et al 2001b The affects of acupuncture at Sibai and Neiting acupoints on gastric peristalsis. Journal of Traditional Chinese Medicine 21: 286–288.

Griffiths V 2000 Traditional Chinese medicine: a case of dysmenorrhoea. Australian Journal of Holistic Nursing 7: 42–43.

Maciocia G 1989 The foundations of Chinese Medicine. Edinburgh: Churchill Livingstone.

MacPherson H, White AR, Cummings M et al 2002 Standards for Reporting Interventions in Controlled Trials of Acupuncture: the STRICTA recommendations. Acupuncture in Medicine 20: 22–25.

Porzio G, Trapasso T, Martelli S et al 2002 Acupuncture in the treatment of menopause-related symptoms in women taking tamoxifen. Tumori 88: 128–130.

Proctor ML, Smith CA, Farquhar CM, Stones RW 2002 Transcutaneous electrical nerve stimulation and acupuncture for primary dysmenorrhoea. Cochrane Database Systematic Reviews 1: CD002123.

Richter A, Herlitz J, Hjalmarson A 1991 Effect of acupuncture in patients with angina pectoris. European Heart Journal 12: 175–178.

Ross J 1995 Acupuncture point combinations. Edinburgh: Churchill Livingstone.

Schiff E, River Y, Oliven A, Odeh M 2002 Acupuncture therapy for persistent hiccups. American Journal of Medical Science 323: 166–168.

Schnyer RN, Allen JJB 2001 Acupuncture in the treatment of depression. A manual for practice and research. Edinburgh: Churchill Livingstone.

Seem M 1987 Acupuncture energetics. A workbook for diagnostics and treatment. Rochester, Vermont: Healing Arts Press.

Sherman KJ, Cherkin DC, Hogeboom CJ 2001 The diagnosis and treatment of patients with chronic low back pain by traditional Chinese medical acupuncturists. Journal of Alternative and Complementary Medicine 7: 641–650.

Smith C, Crowther C, Beilby J 2002 Acupuncture to treat nausea and vomiting in early pregnancy: a randomised controlled trial. Birth 29: 1–9.

Williams JE 1992 Liver and Gall Bladder Damp Heat syndrome. American Journal of Acupuncture 20: 205–211.

<table>
<tr><td>

CHAPTER

9

</td><td>

Possible acupuncture mechanisms

</td></tr>
</table>

KEY CONCEPTS

- The original research work was done with acupuncture analgesia.
- Much of the research has been done on small rodents.
- The 'gate' theory was the original explanation and this, linked to segmental theories and opioid neurohumoral transmitters, is the explanation for much of the effect of acupuncture.
- The involvement of the higher centres is more difficult to research and understand, and the picture is not yet complete.
- Increased or decreased sympathetic activity is implicated in some of the documented acupuncture effects.
- There are other mechanisms involved in the effect of acupuncture on blood circulation, immune systems, the viscera, muscle tone and strength, and mood and motivation.
- Perhaps some points really do have a stronger effect than others.
- A combination of segmental acupuncture and sympathetic stimulation may be the most 'scientific' form of treatment.

Introduction

How does acupuncture work? What is happening in the body when needles are inserted? Must the needles be inserted into designated acupoints? Is a treatment necessarily point-specific?

It is clear, clinically, that in certain specific areas something is happening, but at present it is not understood exactly what. There is a substantial body of research suggesting the mechanism of action of acupuncture with regard to pain. There are many theories, but they are often contradictory, contributing only a part of the – as yet elusive – complete answer.

In this chapter the most important research in acupuncture analgesia will be briefly discussed. This field is rapidly expanding and becoming ever more complex, and is likely to have changed again before this book is published, but some of the basic research findings could be indicators of possible mechanisms for acupuncture in the treatment of systemic and neurological disease, as well as in pain. A brief review of the research into the existence of meridians and the acupuncture points situated on them follows, linking with Chapter 1.

Acupuncture and pain

If we consider the basic mechanism of acupuncture in terms of Traditional Chinese Medicine (TCM), it is described simply as the 'movement of Qi', but such an explanation will never be acceptable to a critical scientist. However, the other important TCM idea, that of Yin and Yang, may have some echo within Western medicine, even if not expressed in the same way. Han (2001, p 51) states: '... one concept shared by both medical systems is that most if not all physiological functions are regulated by activities possessing opposite effects'. Blood sugar concentration is decreased by insulin and increased by glucagon. Sympathetic and parasympathetic systems tend to have opposing or contrasting functions in regulating internal physiology. The homeostasis of Western medicine can perhaps be equated with the dynamic balance found within TCM, but this is not specific enough to explain the mechanisms involved in acupuncture.

The visit of Richard Nixon to China in 1972 began the investigations into acupuncture mechanisms by providing an impetus to look at pain relief. Media exposure of the replacement of anaesthetics by acupuncture during surgery meant that early Western acupuncture research became an effort to map and measure pain, and to investigate the mechanisms that would explain acupuncture analgesia.

Overview of physiological aspects of acupuncture analgesia

Acupuncture is a potent form of sensory stimulation. The insertion of a needle into the skin and underlying tissues produces a clear pattern of afferent responses in peripheral nerves. The basic science of acupuncture has been subject to research, with regard to the analgesic effect, and the studies have mainly examined the effect of acupuncture on the central, peripheral and autonomic nervous systems together with related neurohumoral effects and changes in blood biochemicals. Other effects, such as the effect on the vascular system, have also been investigated and these are discussed in the next section.

The first research studies looked at the effect of acupuncture on the nervous system, and the model proposed by Pomeranz indicated how acupuncture could affect the nervous system, increasing the secretion of neuropeptides and monoamines in the bloodstream or cerebrospinal fluid. These include the endorphins, enkephalins, dynorphins, serotonin and adrenaline (epinephrine). In his presentations and publications, Pomeranz has documented 17 convergent lines of evidence supporting the claim that acupuncture releases endorphins, producing acupuncture analgesia that is naloxone reversible (Pomeranz 1996). This work played a major part in convincing the Consensus Development Conference of the US National Institutes of Health of the scientific credibility of acupuncture for pain relief in 1997 (NIH Consensus Development Panel on Acupuncture 1998).

Some of this work was done on mice and rats (Han & Terenius 1982) and, although the biochemical effects achieved are convincing, it must be noted that an acupuncture needle into an acupoint in such small animals will result in a considerably greater traumatic effect than the same needle in a human being. Much acupuncture, while obtaining the 'DeQi' or needling sensation in order to work, is really quite a gentle stimulation and the opioid neurotransmitters may not be the only mechanism involved.

True acupuncture is characterized by sensations of heaviness, numbness and soreness. Briefly, the mechanism now widely accepted is that the acupuncture stimulus is transmitted from the sensory receptors of small afferent nerve fibres of Aδ, Aγ and C sizes through the contralateral, anterolateral spinothalamic tract to the dorsal central periaqueductal grey matter, and moves upwards to reach the medial part of the hypothalamic arcuate nucleus. Non-acupuncture stimuli are thought to be transmitted to the anterior part of the hypothalamic arcuate nucleus (Takeshige 2001).

The hypothalamus is located in the centre of the brain and has important connections to the limbic system, thalamus, cerebral cortex and brainstem. The limbic system is where emotional and affective responses to pain are integrated with the sensory experience. The hypothalamus integrates humoral and endocrine function, neurochemical production and, effectively, autonomic responses. The hypothalamus controls autonomic outflow via the vasomotor centre in the medulla; thus acupuncture can have a real effect on central sympathetic responses. It activates the descending inhibitory pain pathways, producing analgesia via the spinal cord. It has been suggested that acupuncture simply activates the hypothalamus, which automatically regulates the body environment, heat and body temperature, hunger and satiety, and water balance, thus improving general well-being, with the implication that point specificity is unimportant. Teasing out the answer to this is likely to be very difficult.

The effect of acupuncture on the limbic system appears to be less clear than originally thought. Electroacupuncture to St 36, LI 4 and GB 34 has been shown to deactivate structures associated with this area (Hsieh et al 2001), but another study (Biella et al 2001) using manual acupuncture for a considerably longer treatment time found the limbic areas were activated. It would appear that there is some response to the acupuncture, but it is not clear how this is to be controlled and how much clinical use it is to a patient with chronic pain.

This activity is shown in Figure 9.1. Dopamine is involved in the transmission between the anterior hypothalamic arcuate nucleus (A-HARN) and the posterior hypothalamic arcuate nucleus (P-HARN); adrenocorticotrophic hormone (ACTH) released from the pituitary gland is thought to be essential for this.

β-Endorphin, shown to be released by acupuncture stimulation, influences a number of hypothalamic reactions including body temperature, respiration and cardiovascular function (Holaday 1983). β-Endorphin is produced and released from the hypothalamic nucleus and the arcuate nucleus.

There is also a β-endorphin system in the pituitary. The hypothalamic β-endorphinergic system and neuronal network project to the midbrain and to periaqueductal grey matter and the nucleus raphe magnus, which in turn activate two pain-alleviating descending neuronal pathways, the serotonergic and noradrenergic systems.

The reverse mechanism is shown in Figure 9.2. Synaptic transmission from the P-HARN to the hypothalamic ventromedian nucleus (HVN) is apparently dopaminergic, as it can be blocked by dopamine antagonists or lesions of the HVN.

The role of opioid peptides in the analgesia produced by acupuncture has not gone unchallenged; Bossut & Mayer (1991), who replicated Han's

Figure 9.1 Afferent pathway for acupuncture and non-acupuncture analgesia. ACTH, adrenocorticotrophic hormone; A-HARN, M-HARN and P-HARN, anterior, medial and posterior hypothalamic arcuate nucleus. (Redrawn from Takeshige 2001.)

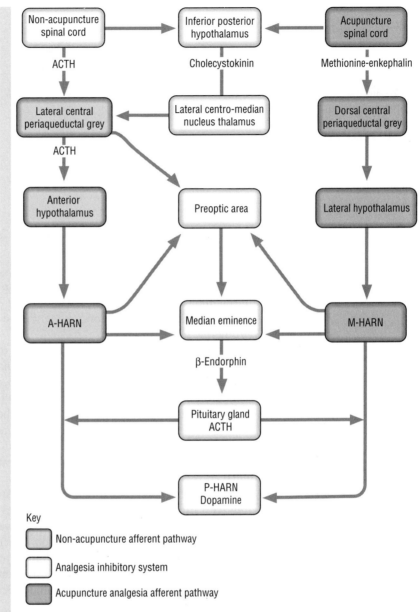

experiments, claimed that opioid peptides were neither sufficient to explain acupuncture analgesia nor essential to the phenomenon. However, they are clearly part of the answer.

Segmental acupuncture, where treatment is given only in the clearly defined area of a particular nerve root supply, operates through a circuit involving inhibitory enkephalinergic stalked cells in the outer part of lamina II of the spinal grey matter, contacted directly by the Aδ/group III primary afferents. This was previously described as the 'gate mechanism' and formed the basis of the original theories on the mechanism of acupuncture.

The mechanism of heterosegmental acupuncture analgesia is generally said to be brought about by the release of β-endorphin and met-enkephalin,

Figure 9.2 Efferent pathway of the descending pain inhibitory system. D-raphe, dorsal raphe nucleus; HVN, hypothalamic ventromedian nucleus; P-HARN, posterior hypothalamic arcuate nucleus; RPCN, reticular paragiganto cellular nucleus. (Redrawn from Takeshige 2001.)

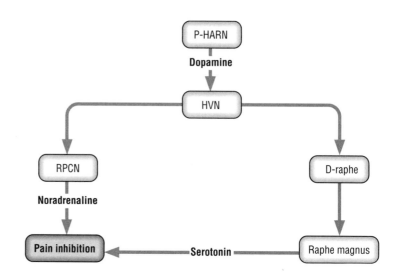

a generalized neurohormonal mechanism, and by activation of the descending pain inhibitory system through specific pathways connected to the acupoints while allowing maintenance of consciousness. The two descending inhibitory systems, as mentioned above, are serotonergic and adrenergic in nature.

The stimulus that provokes the release of opioid peptides also provokes the release of cholecystokinin (CCK), an antagonist. It is suggested that acupuncture tolerance, produced after repeated treatments, may have something to do with increased CCK activity (White 1999).

The situation is further complicated by the fact that a needle inserted anywhere within the body, other than at an acupoint, will also produce a reaction. This is termed diffuse noxious inhibitory control (DNIC), and may contribute in a minor way to the acupuncture effect (Le Bars et al 1991). It is also a pain-suppressing system, and Le Bars has shown that it is an opioidergic mechanism acting on the spinal cord neurons transmitting pain information to the brain, but it has been demonstrated to have only a short-term effect (Hashimoto & Aikawa 1993).

As DNIC is activated by stimulation of acupoints or non-acupoints, it leads to non-specific inhibition of different interconnected pathways. This means that it may be possible to distinguish between the effect of acupoints and non-acupoints by their anatomically distinct brain pathways (Takeshige 2001) (Fig. 9.3).

The analgesic activity of non-acupuncture points is actually self-inhibiting at the lateral central periaqueductal grey matter (LPAG) level (see Fig. 9.1). Lesions of the lateral centromedian nucleus of the thalamus at the level of the LPAG result in analgesia produced by needling non-points, thus partly confirming the specific action of acupuncture points (Takeshige 2001).

The main support for these theories suggesting neural pathways comes from work done on rats and rabbits. Acupuncture points can be identified on these animals, chiefly St 36 Zusanli and LI 4 Hegu, and low-frequency electroacupuncture is used to produce the analgesic response. This can be compared to the action of intraperitoneal morphine (0.5 mg/kg), which gives a similar form of analgesia that is also abolished by naloxone (Takeshige et al 1993).

Figure 9.3 Differentiation of acupuncture and non-acupuncture points by the analgesia inhibitory system. I-PH, inferior posterior hypothalamus; L-CM, lateral centromedian nucleus of the thalamus. (Redrawn from Takeshige 2001.)

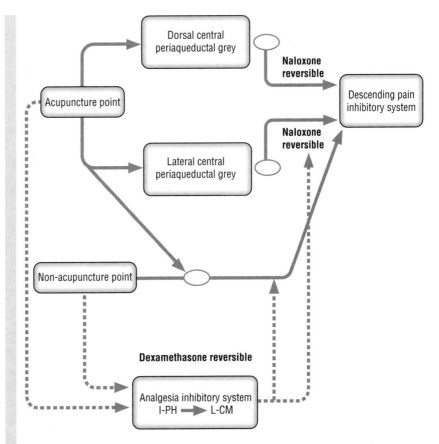

As much of the research into the physiological mechanisms of acupuncture has been performed on small animals, the studies have inherent flaws and are of doubtful clinical relevance, while demonstrating some basic ideas. Most animal behavioural models are set up to investigate whether the length of time for which an experimental animal will tolerate a painful stimulus can be lengthened. In essence, this means that only acute pain is being investigated, whereas acupuncture is more commonly used in the clinical setting to treat chronic pain. The mechanisms involved in chronic and acute pain are different.

In addition, the animals are restrained while a painful stimulus is applied, and this could cause stress-induced analgesia, thus confounding the results. Electroacupuncture is commonly used because it is easier to standardize a 'dose', leading to greater ease in reproduction of investigative work, but the doses given to animal subjects are often much higher than those used in clinical practice. It has been observed that the analgesic effects of electroacupuncture diminish rapidly, within 10–20 minutes (Han 1986). This is at odds with clinical experience in human patients, where acupuncture is recognized as often having a cumulative and long-lasting effect.

Segmental theories

Segmental applications, acupuncture, transcutaneous electrical nerve stimulation (TENS) and manual therapy utilize the characteristic functional differences between the large and smaller nerve fibres. In general, the aim is selectively to stimulate the larger fibres, which are generally more sensitive to pressure, in order to inhibit the effects of the smaller fibres, thus suppressing segmental effects such as pain, autonomic disturbances and raised muscle tone.

Mild acupuncture will stimulate only the large fibres, more painful needling only the smaller fibres, and manipulation of the needle, tending to wrap the muscle fibres around it, will stimulate both. Low-intensity, high-frequency electrical stimulation (50–100 Hz) will stimulate mainly the large fibres, whereas a high-intensity, low-frequency application will stimulate mainly the smaller fibres (1–4 Hz).

Increased and prolonged activation of the small C fibres by mechanical stimuli is one of the causes of increased sympathetic activity affecting vasoconstrictor nerve fibres. In time, these longer-lasting abnormal reflexes can achieve a degree of permanency in the spinal cord and brainstem. Sympathetic fibres have been shown to be affected by the stimulation of somatoafferent fibres (Sato & Schmidt 1973), and an existing increased activity of sympathetic fibres in the same segment can be inhibited after a short initial stimulus, thereby diminishing pain and other abnormal autonomic effects. Thus the acupuncture treatment as a nociceptive stimulus in one part of a segment can affect all the other parts of the same segment, resulting in changes in symptoms such as referred pain, hyperalgesia, increased muscle tone and activated myofascial trigger points, and autonomic symptoms such as vasomotor and trophic changes. Segmental activity is also subject to modulation from two main supraspinal centres, the reticular formation in the brainstem and the limbic area (thalamus and hypothalamus), as explained previously.

A long-lasting painful shoulder is more likely to give additional cervical complaints, especially when the patient is overanxious or mentally stressed. In this case the patient may have an increased sense of pain owing to insufficient central inhibition by the pain-modulating tracts from the nucleus raphe magnus. The patient will be in a state of continual alert, and the descending reticular activating system will raise the tone of the skeletal muscles, particularly trapezius (one of the 'stress' muscles), thus establishing a vicious circle of chronic pain.

The application of segmental acupuncture to both muscular and visceral pain has been well described by Bekkring & van Bussel (1998), and the linking of palpable signs in the dermatome is useful and familiar to physiotherapists. Signs such as increased sweat, dry skin, pitting and areas of goose flesh can all help to indicate the segmental origin of the problem.

Acupuncture meridians

Many researchers have sought proof of the existence of meridians, but the evidence is by no means conclusive. The possible relationship between the meridian system and the development of the embryo was noted some time ago (Mann 1971), but this has not been investigated.

Propagated channel sensation (PCS) has been investigated extensively by many Chinese authors. PCS refers to the sensations experienced by a small proportion of individuals when acupuncture points are needled. These sensations of a deep ache, warmth or heaviness tend to run along the acupuncture meridians, although it is not clear whether the subjects, who are presumably all Chinese, know in advance where the meridian pathways are supposed to be (Bensoussan 1991). No useful research of this type has been done in the West.

Changes in skin resistance and temperature have also been suggested as providing evidence for the existence of meridians (Zhaowei et al 1985). Reviewing this work, Macdonald (1989) acknowledged that sensations may follow meridian lines, but suggested that such phenomena can be explained without postulating the existence of a meridian system. Other Western physicians, notably Felix Mann (1992), have suggested that the acupoints do not exist, as such, offering large acupuncture areas with variable positions instead.

Darras et al (1993) concluded that meridian pathways could be marked by injecting radioactively labelled technetium into acupuncture points and finding that these pathways were separate from lymph vessels and identifiable parts of the circulatory or nervous systems. In China, research on the meridian phenomena continues, but most Western researchers would probably dismiss the idea of a meridian system. At the very least, it must be concluded on current evidence that the existence of the meridians remains interesting but unproven. However, the work of Cho et al (1999) and Wu et al (1999), discussed under the location of points later in this chapter, may indicate linking between the acupoints under test and the brain tissue that is as yet unexplained by either science or anatomy.

Acupuncture points

Research on acupuncture points, however, has been more fruitful. There are definite links between the observations made by acupuncturists and phenomena observed by other clinicians and scientists. The existence and location of acupuncture points are crucial for a proper evaluation of clinical studies.

Macdonald (1989) has made a number of comments. First, it is difficult to be precise about the location of acupuncture points. Their position is usually assessed according to the size and shape of the patient and, although there is reasonable agreement about the locations of many fundamental points (Vincent & Richardson 1986), the number of points continues to grow. Second, there is evidence that the points become tender when a patient is sick, and there is considerable overlap with the independently developed concept of trigger points (Melzack et al 1977). Third, it is possible that acupuncture point locations have some kind of neurophysiological basis, perhaps corresponding to the termination of peripheral nerve endings.

There is no reason contained within the neurohumoral hypothesis as to why acupuncture works well at a particular locus or possesses specific therapeutic indications there, yet may induce a negligible change just 1 cm away, even though the sham locus is within the same area of nerve distribution. The sham locus may be even richer in blood vessels and nerve distribution (Bensoussan 1991). It is therefore important to realize that, although acupuncture point locations may provide useful therapeutic guidelines, they are unlikely to have a precise and constant location.

However, the situation is complicated by the existence of points that appear to have a stronger effect than others. These correspond mostly with TCM-designated He Sea points (see Ch. 5), supporting the idea that a greater effect can be obtained from these points, or are found on the head and face. It may be that needling these points vigorously and repeatedly influences the peripheral circulation via the sympathetic reflexes. Certainly minimal acupuncture does not show the same response either locally or in the pain-processing areas of the brain (Wu et al 2002).

The situation is further complicated by the existence of trigger points, which have a clear anatomical location, often palpable within the muscle tissue, whereas true acupuncture points are associated with the ancient concept of meridians. However, it is reasonable to assume that the empirical observation – that pressure on certain points can be associated with defined pain referral patterns and the pain subsequently decreased by a stimulus such as pressure or insertion of a needle – led to the use of these points as either acupoints or adjuncts to the therapy, the so-called Ah Shi points. Certainly Melzack et al (1977) described a 71% correlation between these known trigger points and acupuncture points, suggesting that the response of trigger points is part of the acupuncture mechanism, although this figure has been questioned and revised downwards by Birch (2003).

Finally, the location of acupuncture points is not as accurate as practitioners claim: comparison of one textbook or atlas with another can produce anomalies with variations in the precise locations or the anatomical descriptions. One such is GB 39 Xuanzhong, found on the posterior border of the fibula in some texts and on the anterior border in others. It is, however, probably still in the same dermatome.

Clinical experience suggests that certain points do have specific actions in Chinese Medicine, but the most significant research has been done on only one of these points, Pe 6 Neiguan, which is used for treating sickness and nausea (Dundee & Ghaly 1991, Dundee et al 1986). This point has been researched extensively because it has a clearly demonstrable action, that of decreasing nausea and vomiting, which it does not appear to share with any other acupoint.

The Chinese have studied needling sensation, or 'DeQi', quite intensively and found that needling sensation does not occur in patients with syringomyelia; consequently they have suggested that it is mediated through the spinothalamic tracts (Bensoussan 1991). However, one of the earliest and most clearcut papers on needling sensation was published by Chiang et al (1973). These authors showed that in order to produce analgesia it was essential to elicit DeQi. Subcutaneous injection of local anaesthetic did not block DeQi, but intramuscular procaine did. Moreover, when DeQi was blocked, so was acupuncture analgesia, although this was not in itself target specific. When acupuncture points in the arm were stimulated to produce DeQi, they appeared to produce the same amount of analgesia in all parts of the body (Andersson 1979).

This research has led Pomeranz (1991) to suggest that acupuncture maps are essential for locating the sites where DeQi can be best achieved. He suggests that this is as near as possible to type II and type III muscle afferents. Probably the best experiments supporting the importance of DeQi have been done in humans with direct microelectrode recording from single fibres in the median nerve while acupuncture was performed distally (Wang et al 1985). When the patient experienced DeQi, type II muscle afferents produced numbness, type III gave sensations of heaviness, distension and aching, and the type IV unmyelinated fibres gave a feeling of soreness. Soreness is an uncommon aspect of DeQi; the sensations most commonly experienced are those that we know to be related to type II and type III afferents (the small myelinated afferents from muscle). It would appear, therefore, that the ancient Chinese observation that it is necessary to obtain DeQi in order to have effective acupuncture is at least in part supported by conventional neurophysiology.

Acupuncture research using magnetic resonance imaging

Using the newer functional magnetic resonance imaging (fMRI) techniques to scan the brain and localize activity, Cho et al (1998) have demonstrated that needling a point on the foot can affect the brain tissue. This is an important step forward in the search for definitive mechanisms as some of the, so far untested, TCM meridian theories can now be examined.

A group of healthy students were selected and three points on the outer border of the foot, UB 65, UB 66 and UB 67, said by TCM theory to have an effect on vision, were needled while the visual cortex was scanned. Activity similar to that found when the eyes were opened in the light was observed, although the eyes remained closed. The experiment was controlled by needling non-acupoints 2–5 cm away on the surface of the foot, without the same effect in the visual cortex. This evidence is fascinating and perhaps gives some credence to the idea of meridians or, at least, a transmission mechanism that is not yet fully understood. This original study was complicated by an attempt to differentiate between Yin and Yang with different types of needling, which detracts from the overall validity. However, further studies have been done without this complication and similar results were obtained when response in the auditory cortex to body acupuncture points affecting the ear was explored (Cho et al 1999). This work shows a clear cortical response to the needling stimulus.

The most recent work is even more interesting, and involves the general pain response mechanism of the body. Cho has identified the limbic system as being the most reactive in cases of pain, and isolated this area in the brain, particularly the cingulate gyrus. Volunteers were subjected to a painful stimulus – immersion of their hand into hot water – and the brain was scanned for areas of activity. The classical TCM bilateral acupoint combination of LI 4 and Liv 3, known as the 'Four Gates' and traditionally used to relieve pain, calm and relax the patient, was then used. Cho and his colleagues noted a decrease in the limbic activity, as seen on the fMRI scan, indicating a different reaction to this form of needling (ZH Cho 2001, personal communication). Explanations for this phenomenon are not available yet, but it adds some credence to a very ancient pain relief technique.

Wu et al (1999) did the original work on this aspect. Specific points were selected and activated, and the corresponding areas of the brain to be stimulated were noted carefully. This work is less precise than that of Cho, and the numbers of volunteers in each group were smaller, but the two seem broadly to agree. Wu stimulated St 36 and LI 4, both considered 'strong' and influential points in Chinese Medicine, and produced evidence of activity in the structures of the descending antinociceptive pathways and less clear evidence of activity of the limbic areas associated with pain response. This was a controlled trial with minimal acupuncture – pricking only, with no DeQi or needling sensation in the limb – given to the control subjects. Autonomic responses were assessed and acupuncture at the genuine acupoints resulted in significantly higher scores for DeQi and bradycardia. The control stimulation did not produce the physiological responses or the changes in brain tissue activity.

Figure 9.4 is a simplified summary of current ideas on the pain relief mechanisms of acupuncture.

Mechanisms of acupuncture with effects beyond those of pain control

Although we have a relatively good understanding of how acupuncture may be working in pain, our understanding of the overall effects is far more fragmented. We are aware that acupuncture may be having an effect on the circulation in general, including both the microcirculation and the cerebral circulation. We are also aware that acupuncture may influence recovery from neurological damage and may have direct effects on muscle tissue as well as mood. However, there is no coherent physiological or immunological theory that unites these various disparate observations. Furthermore, much of the research in this area is limited and has not been reproduced independently; some of the science, particularly from the Chinese studies, is poor. The following are some speculative ideas that explore how acupuncture might be working in the context of neurological damage,

Figure 9.4 Basic mechanisms of acupuncture pain relief. ACTH, adrenocorticotrophic hormone; CSF, cerebrospinal fluid; PAG, periaqueductal grey matter.

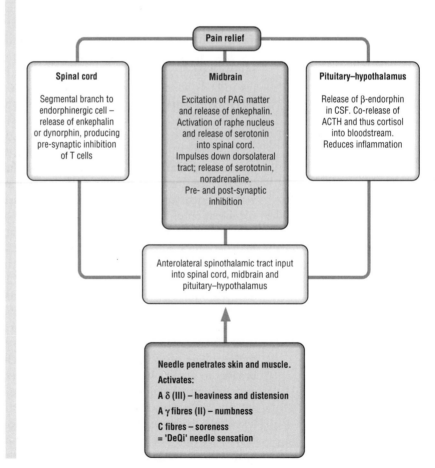

although the main emphasis of this section is to look at how acupuncture may be acting clinically rather than in terms of its basic mechanisms.

General circulation

The Chinese have long claimed that acupuncture produces changes in circulation, but tend to assert that these are only a normalization process, restoring the characteristics of healthy circulation in terms of mechanical flow and the state of blood cells. Research into acupuncture and the cardiovascular system has the advantage that the cardiovascular system is capable of reliable and relatively convenient monitoring.

Patients frequently comment that they feel warm after acupuncture (Filshie & White 1998). Indeed Cao et al (1983), measuring changes in skin temperature and assessing blood flow by finger plethysmography, suggested that patients who responded to acupuncture analgesia tended to show a measurable increase in the skin temperature of the palms. Ballegaard et al (1993) showed that the effect of acupuncture on skin temperature depended on baseline temperature. In controlled experiments they showed that electroacupuncture reduced the skin temperature in those whose temperature was, initially, higher than normal, increased it in those with a low temperature, and had little effect on mid-range patients, thus reinforcing the TCM theory that acupuncture restores 'balance' or normality.

A more recent study (Dyrehag et al 1997) indicated that the local skin temperature changed in a group of 12 patients after 4 weeks of electroacupuncture. These patients were all being treated for long-standing nociceptive pain conditions. The skin temperature actually dropped after the first 30-minute treatment, indicating an increase in skin vasoconstrictor sympathetic activity; however, the temperature was significantly higher after the full treatment period and remained that way for 3 months. This was only a small group of patients, but the changes were significant. Skin temperature changes were measured in four different locations, two on the hand (volar and dorsal sides), elbow and forehead. This study indicates either an inhibition of skin sympathetic activity or a release of vasodilatory substances. The latter could be supposed to affect the whole circulation.

These results were not reproduced completely by Litscher & Wang (1999), who noted the short-term cooling effect on the hand immediately after needling in all of six of the subjects in their study, but produced the warming effect (a rise of 2°C) in only three; the others showed further cooling. All of these investigations took place on the same day, so the long-term effects were not examined.

Some recent work on acupuncture for reflex sympathetic dystrophy has investigated the reported sensation of warmth when acupuncture is given for this condition. Ten healthy, age- and sex-matched patients were used as controls. The ten patients received acupuncture to the affected limb: LI 4, LI 10 and LI 11 for the upper limb and St 29, St 36 and St 41 on the lower limb. The control group were matched for limb and side. Blood flow was measured by duplex sonography of either the brachial or the femoral artery before, during and after the third session of acupuncture. Ten treatments were given in total. Blood flow increased significantly in patients' affected limbs compared with the untreated (unaffected) limb. All but one patient reported an improvement in symptoms. Interestingly, only an improvement in subjective function, not subjective pain, was positively correlated to the increase in blood volume flow (Bar et al 2002).

Acupuncture appears to have the ability to correct abnormally low blood pressure in experimental animals (Sun et al 1983a). These researchers lowered the blood pressure of rats by withdrawing blood. Electroacupuncture was applied to the sciatic nerve simultaneously in the treatment group. This reduced the fall in blood pressure compared with that in untreated controls.

This response has also been investigated in human subjects by several researchers, one of the earliest being Tam & Yiu (1975). In this study 28 patients with essential hypertension were treated with acupuncture: 16 showed excellent improvement in terms of the lowering of blood pressure to normal and the disappearance of original symptoms, eight had a moderate improvement and four showed no response. The results of treatment seem to indicate that improvement is closely related to the duration of disease and history of drug treatment. The selection of acupuncture loci and the techniques of needle insertion and manipulation were discussed in detail, but there was no control group. Also, the descriptions of the results as 'excellent', 'moderate', etc. were not sufficiently objective to draw any definite conclusions.

A more rigorous recent study (Ballegaard et al 1993) found that acupuncture tends to regulate responses towards the norm: high blood pressure is lowered, possibly due to the release of endorphins and serotonin, and low blood pressure is raised, possibly through the release of central acetycholine and vasopressin. These results were highly significant in comparison to placebo. This type of finding tends to support the original Chinese theories that acupuncture has no effect in a healthy person.

Auricular acupuncture has also been shown to have an effect on blood pressure (Gaponjuk & Sherkovina 1994). In a study of 104 patients the haemodynamic influence of each of 16 pairs of auricular acupuncture points was observed in hypertensive patients. Changes in heart rate, stroke output and peripheral vascular resistance were measured, so that the degree of change could be charted for each acupuncture point. It became clear that certain groups of ear points induced a fall in blood pressure by influencing changes in one or more of these cardiac perimeters. The ear has a particularly rich nerve supply derived from several cranial and upper cranial nerves, and it is possible to explain the hypotensive action of specific groups of acupuncture points by reference to their innervation. Branches of the trigeminal, facial, glossopharyngeal, vagus and cervical nerves are all present on the surface of the ear. The researchers claimed that the most effective auricular acupuncture points for hypertensive patients could thus be predicted accurately.

Another study (published in English earlier than the original work) by Gaponjuk et al (1993) involved a simple course of auricular acupuncture performed on 78 patients with stage I–II essential hypertension. A control group of 20 underwent sham electrostimulation. The analysis, according to multiple criteria, which included haemodynamic norms, tolerance to physical load using a static bicycle and arterial pressure, showed reduced symptoms and drug consumption for the electroacupuncture group. This was claimed as further proof of the accuracy of the auricular points identified.

More recently Stener-Victorin et al (1996) used repeated electro-acupuncture treatments applied to points sharing the same segmental innervation as the uterus. This was found to significantly reduce blood flow impedance, suggesting that the effects were due to alterations in sympathetic outflow causing vasodilatation in the uterine vessels.

Cerebral circulation

Litscher et al (1998a) also demonstrated a change in blood flow velocity produced in a cerebral artery in response to acupuncture. Using 12 healthy volunteers, a form of body acupuncture designed to increase Qi, or energy, was given. Measurements were taken before, during and after treatment by means of transcranial Doppler ultrasonography (TCD). The sonography probes allowed three-dimensional imaging and, by using multiscan methods, a significant increase in mean blood flow velocity was measured at different depths of the cerebral artery. This measuring technique has also been used to demonstrate small increases in regional cerebral oxygenation (Litscher et al 1998b).

TCD technology was used in another study in which the effect of a single acupoint on cerebral circulation was measured (Yuan et al 1998). The point in question was GB 20 Fengchi, a point commonly used in the treatment of stroke and stroke sequelae. The blood velocity in the vertebral and basilar arteries was measured in 97 patients before and after bilateral acupuncture at the Fengchi points. In the treatment group of 82 patients, some differentiation was made between patients suffering from different problems: those with high blood flow were given strong stimulation at this point and those with low blood flow were given only mild stimulation. This is in accord with TCM theory. The healthy control group of 15 subjects received acupuncture using a neutral technique. There was a significant difference between the blood flow rates, before and after treatment, in patients with either a high blood flow (mean velocity reduced by 12 cm/s) or a low blood flow (increased by 4.5 cm/s). There was no significant difference in the control group. It would have been interesting to see whether similar changes could be produced by testing other specific acupuncture points, perhaps some of those not indicated by the TCM literature as effective in treating congested cerebral circulation.

Several studies have been performed in China to show the effect of acupuncture on the circulation and composition of blood (Ji et al 1987, Qi 1990, Sun et al 1983b, Zhang 1991). These studies all investigated the action of acupuncture on stroke, and are usually rejected in that context because they were not adequately controlled, using in the main different forms of acupuncture as control. However, the investigations on blood composition, viscosity, flow rate and pressure before and after acupuncture treatment remain valid, showing clear changes and providing food for thought.

Various tests were used: Ji et al (1987) employed an onychographic procedure to look at the microcirculation around the joints of the third finger on both hands in 26 patients. Thirteen of these patients showed signs of stasis and haemorrhage around the joints before treatment; this resolved completely in nine and improved in four. Rheoencephalography showed a reduction in blood clotting factors after treatment, which, the authors suggest, could reduce the risk of microemboli. Blood pressure was also shown to be reduced after a mixture of scalp and body acupuncture treatment.

Other Chinese researchers, Jiao et al (1992), were responsible for a large study of 334 cases of stroke. These were identified as mainly belonging to the TCM syndrome group of 'blood stasis', and the subsequent investigations were aimed at demonstrating changes in circulation that would facilitate a decrease in this 'stagnation' of blood circulation. The viscosity was significantly lower after acupuncture, as was the fibrinogen concentration. Jiao et al examined the microcirculation in the nail folds and demonstrated an improved speed and quantity of blood flow.

Qi (1990) also examined these parameters and observed a significant improvement in blood viscosity with decreased fibrinogen levels after acupuncture. He also noted changes in cholesterol and triglyceride levels in the blood, with a drop after acupuncture. There were 322 subjects in the total study group, but the blood indices were examined only in a matched group of 46 defined as having 'cerebral occlusion'. It is worth noting, however, that these patients received all 45 treatments – a lengthy course of daily treatment, even by Chinese standards.

It is not clear how recent the strokes were in any of the above studies, but it is reasonable to assume that the acupuncture intervention was at least started while the stroke was subacute, probably after 1–2 weeks.

Rian (1993) gave more information on the time since stroke, which ranged from less than 1 month to over 3 years. The 100 patients nearly all improved, but the study compared two forms of acupuncture – body acupuncture and a form of temporal needling – so there was no untreated group as control. Blood rheology was used to determine whole blood viscosity, plasma viscosity, red blood cell electrophoresis and blood sedimentation changes before and after acupuncture treatment. Significant changes ($P < 0.001$) were found in whole blood viscosity, plasma viscosity and white blood cell iontophoresis, with the values tending to normalize. Rian (1993) concluded that acupuncture has an effect on TCM 'blood stasis' and that these results are also interesting from a Western medical point of view, with possible effects on reperfusion of the penumbra.

Neurological damage

Whether acupuncture can affect the spasticity often present in muscles after neurological damage is as yet unknown, but a single interesting study has looked at the effect on spinal motor neuron excitability (Yu et al 1995). The investigation took 16 stroke patients with spastic hemiparesis and evaluated their spinal neuron excitability by measuring the H-reflex recovery time and H-reflex recovery curve. Eleven age-matched normal volunteers were used as a control group. The measures showed that there was increased spinal motor neuron excitability in the paretic limbs in stroke patients, and this decreased significantly after acupuncture, approximating that of the normal controls.

There would appear, as usual, to have been more research on rats and mice than on humans in this field, although one paper discusses both (Si et al 1998). In two studies that ran concurrently, these authors looked at the effect of electroacupuncture on patients with acute cerebral ischaemia and also on rats with middle cerebral arterial occlusion. As this was a controlled trial, the good results obtained clinically with the patients are discussed in the literature review chapter (see Ch. 10). Middle cerebral artery occlusion was accomplished surgically in the 14 rats and the subsequent recovery time of the sensory evoked potential (SEP) measured. Results in the rats suggest that the sooner the electroacupuncture is given after the stroke, the sooner the SEP begins to recover. The SEP in the treated group recovered significantly faster than that of the other group. Si et al (1998) suggest that these results may be extended to humans, but there is a difficulty in transposing acupuncture results from rats to humans because the insertion of acupuncture needles in these small animals is much more traumatic.

The evidence regarding the existence of acupuncture meridians has always been equivocal. The meridians have no morphological counterpart in the peripheral structures, although they may have a functional basis in referred and projected sensations elicited by the stimulation of afferent nerve fibres. The most convincing study was mentioned in Chapter 1, and investigated the pathways of acupuncture meridians by injecting radioactive tracers at acupuncture points (Darras et al 1993). This might indicate that an intact nervous system is not essential for transmission of the acupuncture effect, but no further work has been done on this to date.

The work carried out by both Cho et al (1998) and Wu et al (1999), mentioned in this chapter, indicates links between peripheral acupoints and brain tissue, and reinforces some of the TCM theories. However, more individual points need to be investigated to see whether the response to each point is truly unique or is in fact non-specific.

Effect of acupuncture on muscle tissue

There is a scarcity of evidence that acupuncture has an effect on muscle strength, other than a single German trial (Ludwig 2000). Forty-two sportsmen were examined in an isometric strength test on an isokinetic system linked up with electromyography (EMG); 14 persons received true acupuncture. After tonifying stimulation of two acupuncture points (St 32 Futu and St 36 Zusanli), the quadriceps femoris muscle showed a significant increase in EMG amplitude (on average 29%) and maximum strength (10%) values in the retest. A second group received placebo acupuncture. A control group received no treatment. Both of these groups showed no improvement in the retest. Acupuncture appeared to produce better excitability in tonifying muscle function and enabled the quadriceps muscles to produce a higher performance. However, the statistical analysis of this study was poorly described and baseline differences between the groups were in some instances larger than differences before and after acupuncture. It has been suggested that the circulatory effects of acupuncture may be what contributes to the muscle recovery of affected limbs after stroke (Omura 1975).

Tanaka, who suggested that acupuncture might be beneficial for decreasing functional muscular distortion and improving synergistic coordination, did further work using EMG measures in 30 healthy subjects. However, as only ten subjects in this group actually exhibited asymmetrical paravertebral muscle activity before acupuncture, the conclusion that acupuncture reduced EMG activity in muscles associated with tension headache applies only to this small group (Tanaka et al 1998). A study by Toma et al (1998) assessed the effect of needle stimulation on grip strength as well as on hamstring activity, and claimed a significant increase in EMG responses. However, the methodology was poorly described and the statistical analysis was inadequate.

A few other acupuncture studies have used muscle power as an outcome measure. Two examples are the studies of Hopwood & Lewith (1997) and Naeser et al (1992), who treated chronic stroke patients, although neither produced significant results. Hopwood & Lewith (1997) treated only six chronic stroke patients in a series of case studies, and Naeser et al (1992) treated only 20; both observed an increase in measured muscle power after acupuncture treatment. Hopwood used the Motricity Index, based on the Oxford scale of muscle power, and Naeser used the Boston Motor Inventory test to measure changes in motor power. Naeser also observed the motor pathway areas (the motor cortex and subcortical periventricular white matter area) on computed tomography, and stated that patients in whom these pathways were totally occluded did not improve, whereas those who had only partial occlusion did well with acupuncture treatment. These findings are interesting but, because of the small numbers, not generalizable.

Effect of acupuncture on mood

One of the most troubling side-effects of any illness is clinical depression, particularly in patients with stroke, in whom depression is often thought to delay rehabilitation because motivation is absent (Clark & Smith 1997). Several researchers have investigated the action of acupuncture in general depression. In one of these studies (Luo et al 1985), 47 patients suffering from depression were observed, of whom 27 were treated by electroacupuncture and 20 by the tricyclic antidepressant amitriptyline. Statistical analysis showed the curative effect achieved in the electroacupuncture group to be equal to that in the drug group. Hamilton's Depression Scale was the main outcome measure used. It was notable that no side-effects were observed in the acupuncture group.

Han (1986) showed that the impaired function of monoamine - neurotransmitters in the central nervous system is a major factor in the development of depression. He demonstrated that stimulation with electroacupuncture accelerates the synthesis and release of serotonin, and that the action of acupuncture was similar to that of amitriptyline in depression, with patients treated by acupuncture doing as well as those treated with the drug. He did not observe a significant difference between the two treatments, but remarked that the acupuncture had far fewer side-effects.

As depression is increasingly common in Western society, the use of a modality with an effect similar to amitriptyline without major side-effects could be of considerable clinical use. Another study (Dong 1993) measured Hospital Anxiety and Depression (HAD) scales in 68 patients with chronic conditions before and after 1 month of acupuncture treatment; 42 of 60 anxiety scores and 45 of 50 depression scores returned to normal. These results were statistically significant. There are few details about the actual conditions in this study, but the author recommended the use of acupuncture for psychoemotional problems, making the strong point that acupuncture carries few, if any, side-effects in comparison to the type of drug therapy usually applied to this type of patient.

A more recent study has shown similar results, using acupuncture to treat patients with anxiety disorders or minor depression (Eich et al 2000). However, this study appears to have been seriously underpowered, only using 60 patients in total, when depression and anxiety can take such varying forms. It showed acupuncture as producing a significant clinical improvement, although a form of sham acupuncture was used as a control, suggesting that the effect might have been greater if the non-specific effects of needling could have been ruled out.

Johansson (1995) postulated that the significant results obtained in her acupuncture study of stroke patients might have had more to do with the improvement in patients' mood than any other acupuncture effect. This is certainly a possibility, but because the study was poorly controlled, with the acupuncture patients receiving what they might have perceived to be favoured treatment while the control group had only normal care, it is difficult to be certain.

Andersson (1997), who compares acupuncture to the effect of exercise on the endocrine system and believes that the physiological changes occurring during exercise should help with understanding those of acupuncture, links the effect of acupuncture on mood directly to the increase in endorphin levels. In normal conditions, no or only small effects are seen. 'The natural counterpart to acupuncture is long-lasting physical exercise, which is a stressful situation requiring the body to continually readjust to keep the correct homeostasis.' (Andersson 1997, p 36). According to Andersson, an increase in the β-endorphin level has been observed in brain tissue of animals after both acupuncture and muscle exercise. This endogenous opioid is associated with pain control as well as the regulation of blood pressure and body temperature. It may influence pain sensitivity as well as autonomic functions, eliciting decreased sympathetic tone with vasodilatation and a decreased drive on the heart following the initial excitation.

Serotonin, or 5-HT, release mediates descending pain-inhibiting pathways and may provide an explanation for the longer-lasting effects of acupuncture. Interestingly the analgesic effect of acupuncture is reduced when 5-HT is depleted (Chiang et al 1979), suggesting that when a patient is depressed pain relief acupuncture works less well. However, acupuncture may itself be used to treat that depression (Han 1986).

Another area of research that may impinge on mood is that of oxytocin production during acupuncture. There is little published work on this, but it has been suggested that the known effects of oxytocin release – anxiolytic and sedative effects, reduction in blood pressure, increased pain threshold and a rise in the level of other hormones such as corticosteroids and insulin – closely mirror the changes seen following acupuncture treatment (Uvnas-Moberg et al 1993). These authors further suggest that the autonomic effects of acupuncture could be linked to oxytocin production. As an increased oxytocin concentration is present in situations where human bonding occurs (breastfeeding, for example, or even social drinking with friends), it is reasonable to expect this to have an effect on patient compliance with acupuncture treatment.

Conclusion

Acupuncture is a method of utilizing endogenous mechanisms to influence a variety of body functions. Its effects are often unreliable, because our present knowledge of the control mechanisms is limited and the practice of the method currently rests on tradition rather than on a solid body of scientific research. Certainly, some of the observed reactions including:

- an increase in cerebral blood supply
- decreasing whole-blood viscosity
- an improvement in mood and, possibly, motivation
- change in muscle response
- relief of pain

indicate mechanisms that could be influential in many diseases.

Our understanding of the mechanisms should allow some confidence in treating nociceptive pain segmentally. With more complex pain problems, more focused attempts to influence the sympathetic nervous system may be the answer and may help to explain the success of some TCM prescriptions.

There is considerable scope for further experimental research on the mechanisms and the optimum time for their application before these acupuncture effects can be confidently incorporated into clinical practice. In the meantime, there are grounds for setting up large controlled studies to investigate efficacy further.

Acupuncture analgesia in both animals and humans involves the release of opioid peptides, but they do not appear to be the only transmitter involved – and may not even be the most important. Descending inhibitory control systems employ serotonin at certain stages. However, it does not seem likely that these short-term mechanisms will explain the effect of acupuncture on chronic clinical pain.

Many elegant neurology maps have been suggested to explain the routing of the acupuncture stimulus and most of this research has centred on pain relief. Slowly, the jigsaw puzzle is being assembled with meticulous research into the production and distribution of the known opioid neurotransmitters. So far, there is no single explanation that can be applied to all the acupuncture effects described in clinical practice. This less than precise grasp of the mechanism has a bearing on clinical acupuncture research, ultimately influencing the choice of control in controlled clinical trials.

References

Andersson SA 1979 Pain control by sensory stimulation. In: Bonica JJ, ed. Advances in pain research and therapy, vol. 3. New York: Raven Press; 561–585.

Andersson S 1997 Physiological mechanisms in acupuncture. In: Hopwood V, Lovesey M, Mokone S, eds. Acupuncture and related techniques in physiotherapy. London: Churchill Livingstone; 19–39.

Ballegaard S, Muteki T, Harada H et al 1993 Modulatory effects of acupuncture on the cardiovascular system: a crossover study. Acupuncture and Electro-Therapeutics Research International Journal 18: 103–115.

Bar A, Li Y, Eichlisberger R et al 2002 Acupuncture improves peripheral perfusion in patients with reflex sympathetic dystrophy. Journal of Clinical Rheumatology 8: 6–12.

Bekkring R, van Bussel R 1998 Segmental acupuncture. In: Filshie J, White AR, eds. Medical acupuncture. Edinburgh: Churchill Livingstone; 105–135.

Bensoussan A 1991 The vital meridian, a modern exploration of acupuncture. Melbourne: Churchill Livingstone.

Biella B, Sotgiu M, Pellegata G et al 2001 Acupuncture produces central activations in pain regions. Neuroimage 14: 60–66.

Birch S 2003 Trigger point–acupuncture point correlations revisited. Journal of Alternative and Complementary Medicine 9: 91–103.

Bossut DF, Mayer DJ 1991 Electroacupuncture analgesia in rats: naltrexone antagonism is dependent on previous exposure. Brain Research 549: 47–51.

Cao X, Xu S, Lu W 1983 Inhibition of sympathetic nervous system by acupuncture. Acupuncture and Electro-Therapeutics Research International Journal 8: 25–35.

Chiang CY, Chang CT, Chu HL, Yang LF 1973 Peripheral afferent pathway for acupuncture analgesia. Scientia Sinica 16: 210–217.

Chiang CY, Tu HX, Chao YF et al 1979 Effect of electrolytic or intracerebral injections of 5,6 dihydroxytryptamine in raphe nuclei on acupuncture analgesia in rats. Chinese Medical Journal 92: 129–136.

Cho ZH, Chung SC, Jones JP et al 1998 New findings of the correlation between acupoints and corresponding brain cortices using functional MRI. Proceedings of the National Academy of Sciences USA 95: 2670–2673.

Cho ZH, Lee SH, Hong IK et al 1999 Further evidence for the correlation between acupuncture stimulation and cortical activation. Workshop at New Directions in the Scientific Exploration of Acupuncture, Society for Acupuncture Research, University of California, Irvine, 22 May 1999, pp 1–8.

Clark MS, Smith DN 1997 Abnormal illness behaviour in rehabilitation from stroke. Clinical Rehabilitation 11: 162–170.

Darras JC, Albarede P, de Vernejoul P 1993 Nuclear medicine investigation of transmission of acupuncture information. Acupuncture in Medicine 11: 22–28.

Dong JT 1993 Research on the reduction of anxiety and depression with acupuncture. American Journal of Acupuncture 21: 327–329.

Dundee JW, Ghaly G 1991 Local anaesthesia blocks the antiemetic action of P6 acupuncture. Clinical Pharmacology and Therapeutics 50: 78–80.

Dundee JW, Chestnutt WN, Ghaly RG, Lynas AGA 1986 Traditional Chinese acupuncture: a potentially useful antiemetic? British Medical Journal 293: 583–584.

Dyrehag LE, Widerstrom-Noga EG, Carlsson SG, Andersson SA 1997 Effects of repeated sensory stimulation sessions (electro-acupuncture) on skin temperature in chronic pain patients. Scandinavian Journal of Rehabilitation Medicine 29: 243–250.

Eich H, Agelink MW, Lehmann E et al 2000 Acupuncture in patients with minor depressive episodes and generalised anxiety. Fortschritte der Neurologie-Psychiatrie 68: 137–144.

Filshie J, White A 1998 Medical acupuncture, a Western scientific approach. Edinburgh: Churchill Livingstone.

Gaponjuk PJ, Sherkovina TJ 1994 The clinical and physiological foundation of auricular acupuncture therapy in patients with hypertensive disease. Acupuncture in Medicine 12: 2–5.

Gaponjuk PJ, Sherkovina TJ, Leonova MV 1993 Clinical effectiveness of auricular acupuncture treatment of patients with hypertensive disease. Acupuncture in Medicine 11: 29–31.

Han JS 1986 Electroacupuncture: an alternative to antidepressents for treating affective diseases? International Journal of Neuroscience 29: 79–92.

Han JS 2001 Opioid and antiopioid peptides: a model of Yin–Yang balance in acupuncture mechanisms of pain modulation. In Stux G, Hammerschlag R, eds. Clinical acupuncture, scientific basis. Berlin: Springer; 51–68.

Han JS, Terenius L 1982 Neurochemical basis of acupuncture analgesia. Annual Review of Pharmacology and Toxicology 22: 193–220.

Hashimoto T, Aikawa S 1993 Needling effects on nociceptive neurons in rat spinal cord. Proceedings of the Seventh World Congress on Pain, IASP, p 428.

Holaday JW 1983 Cardiovascular effects of endogenous opiate systems. Annual Review of Pharmalogy and Toxicology 23: 541–591.

Hopwood V, Lewith G 1997 The effect of acupuncture on the motor recovery of the upper limb after stroke. Physiotherapy 83: 614–619.

Hsieh JC, Tu CH, Chen FP et al 2001 Activation of the hypothalamus characterizes the acupuncture stimulation at the analgesic point in human: a positron emission tomography study. Neuroscience Letters 307: 105–108.

Ji N, Xian Y, Ran X et al 1987 A study on the mechanism of acupuncture therapy in the treatment of sequelae of cerebrovascular accident or cerebral injury. Journal of Traditional Chinese Medicine 7: 165–168.

Jiao X, Chang X, Yin K, Gao Y 1992 Clinical and experimental studies on acupuncture therapy of stroke-related blood stasis. International Journal of Clinical Acupuncture 3: 231–241.

Johansson BB 1995 Acupuncture in stroke rehabilitation. Acupuncture in Medicine 13: 81–85.

Le Bars D, Villaneuva L, Willer JC, Bouhassira D 1991 Diffuse noxious inhibitory control (DNIC) in man and animals. Acupuncture in Medicine 9: 47–57.

Litscher G, Wang L 1999 Thermographic visualisation of changes in peripheral perfusion during acupuncture. Biomedizinische Technik (Berlin) 44: 129–134.

Litscher G, Schwarz G, Sandner-Kiesling A, Hadolt I 1998a Robotic transcranial Doppler sonography probes and acupuncture. International Journal of Neuroscience 95: 1–15.

Litscher G, Schwarz G, Sandner-Kiesling A et al 1998b Effects of acupuncture on the oxygenation of cerebral tissue. Neurological Research 20 (Suppl 1): 528–532.

Ludwig M 2000 Influence of acupuncture on the performance of the quadriceps muscle. Deutsche Zeitschrift fur Akupunktur 43: 104–107.

Luo H, Jia Y, Zhan L 1985 Electro-acupuncture VS. Amitriptyline in the treatment of depressive states. Journal of Traditional Chinese Medicine 5: 3–8.

Macdonald A 1989 Acupuncture analgesia and therapy. In: Wall PD, Melzack R, eds. Textbook of pain, 2nd edn. London: Churchill Livingstone; 906–919.

Mann F 1971 Acupuncture. Random House.

Mann F 1992 Re-inventing acupuncture: a new concept of Ancient Medicine. Oxford: Butterworth-Heinemann.

Melzack R, Stillwell DM, Fox EJ 1977 Trigger points and acupuncture points for pain: correlations and implications. Pain 3: 3–23.

Naeser MA, Alexander M, Stiassny-Eder D et al 1992 Real versus sham acupuncture in the treatment of paralysis in acute stroke patients: a CT scan lesion site study. Journal of Neurologic Rehabilitation 6: 163–173.

NIH Consensus Development Panel on Acupuncture 1998 Acupuncture. Journal of the American Medical Association 280: 1518–1524.

Omura Y 1975 Pathophysiology of acupuncture treatment: effects of acupuncture on cardiovascular and nervous systems. Acupuncture and Electro-Therapeutics Research International Journal 1: 51–141.

Pomeranz B 1991 The scientific basis of acupuncture. In: Stux G, Pomeranz B, eds. Basics of acupuncture. Berlin: Springer; 5–55.

Pomeranz B 1996 Scientific research into acupuncture for the relief of pain. Journal of Alternative and Complementary Medicine 2: 53–60.

Qi LY 1990 Observation on acupuncture treatment of 322 cases of cerebral infarction and changes in serum HDL-C fibrinogen, FDP, hemorrheological indices etc during treatment. International Journal of Clinical Acupuncture 1: 39–46.

Rian L 1993 Clinical observation and experimental studies on the treatment of sequelae of stroke by needling temporal points. International Journal of Clinical Acupuncture 4: 19–26.

Sato A, Schmidt RF 1973 Somatosympathetic reflexes: afferent fibers, central pathways, discharge characteristics. Physiological Reviews 53: 916–947.

Si Q, Wu G, Cao X 1998 Effects of electro-acupuncture on acute cerebral infarction. Acupuncture and Electro-Therapeutics Research International Journal 23: 117–124.

Stener-Victorin E, Waldenstrom U, Andersson S, Wikland M 1996 Reduction of blood flow impedance in the uterine arteries of infertile women with electro-acupuncture. Human Reproduction 11: 1314–1317.

Sun XY, Yu J, Yao T 1983a Pressor effect produced by stimulation of somatic nerve on hemorrhagic hypotension in conscious rats. Acta Physiologica Sinica 35: 264–270.

Sun S, Li S, Zhu Y et al 1983b Clinical study on 500 cases of cerebro-vascular hemiplegia treated by acupuncture through Baihui to Qubin. Journal of Traditional Chinese Medicine 5: 167–170.

Takeshige C 2001 Mechanisms of acupuncture analgesia produced by low frequency electrical stimulation. In: Stux G, Hammerschlag R, eds. Clinical acupuncture, scientific basis. Berlin: Springer; 29–50.

Takeshige C, Oka K, Mizuno T et al 1993 The acupuncture point and its connecting central pathway for producing acupuncture analgesia. Brain Research Bulletin 30: 53–67.

Tam KC, Yiu HH 1975 The effect of acupuncture on essential hypertension. Americal Journal of Chinese Medicine 3: 369–375.

Tanaka TH, Leisman G, Nishijo K 1998 Dynamic electromyographic response following acupuncture: possible influence on synergistic coordination. International Journal of Neuroscience 95: 51–61.

Toma K, Conatser RR, Gilders RM, Hagerman FC 1998 The effects of acupuncture needle stimulation on skeletal muscle activity and performance. Journal of Strength and Conditioning Research 12: 253–257.

Uvnas-Moberg K, Bruzelius G, Alster P, Lundeberg T 1993 The antinociceptive effect of non-noxious sensory stimulation is mediated partly through oxytocinergic mechanisms. Acta Physiologica Scandinavica 149: 199–204.

Vincent CA, Richardson PH 1986 The evaluation of therapeutic acupuncture. Concepts and method. Pain 24: 1–13.

Wang KM, Yao SM, Xian YL, Hou Z 1985 A study of the receptive field of acupoints and the relationship between characteristics of needling sensation and groups of afferent fibres. Scientia Sinica 28: 963–971.

White A 1999 Neurophysiology of acupuncture analgesia. In: Ernst E, White A, eds. Acupuncture: a scientific appraisal. Oxford: Butterworth Heinemann; 60–92.

Wu MT, Hsieh JC, Xiong J et al 1999 Central nervous pathway for acupuncture stimulation: localisation of processing with functional MR imaging of the brain – preliminary experience. Radiology 212: 133–141.

Wu M, Sheen J, Chuang K et al 2002 Neuronal specificity of acupuncture response: a fMRI study with electroacupuncture. Neuroimage 16: 1028.

Yu Y, Wang H, Wang Z 1995 The effect of acupuncture on spinal motor neuron excitability in stroke patients. Chinese Medical Journal (Taipei) 56: 258–263.

Yuan X, Hao Z, Lai H et al 1998 Effects of acupuncture at Fengchi point (GB 20) on cerebral blood flow. Journal of Traditional Chinese Medicine 18: 102–105.

Zhang D 1991 Effects of moxibustion on impedance rhoencephalogram and blood pressure in patients with hemiplegia due to apoplexy. International Journal of Clinical Acupuncture 2: 137–140.

Zhaowei M, Zongxiang Z, Xianglong H 1985 Progress in the research of meridian phenomena in China during the last five years. Journal of Traditional Chinese Medicine 5: 145–152.

Acupuncture trials and methodological considerations

KEY CONCEPTS

☯ Acupuncture research is not always straightforward.
☯ Formulating the question clearly is vital.
☯ The exact question dictates the methodology (qualitative or quantitative) and the type of control in the quantitative research.
☯ Specifying the precise type of traditionally based acupuncture is essential to ensure the possibility of replication.
☯ When reading or writing papers, the STRICTA recommendations should be borne in mind.
☯ There is no fundamental reason why careful acupuncture research should not be scientifically acceptable.

Introduction

Acupuncture has a rich and lengthy history, and an extensive body of literature that began around 200 BC, continuing to the present day. Much practice in China and the West has been based largely on the ancient published texts, principally Huang Di Nei Jing Su Wen ('The Classic of the Yellow Emperor'), Huang Di Nei Jing Ling Shu ('Pivotal Questions') and the Nan Jing (circa AD 100) and their many commentaries.

It would be wrong to categorize these approaches as unquestioning acceptance of archaic beliefs. Indeed, the essence of written Traditional Chinese Medicine (TCM) is question and answer, continually extending a debate as to the action of the various points, meridians and techniques. It could be considered a 'consensus medicine'. This has not been good enough to gain unquestioning acceptance in the West, but the vast legacy of empirical data has inspired enthusiastic research in recent years. Nevertheless, nearly 30 years of acupuncture research have failed to demonstrate clinical efficacy beyond doubt (Moroz 1999). This is not because there has been little research – on the contrary, there has been a great deal of research, some of a good standard – but because the essential characteristics of this form of therapy make it difficult to assess its specific effect in experimental clinical studies.

Problems with research methodology have been an important reason for the slow acceptance of acupuncture in the West. The accepted 'gold standard' – the double-blind placebo-controlled randomized clinical trial – is fraught with complications as far as acupuncture is concerned. One of

A version of this chapter was first published in Hopwood & Lewith (2003). Acknowledgements are due to Dr George Lewith for his contribution.

the main difficulties arises from the fact that acupuncture treatment is rooted in a very different tradition, involving different concepts of physiology and diagnostics (Zang Fu, Eight Principles). For instance, the diagnostic process in Oriental Medicine often defines several subgroup patterns within one recognized medical condition, which may or may not correspond to that defined in Western medicine. Each subgroup or syndrome is said to require a slightly different combination of acupuncture points. Good traditional acupuncture would be expected to modify point selection further as the condition progressed or improved, possibly also modifying the needling technique and adding allied techniques such as electro-acupuncture and moxibustion.

Acupuncture treatment, like many of the treatments employed within complementary and alternative medicine, is individualized. This necessarily makes the evaluation of such treatments difficult, but not impossible, within the context of randomized controlled trials. Blinding (both patients and practitioners), randomization and the use of an appropriate placebo or control are fundamental to the structure of good-quality explanatory clinical trials that differentiate specific from non-specific treatment effects. These both have enormous problems for the development of acupuncture research, some of which may be almost insoluble. This chapter explores some of the issues, focusing particularly on the problem of acupuncture controls and types of trial design.

General considerations

What is good acupuncture?

If one is examining the effect of 'good' acupuncture, it becomes necessary to avoid a rigid recipe of points for a single biomedical diagnosis because the dynamic nature of the therapy would preclude this kind of application. 'Clinical trial designs cannot easily accommodate individualised treatments, yet requiring all patients to be treated at the same set of acupuncture points may seriously under-evaluate the efficacy of the treatment being assessed.' (Hammerschlag 1998, p 160).

The application of scientific protocols to acupuncture research brings, as a logical consequence, a dependence on easily repeatable 'formulae' and therefore an emphasis on musculoskeletal pain problems, as these are most frequently treated in a formulaic manner. This has also led to the avoidance of conditions for which these formulae are not so applicable, because the practised acupuncturist would expect to be changing the prescription at almost every treatment. As the relatively simple musculoskeletal approach is most effective in pain management, this partly explains why the bulk of research has been into pain alleviation. Another possible reason for the popularity of research into this type of problem is that the fundamental outcome measure (i.e. pain or no pain) is relatively easy to quantify compared with the slow and fluctuating progress in a neurological disorder such as stroke where there are many more variables. Clinical work on acupuncture and pain relief has also been underpinned by the discovery of the naloxone-reversible production of endorphins in acupuncture analgesia (Cheng & Pomeranz 1980) (see Ch. 9).

Most practitioners now agree that the acupuncture points are probably not fixed entities, but simply areas where the nervous system is signalling that it needs to be stimulated. Points are not always selected for treatment on the basis of an energy 'imbalance' or 'blockage', but sometimes because they lie over known trigger points or are in a particular segment. However, some points still have only empirical evidence and clinical experience to substantiate the claims made for their actions, with no physiological explanation as yet discovered (e.g. St 38 for chronic shoulder pain). Functional magnetic resonance imaging may be a rich future source of evidence here (Cho et al 1998).

Traditionally based systems of acupuncture, as defined by Stephen Birch (1997, p 148) 'utilize the languages and concepts derived from the historical texts of acupuncture. Terms and concepts such as "yin-yang", "jing-luo", "xang-fu" and "qi" are used by each system but in different patterns, to describe both normal and abnormal physiology, treatment principles and targets.' Thus, it is also necessary to define precisely which traditional system (and which technique) is being evaluated, in order to avoid subsequent confusion among practitioners and ensure precise repeatability.

Placebos

Most medical research programmes involve the rigorous testing of pharmaceuticals. It is usually possible to construct double-blinded situations where neither the patient nor the assessor is aware which is the placebo intervention or drug, thus ensuring that patient and practitioner expectations are not a confounding factor. Obviously this is much more difficult in acupuncture because, as the name itself implies, the most evident thing about an acupuncture treatment is the actual insertion of needles into the body. It would, indeed, be possible to grade the depth of insertion, given that a deep insertion with a definite accompanying sensation is required by traditional acupuncture, were it not for the fact that any kind of needle insertion will trigger off the reactions in the skin and tissues that result in part of the acupuncture effect. This is termed 'diffuse noxious inhibitory control' (Le Bars et al 1991). Not enough is yet known about the reactions initiated by this form of sensory stimulation to be able to isolate the individual effects or, in fact, guarantee that any intervention involving skin contact would be sufficiently inert to produce no response at all. The Japanese style of acupuncture offers a further complication. Apparently excellent results are obtained with only a subdermal insertion within this acupuncture tradition.

It would be valuable to have a clearer idea of 'dosage', but little work has been done in this field. A formula for calculating this, correlating to the inflammatory response, was put forward by Marcus (1994), but remains speculative. Marcus acknowledges the difficulty of taking into account the variations of technique and depth of insertion, and does not tackle the thorny issue of DeQi, or needling sensation.

Blinding

Blinding is problematic in acupuncture trials. Single-blind clinical trials do not eliminate the Rosenthal effect (Rosenthal 1976). The use of sham acupuncture, either with or without skin penetration, as a control is probably effective in maintaining the 'blind' status of patients, but not that of the non-blinded researcher, who may still influence the outcome. Furthermore, although it is theoretically possible to blind the therapist to the validity, or otherwise, of the acupuncture, this may confound the result because the patient–practitioner relationship may be compromised. This relationship may be an important one, influencing the treatment outcome. This has been done in some unpublished trials where untrained therapists were told which points to needle after the patient had been examined by a qualified acupuncturist. The potential of this could be explored further.

Blinding can be applied to four components in a randomized controlled clinical trial: the patient, the operator, the assessor and the statistician. The Jadad scale, frequently applied in systematic reviews, evaluates blinding solely for the patient–therapist interface, the typical situation in a drug trial. However, there is an argument for stating all the blinding achievable within an acupuncture trial and perhaps assessing the quality more completely in relation to those variables.

Crossover

A further complication arises when controlled crossover trials are planned. Acupuncture appears to continue to work after the needles are extracted and often for some time after the completion of treatment. Where a course of acupuncture treatment is given under research conditions, sufficient time must be allowed after this for the effect to diminish naturally before commencing with the control intervention. An early trial assessing the effect of acupuncture on chronic facial pain (Hansen & Hansen 1983) took this into account with an initial pretreatment period of 4 weeks, acupuncture treatment for 2 weeks and then a 'washout' period of 4 weeks before using placebo acupuncture for 2 weeks followed by a further 4 weeks' post-treatment. The study showed the acupuncture to have a clear positive effect.

Chinese research

There is, indeed, a vast wealth of acupuncture research material available from Chinese researchers. Many clinical trials have been conducted in China to evaluate the effectiveness of TCM, but much of the information is inaccessible to Western doctors. A recent review of this body of work, 2938 randomized controlled clinical trials in total, was undertaken (Tang et al 1999), but the overall quality was found to be poor, many being published only as reports with no detail. Effectiveness was rarely expressed quantitatively, blinding was rare, and only short-term outcomes were reported.

Most Chinese trials are very large and could be expected to contribute greatly to our knowledge were it not for the fact that they rarely use a control. It is considered unethical to withhold acupuncture in circumstances where clinical experience indicates that it is effective. Hence most acupuncture trials in China compare different forms of acupuncture, but do not have a group that does not receive it. Any results would become truly significant only if it could be shown that this did not happen without either type of acupuncture intervention.

Some possible solutions

Selection of controls

It is useful to consider the varying types of acupuncture research projects published to date and examine the structures and inherent problems shown, particularly with regard to the many different types of control selected. These can be broadly identified as:

- no treatment, or waiting list
- normal treatment
- some other tested and validated modality
- sham acupuncture, no penetration
- true acupuncture at alternative sites
- superficial or inappropriate needling
- deactivated alternatives.

No treatment, or waiting list

A patient population on a documented and controlled waiting list has been seen as ideal for testing many treatment modalities, but is justifiable only when the condition under test is a chronic, relatively stable, one. It will certainly be useful for assessing the level of spontaneous remission and is considered as an ethical alternative to a controlled trial where treatment is sometimes withheld. Acupuncture trials using this form of control have dealt with non-life-threatening conditions such as low back pain (Coan et al 1980), neck pain (Coan et al 1982) and osteoarthritis (Christensen et al 1992). In the first trial (Coan et al 1980) an attempt was made to control for possible spontaneous remission by offering acupuncture treatment after 8 weeks to the waiting list group, and comparing the outcome in both groups to that in patients who had no intervention.

The main problem with this type of design is that it does not control for placebo effects or for non-specific responses to needling. An additional problem is that nocebo effects (possible patient-engendered negative effects) are also not controlled. In addition, it is not possible to compare the effects of acupuncture with those of other treatments.

Alternative treatment

This type of clinical research design is sometimes called a positive control trial. In this type of study acupuncture treatment is compared to another form of biomedical intervention; this could be as precise as a transcutaneous electrical nerve stimulation (TENS) to the same points as are needled in the acupuncture, or as generically vague as 'physiotherapy' which could, in practice, be any one of a number of modalities, some of which may work through similar mechanisms to those of acupuncture. It is necessary for this other form of intervention to have been shown previously to be more effective than placebo; the effects must have been researched, measured and established. In this case, a control group for the acupuncture is not required. There is considerable ethical appeal in this form of trial, as all patients are seen to receive treatment. One drawback with this option is the possibility that differences in results between the compared modalities would not be large and therefore a considerable number of participants would be required for the study results to achieve statistical significance (Moore et al 1998).

The demonstration of acupuncture efficacy in this type of trial lies not in outperforming a control intervention but in performing at least as well as standard care and, possibly, demonstrating advantages over it. Perhaps the greatest disadvantage of this type of trial is that neither the patients nor the practitioners can be blinded, so the success of the trial will rely on the fact that the assessors are not aware of the form of treatment given. Great care must therefore be taken with the structure of assessment sessions, with patients being prevented from entering into conversation with the assessors with regard to the form of treatment received. Expectations of patients may also be involved in this type of trial (Shen et al 1997). On becoming aware that they have been selected for 'normal' care and not the modality under test, there may be disappointment. This can be tackled by offering treatment to all patients at the end of the study. Then the ethical issue is only whether the patient's condition is likely to deteriorate seriously.

It is possible to make direct comparisons with the conventional treatment with regard to cost, side-effects, duration of treatment and time of onset. A systematic review of this type of trial showed generally poor results for acupuncture, but acknowledged the difficulty of comparing widely varying research protocols (Hammerschlag & Morris 1997). In the 23 studies selected for the review, many forms of control intervention were used: TENS was used in seven studies, drug therapy in 11, standard physiotherapy or occupational therapy in one, and several forms of dental splint in three studies on facial or dental pain.

A good example of this type of trial (Berman et al 1999) investigated 73 patients with osteoarthritis of the knee who were randomized into two groups, one of which was given 'standard care' and the other acupuncture in addition to the standard care. After 12 weeks patients in the control group were offered acupuncture, and the results were compared with those of the original experimental group. This is ethically satisfactory as both groups received treatment and both were, eventually, treated with acupuncture if they desired it. No placebo control group was used, however, and this did not enable the study to explore non-specific effects, such as physician attention, interest and concern. One advantage of this type of trial, where the design is A + B versus B alone, is the ease with which it can be modified into a three-arm trial.

A controlled study of acupuncture in relation to medication for chemotherapy-induced nausea (Shen et al 1997) showed that the acupuncture group did best; however, a third group receiving sham acupuncture plus medication benefited to an intermediate extent. This allows a measure to be made of the total benefit of the acupuncture treatment.

Another way of tackling this problem has been demonstrated in Japan. Here, the patients use their acupuncturist on a regular basis and withholding acupuncture treatment is not an ethical option, as in the Republic of China. A recent trial (Kawakita 2001) screened large numbers of patients for a specific acupuncture diagnosis and randomized identified patients to a treatment group. The remainder were treated for whatever else was wrong with them. This is not an ideal trial construction, but it does allow measures to be made on a control population also receiving acupuncture and, presumably, showing physiological changes too, even if not within the precise parameters of the core trial group.

Sham acupuncture

Sham acupuncture is a somewhat misleading term as a needle is either inserted into the skin or it is not, so that it is obvious whether or not acu*puncture* has occurred. Sham acupuncture is considered under this heading as a non-invasive technique.

For obvious reasons it is possible to use sham acupuncture as a control only in acupuncture-naive patients. It is also much better to use it when the patient is not able to see the area of skin being treated, and this technique has therefore been proposed for the treatment of back and neck problems. Some light stimulation of the skin is involved: a light tap over a bony area or gentle pressure on the skin from a blunt object. A relatively recent example is the study published by White et al (1996), in which a blunted cocktail stick was used in an acupuncture guide tube in a study of head and neck pain. The immediate drawback of this study design is that any true acupuncture treatment of pain in these areas should involve the use of visible distal points on the hands or feet, so the acupuncture itself will be artificially limited to points that are are out of view.

One way to overcome this is to blindfold the patient for the duration of the treatment (Lao et al 1995). In this study of pain after dental extraction the true acupuncture was administered by using needles with a guide tube, and the control involved merely tapping with the same type of tube. Both the needle and the tube were subsequently lightly taped in place. As the patients were unable to see what was happening, they rated this as a credible form of treatment, with a high proportion of control patients guessing that they had received acupuncture.

Other forms of 'sham' acupuncture that have been proposed include tapping a toothpick on the skin, using just a plastic applicator tube (with an unsighted patient) or using a press needle with the point removed. If the latter is pressed on to the skin and secured with a piece of opaque plaster, the slight sensation is quite convincing to the patient (Filshie & Cummings 1999).

The concept of a non-acupuncture needle has resulted in some interesting ideas. Streitberger & Kleinhenz (1998) developed a 'placebo' acupuncture needle using insertion tubes and a shortened needle. The blunted needle retreats partially into the handle, rather like a stage dagger. This, like the modified press needle, is yet to be used in a major acupuncture trial, although some interesting work has been published on rotator cuff shoulder injuries in athletes. In this study, true needling was shown to be more effective than the sham needling, although the patients were not aware of the different needles used (Kleinhenz et al 1999). Another needle that operates on the same principles but with a much smaller adhesive base is the Park acupuncture needle (Park et al 1999). This needle is also not yet fully validated but shows promising results where patients appear unable to distinguish between this and an invasive needle.

Minimal acupuncture or selected points

This is the use of invasive but inappropriate needling. It may be of a different type (e.g. shallow as opposed to deep needling) or may just be in another part of the body. It may utilize known acupuncture points, either out of the area or with different recorded clinical effects, or areas of skin that are not designated acupuncture points or not situated on the course of the meridians. It is also, as mentioned previously, frequently confused with sham needling. In a survey of 70 clinical trials (Hammerschlag 1998), 22 used what was termed 'sham' needling, varying the site and depth of the needles. This is more logically defined as inappropriate or alternative needling.

A good example of this is the study of tension headache undertaken by Tavola et al (1992). In the treatment group of 15 patients six to ten needles were inserted 10–20 mm into points established by 'energy status' according to TCM, and in the placebo group the same number of needles was used but inserted only 2–4 mm in the same regions but not into defined acupuncture points. The frequency of the headaches and the analgesic consumption in both groups decreased significantly over time, but not the duration or intensity of the headaches. However, there was no significant difference between the true acupuncture and the placebo, indicating the difficulty of ruling out associated effects from any form of needling (Tavola et al 1992).

The most obvious drawback with this type of control is that the use of previously untested 'sham' points could result in false conclusions and misrepresentation of the real efficacy of acupuncture. Assuming that the placebo effect is the same for both treatment and control groups, but that the effect of the alternative needling points was negative to the effect being researched, a perceived positive effect for the true acupuncture could be masked. It is essential that the effects of minimal or inappropriate acupuncture on the variables measured are known before the trial.

Use of shallow needling was demonstrated to be less effective than classical deep needling in a study on epicondylalgia (Haker & Lundeberg 1990). This form of minimal needling triggers all the non-specific effects but could be supposed to minimize the specific actions of acupuncture points. It is certainly rated by patients as a credible form of control, as they are not likely to be aware of the distinction between the two (Vincent 1989).

Using shallow needling for a control has serious drawbacks. Japanese acupuncture techniques are customarily shallow in nature and some 'controls' in major studies would appear to have as good a chance of being a valid treatment as the technique under test, particularly if valid acupuncture points are being treated this way.

This type of control was demonstrated in a study of the acupuncture effect on disabling breathlessness (Jobst et al 1986). In this study both groups received a form of acupuncture, with appropriate chest points needled in the treatment group and sham points over the patella, with no possible effect on the lungs, selected in the control group. It is not possible to rule out the non-specific effects of these points, however. A variation on this type of control used alternative points in the same area of the body – the ear – in both groups of patients (Bullock et al 1989). Here the points used as non-specific points were differentiated by their electrical signature: all the true points registered more than 50 µA and the non-points registered zero when a potential difference detector was applied. This was necessary to distinguish one location from another in such a small body area. A hand point, LI 4 Hegu, was also used in the treatment group, whereas the control group received a non-specific point that was much easier to locate. The treatment group did significantly better than the control group, adding fuel to the debate over whether ear acupuncture is effective only because of the proximity of the points to the vagus nerve.

Table 10.1 shows the essential differences between invasive, inappropriate acupuncture and non-invasive alternatives, with only true acupuncture providing all the possible effects.

Table 10.1 Components of the acupuncture response triggered by placebo or sham controls (after Hammerschlag 1998)

Type of treatment	Placebo effect	Non-specific needle effect	Specific effects of acupuncture
Placebo, non-invasive	✓		
Inappropriate invasive procedures	✓	✓	
Acupuncture	✓	✓	✓

Deactivated alternatives

To assess placebo effects, a non-invasive procedure must be devised that is both credible to the patients and completely inert. The use of TENS machines seems to be successful: adhesive electrodes attached to acupuncture points with a flashing light or buzzing sound is rated as a credible treatment by patients (Vincent & Lewith 1995, Wood & Lewith 1998), and the use of credibility ratings (Borkovec & Nau 1972) is recommended to ensure the acceptability of the placebo intervention (Vincent 1990). Deactivated therapeutic laser units can also be used. Application of the treatment head, provided there is some evidence of activity (light or a sound) to acupuncture points provides a credible alternative to acupuncture treatment for patients in the control group. As these forms of therapy are becoming increasingly familiar to the patient population, this may also enhance their acceptance – not as an exact substitute for acupuncture, but as a credible alternative treatment. There is an ethical dimension to this, however, and informed patient consent may be difficult.

There is also considerable opposition. Ter Riet et al (1990) have stated that this type of control is 'fatally flawed' because it is so obviously different to needling. The use of deactivated alternatives does have some validation, however, and this type of control continues to be used (Lewith & Machin 1983).

Pragmatic trials

A pragmatic acupuncture trial is often considered to be a fairer test of the modality, indicating the effectiveness of day-to-day practice (MacPherson et al 1999). Pragmatic trials seek to assess the effectiveness of the whole treatment process and can be used to answer questions on both the efficacy and the cost-effectiveness in comparison to conventional treatment. The acupuncture is not limited by the constraints of the protocol and more closely resembles that given to patients in real life, outside research programmes. This is also more likely to mirror 'best practice' in TCM terms. It is also possible to tackle more complex, chronic problems with multiple pathology in this way.

One of the disadvantages (or advantages) of the classic randomized clinical trial is that it can be applied more effectively to a simple acute problem with a clear endpoint. Practitioner involvement is also limited, because it is important that all interventions are standardized for easier measurement and subsequent repeatability. In real life, many patients seek acupuncture treatment for chronic conditions without a quick cure.

The patient has a distinct element of choice in this type of trial, and the relationship with the practitioner becomes more important. A pragmatic trial allows the practitioner the freedom to deal professionally with these situations and, if carefully organized, can allow for and analyse the differences between practitioners who are nonetheless working within the same traditionally based system of acupuncture (MacPherson et al 1999).

Local anaesthetic prior to needling

Injections of local anaesthetic given before needling have been shown to block both the anaesthetic (Chiang et al 1973) and the antiemetic (Dundee & Ghaly 1991) effects of acupuncture. Where the effect under test is not point specific, it would be interesting to see whether this would have any bearing on the results: 'If the absorption characteristics of topical anaesthetics for the skin (LA) can be improved, inactive LA cream plus real needling versus active LA cream plus real needling may be a credible design which would take into account the non specific effects of needling' (Filshie & Cummings 1999). This is at present only speculative, and has not been widely used.

Conclusion

The purpose of this chapter was to explore the area of appropriate placebo or controls in the context of explanatory clinical acupuncture research (Table 10.2). It is evident that, so far, there is no universal answer and the specific controls identified above require further evaluation if we wish to

Table 10.2 Summary of acupuncture trials methods and their purposes (after Lewith & Vincent 1998)

Control	Description	Question addressed
No treatment, waiting list	Observation only	Rate of spontaneous remission; does not account for placebo effect
Alternative treatment	Documented modality with action on condition – physiotherapy?	Comparison with control modality; does acupuncture have any advantage?
Sham acupuncture, no penetration	Activity on skin surface only; patient must be unsighted or needles covered	Could the effects be due to either DNIC or acupuncture?
Minimal acupuncture	Superficial insertion	If the effect is due to DNIC there will be no significant difference
Selected points	Points outside area, not lying on meridian or with other action	Is 'true' acupuncture more effective than the control?
Deactivated alternative	Sham TENS or laser, or interferential therapy	Is acupuncture more effective than placebo?
Pragmatic trial	Free choice of points, 'true' acupuncture	Is 'true' acupuncture more effective than other modalities?
Local anaesthetic	Applied locally before needling	Which of the non-specific effects are effective?

DNIC, diffuse noxious inhibitory control.

ask whether acupuncture has a specific effect. It may be that the ideal investigation will need to be divided into stages, answering one question at a time.

In general, when designing a randomized controlled clinical trial in acupuncture, the following points should be considered:

- The question asked should be clear and the study carefully constructed with this in mind. This will have a direct bearing on the form of control chosen.
- It must also be quite clear what the control is intended to do and, if necessary, the non-specific effects must be addressed.
- The outcome measures must have been validated previously, and must allow for the natural evolution of both the condition and the type of treatment.
- Clear, detailed acupuncture protocols should be used to enable exact repetition of the trial. The rationale for the acupuncture approach must be explained.
- Precisely described randomization should be used to balance the treatment groups as far as possible.
- Single-blind trials are essential, as better techniques are found for blinding patients to the reality of acupuncture needling; double-blind trials may be possible.
- The degree of blinding should in any case be clearly stated.
- Adverse reactions and dropouts must be recorded carefully.
- There should be detailed and prolonged follow-up; time should be used as an endpoint variable.

Acupuncturists have recognized the research problems and have been active in combatting them. Systematic reviews with discouraging results have caused much discomfort and the Standards for Reporting Interventions in Controlled Trials of Acupuncture (STRICTA) guidelines have been evolved as a very useful tool for assessing the validity of the acupuncture used (MacPherson et al 2002). These guidelines do not involve evaluation of the other aspects of a study, but do provide a clear framework for reporting the exact acupuncture procedures undertaken. Where the details are lacking or the acupuncture is clearly substandard, the quality of the evidence may be questioned.

The final word goes to Birch & Felt (2000):

Whoever designs these trials designs the future of acupuncture. Acupuncture will become what it can be statistically proved to do. If these trials are accomplished by biomedicine, any of its subspecialities or mid-level professions, parts of acupuncture will almost certainly be subsumed and attached as techniques to biomedicine. Were the procedures thus established to prove cost-effective, the pressure brought to bear by insurers could be intense – remember the figures for chronic pain and that pain is already a common target of insurance and HMO-sponsored clinical trials. So, although there is no present attack on acupuncture's status quo, and it seems very unlikely that there will be any successful challenge to acupuncturist's right to practice, neither is there any obvious guarantee that the present practitioner population will continue to be exclusive providers of acupuncture. Consid-

ering these possibilities, the inescapable need for scientific proof should not be taken as "bad news". It is in the realm of science that acupuncture is most equal. It is there that the rules are most standard for all. It is there that the unfairness of judging one practice by the methods of another can be addressed. It is there that it will be easiest for acupuncture to join to the mainstream. It is there that a single scientific paper can change the minds of many. Compared to the brute force of politics, the vast power of economic interest, the intellectual realm is easily moved. Compared to moving the interests entrenched in the economics of medical treatment, the cost of controlled clinical trials is small. Of all the places in Western culture where acupuncture could be required to compete, medical science is the one where two millennia of marketplace survival make it best prepared.

The dilemma for acupuncture practitioners engaged in research remains. As the research becomes more rigorous, the number of positive studies seems to be diminishing. It is difficult to envisage the history of acupuncture as one long application of placebo; it is more likely that the questions are still not being formulated quite carefully enough. As a scientifically trained acupuncture practitioner, I remain optimistic and I am also sure that some of the answers will surprise us all.

References

Berman BM, Singh BB, Lao L et al 1999 A randomized trial of acupuncture as an adjunctive therapy in osteoarthritis of the knee. Rheumatology 38: 346–354.

Birch S 1997 Testing the claims of traditionally based acupuncture. Complementary Therapies in Medicine 5: 147–151.

Birch S, Felt R 2000 Letter. Journal of Chinese Medicine Online. Available: http://www.jcm.co.uk/bookrevs70.html 17 March 2000.

Borkovec TD, Nau SD 1972 Credibility of analogue therapy rationales. Journal of Behavior Therapy and Experimental Psychiatry 3: 257–260.

Bullock ML, Culliton PD, Olander RT 1989 Controlled trial of acupuncture for severe recidivist alcoholism. Lancet 1: 1435–1439.

Cheng RSS, Pomeranz BH 1980 Electroacupuncture analgesia is mediated by stereo specific opiate receptors and is reversed by antagonists of type I receptors. Life Sciences 26: 631–638.

Chiang CY, Chang CT, Chu HL, Yang LF 1973 Peripheral afferent pathway for acupuncture analgesia. Scientia Sinica 16: 210–217.

Cho ZH, Chung SC, Jones JP et al 1998 New findings of the correlation between acupoints and corresponding brain cortices using functional MRI. Proceedings of the National Academy of Sciences USA 95: 2670–2673.

Christensen BV, Iuhl IU, Vilbek H et al 1992 Acupuncture treatment of severe knee osteoarthrosis: a long-term study. Acta Anaesthesiologica Scandinavica 36: 519–525.

Coan R, Wong G, Ku SL et al 1980 The acupuncture treatment of low back pain: a randomised controlled treatment. American Journal of Chinese Medicine 8: 181–189.

Coan R, Wong G, Coan PL 1982 The acupuncture treatment of neck pain: a randomised controlled study. American Journal of Chinese Medicine 9: 326–332.

Dundee JW, Ghaly G 1991 Local anaesthesia blocks the antiemetic action of P6 acupuncture. Clinical Pharmacology and Therapeutics 50: 78–80.

Filshie J, Cummings M 1999 Western medical acupuncture. In: Ernst E, White A, eds. Acupuncture: a scientific appraisal. Oxford: Butterworth-Heinemann; 31–59.

Haker E, Lundeberg T 1990 Acupuncture treatment in epicondylalgia: a comparative study of two acupuncture techniques. Clinical Journal of Pain 6: 221–226.

Hammerschlag R 1998 Methodological and ethical issues in clinical trials of acupuncture. Journal of Alternative and Complementary Medicine 4: 159–171.

Hammerschlag R, Morris M 1997 Clinical trials comparing acupuncture with biomedical standard care: a criteria-based evaluation of research design and reporting. Complementary Therapies in Medicine 5: 133–140.

Hansen PE, Hansen JH 1983 Acupuncture treatment of chronic facial pain – a controlled cross-over trial. Headache 23: 66–69.

Hopwood V, Lewith G 2003 Acupuncture trials and methodological considerations. Clinical Acupuncture and Oriental Medicine 3: 192–199.

Jobst K, Chen JH, McPherson K, Arrowsmith J 1986 Controlled trial of acupuncture for disabling breathlessness. Lancet 328: 1416–1419.

Kawakita K 2001 Acupuncture in asthma treatment. Acupuncture Research Symposium, Exeter, UK, 2 July 2001.

Kleinhenz J, Streitberger K, Windeler J et al 1999 Randomised clinical trial comparing the effects of acupuncture and a newly designed placebo needle in rotator cuff tendinitis. Pain 83: 235–241.

Lao L, Bergman S, Langenberg P et al 1995 Efficacy of Chinese acupuncture on postoperative oral surgery pain. Oral Surgery, Oral Medicine, Oral Pathology, Oral Radiology, and Endodontics 79: 423–428.

Le Bars D, Villaneuva L, Willer JC, Bouhassira D 1991 Diffuse noxious inhibitory control (DNIC) in man and animals. Acupuncture in Medicine 9: 47–57.

Lewith GT, Machin D 1983 On the evaluation of the clinical effects of acupuncture. Pain 16: 111–127.

Lewith G, Vincent C 1998 The clinical evaluation of acupuncture. In: Filshie J, White A, eds. Medical acupuncture, a Western scientific approach. Edinburgh: Churchill Livingstone; 205–224.

MacPherson H, Gould AJ, Fitter M 1999 Acupuncture for low back pain: results of a pilot study for a randomised controlled trial. Complementary Therapies in Medicine 7: 83–90.

MacPherson H, White AR, Cummings M et al 2002 Standards for Reporting Interventions in Controlled Trials of Acupuncture: the STRICTA recommendations. Acupuncture in Medicine 20: 22–25.

Marcus P 1994 Towards a dose of acupuncture. Acupuncture in Medicine 12: 78–82.

Moore RA, Gavaghan D, Tramer MR et al 1998 Size is everything – large amounts of information are needed to overcome random effects in estimating direction and magnitude of treatment effects. Pain 78: 209–316.

Moroz A 1999 Issues in acupuncture research: the failure of quantitative methodologies and the possibilities for viable alternative solutions. American Journal of Acupuncture 27: 95–103.

Park J, White A, Lee H, Ernst E 1999 Development of a new sham needle. Acupuncture in Medicine 17: 110–112.

Rosenthal R 1976 Experimenter effects in behavioural research. New York: Irvington.

Shen J, Wenger N, Glaspy J et al 1997 Adjunct antiemesis electroacupuncture in stem cell transplantation. Proceedings of the American Society of Clinical Oncology 16: 42A (abstract).

Streitberger K, Kleinhenz J 1998 Introducing a placebo needle into acupuncture research. Lancet 352: 364–365.

Tang J, Zhan S, Ernst E 1999 Review of randomised controlled trials of traditional Chinese medicine. British Medical Journal 319: 160–161.

Tavola T, Gala C, Conte G, Invernizzi G 1992 Traditional Chinese acupuncture in tension type headache. Pain 48: 325–329.

Ter Riet G, Kleijnen J, Knipschild P 1990 Acupuncture and chronic pain: a criteria based meta-analysis. Journal of Clinical Epidemiology 11: 1191–1199.

Vincent CA 1989 A controlled trial of the treatment of migraine by acupuncture. Clinical Journal of Pain 5: 305–312.

Vincent C 1990 Credibility assessments in trials of acupuncture. Complementary Medical Research 4: 305–312.

Vincent C, Lewith G 1995 Placebo controls for acupuncture studies. Journal of the Royal Society of Medicine 88: 199–202.

White AR, Eddleston C, Hardie R et al 1996 A pilot study of acupuncture for tension headache, using a novel placebo. Acupuncture in Medicine 14: 11–14.

Wood R, Lewith G 1998 The credibility of placebo controls in acupuncture studies. Complementary Therapies in Medicine 6: 79–82.

TCM theory in modern medicine

KEY CONCEPTS

- ☯ Syndromes and TCM are still evolving.
- ☯ There are no really new diseases, but there are combinations of symptoms that were, perhaps, not envisaged by the Chinese.
- ☯ Diseases tend to be susceptible to fashion; suddenly everyone is talking and writing about them although the incidence is probably unchanged.
- ☯ Some of the more topical diseases are described here.

Introduction

The evolution of acupuncture is a continuing process and many of the old ideas can be applied to newer situations. This probably explains the fascination that acupuncture holds for so many practitioners. The most interesting thing about studying Traditional Chinese Medicine (TCM) is the frequent glimpse into the ancient recorded patterns and syndromes of a patient seen only last week and immediately identified. The ideas, and the codes that they are translated from, apply widely to the human condition in sickness and in health. It is not necessary to believe the explanations implicitly, but understanding how the symptoms used to be fitted together to make a logical picture allows us to extrapolate and devise new patterns and new treatments.

Several such applications have been mentioned elsewhere in this book. In Chapter 5, a modern application of the extraordinary meridian, Dai Mai, is taken from Pirog (1996). The excess mental activity or day-to-day stresses of living and accompanying poor dietary habits leading to stagnation of Qi result in a division between the upper and lower body, with pathogenic Heat at the top and a Cold deficient situation in the lower part. The treatment of the Dai Mai, or Girdle, meridian seems to be able to relieve this strange imbalance simply by facilitating the flow of Qi between the two halves of the body. The modern classification of the stages of multiple sclerosis suggested by Blackwell & MacPherson (1993) (see Ch. 8) is another illustration of the possibility of applying TCM theory to almost any medical situation. The staging of the disease seen through a TCM filter is very useful, and makes treatment of a complex and highly variable disease a much less daunting task.

Maciocia (1994) also describes what he refers to as 'modern' syndromes, the most important being Liver stagnation and Liver invading Spleen (see Ch. 8).

However, a word of warning is necessary for medical acupuncturists: just because TCM theory fits, this does not make it correct to revert totally to the ancient teachings and abandon the conveniences of modern medical diagnostics. The use of both modalities gives a richness and sophistication that patients will undoubtedly benefit from, and mirrors current medical practice in China.

'Running on empty'

A well known American doctor, Miriam Lee, has also recognized the changing nature of the pattern of disease and has produced a treatment protocol for the situation she terms 'running on empty'. Along with other acupuncture practitioners, she saw that the modern lifestyle encourages poor dietary habits and inflicts heavy levels of stress on the individual. This is not to say that people were never stressed before, but the problem with today's stress is that there appears to be little physical release. Activity is much reduced. Sitting at work in front of a computer screen all day, driving or riding considerable distances to get home, and then falling into a chair to catch up with the rest of the world on television tends to be perfect behaviour for the encouragement of Liver stagnation and the accompanying emotional and physical symptoms.

The description that Lee has taken from the Nanjing is apt, and echoes the problem with the Dai Mai channel:

When the Stomach and Spleen, the central Jiao, are attacked by emotion, pure Qi cannot ascend to the brain, and the evil Qi, the waste, cannot descend. It will remain stuck in the stomach.

Lee's main aim with treatment is to 'unstick' the Qi trapped at the centre. The points she recommends are balanced for Yin and Yang for upper and lower body, and are used bilaterally. The Large Intestine and Stomach meridians have a good supply of both Qi and Blood, and are therefore relatively safe to treat in any individual. The five points are listed in Table 11.1.

Lee writes at length about the characteristics and energetics of these points and her book is a rewarding read for any acupuncturist (Lee 1992). The prescription was never proposed as a cure for all modern ills, but was originally used by her as a baseline treatment from which she could develop a specific combination of points to suit each patient individually. The ten points (used bilaterally) gave a useful place from which to begin and, as such, may be valuable in physiotherapy departments when the patient presents with a complex set of symptoms involving more than a simple pain. This links rather well with the modern idea that acupuncture has similar effects to exercise (Andersson 1997). Perhaps the vigorous stimulation of these strong points is sufficient to nudge the sympathetic system and readjust the neurochemical balance, mobilizing the stagnation and taking the place of an energetic physical workout.

Cellulite

This is not exactly a disease in Western terms, more a cosmetic problem, although some would disagree that it even counts as a problem, being inextricably bound up with our current obsession with body image and not nec-

Table 11.1 Acupuncture for 'running on empty'

Acupuncture point	Comments
St 36 Zusanli	Stomach channel has abundant Qi and Blood Calms the Liver Reinforces digestion Tranquillizes the spirit Supports Lung Qi in cases of infection The best point to free stuck Qi in the middle Jiao
Sp 6 Sanyinjiao	Treats stagnant Liver Qi Supports Kidneys and Spleen Expels Damp Works with St 36
LI 4 Hegu	Large Intestine has abundant Qi and Blood Treats upper part of body, teeth, jaws and throat Opens the Large Intestine Opens the Lungs Adjusts flow of Qi through whole body Major analgesic point
LI 11 Quchi	Helps bowel to move, clearing waste from the intestines Helps with digestion and absorption Expels the Pathogen Wind
Lu 7 Lieque	Tonifies the Lungs for Kidney Xu Clears the brain Luo point Treats head and neck Clears phlegm from the chest Moistens a dry throat or cough Treats intestinal problems

essarily pathological. Cellulite is defined as subcutaneous deposits of fat that produce a superficial dimpling pattern on the buttocks and limbs, so-called 'grapefruit' skin. It is also associated with poor lymphatic drainage.

Cellulite has been classified in TCM terms by an American author, Skya Gardner-Abbate (1996), who explains that the underlying problem is Spleen Qi Xu. (Box 11.1) She suggests that the usual causes for this are dietary: the regular consumption of rich, oily, greasy foods that are difficult for the Spleen to break down. Cold, raw foods, such as salad, also tend to slow down the activity of the Spleen. Another problem associated with modern lifestyle is eating at irregular times, snacking on the way to and from work, and eating large meals in the evening, all of which strain the capacity of the Spleen to provide Qi at appropriate times. The Pathogens known to damage the Spleen – excessive worry, study and obsessive anxiety – combined with a sedentary lifestyle and a poor eating pattern will further drain the person's energy (Fig. 11.1).

This deficiency will lead to a condition of Dampness within the body, manifest in symptoms such as fatigue, a feeling of 'heaviness', poor mus-

Box 11.1   Major Spleen
Qi Xu points

- St 36 Zusanli
- Sp 6 Sanyinjiao
- UB 20 Pishu
- UB 21 Weishu
- Sp 3 Taibai

The effects of these points are given in Chapter 8.

Figure 11.1   Genesis of
cellulite.

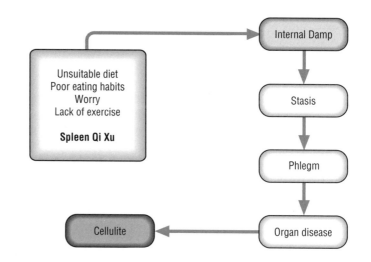

cle tone, abdominal distension after eating and general pallor. There may
also be a slight nausea and a feeling of stuffiness in the chest. Chronic
catarrh is often associated with this condition. The tongue is characteristically pale and swollen.

Although the aetiology is fairly clear from a TCM point of view, treatment should probably not be centred around acupuncture. It is clear that
changes in diet and lifestyle are required, and sometimes weight also
needs to be lost; this regimen will take at least 6 months. Acupuncture to
support the function of the Spleen and Stomach would be useful, and local
points to help with expelling the Pathogen Damp could also be used for visible oedema. As the Kidney is influential with regard to Body fluids, it is
also likely to be involved, probably due to a deficiency of Yang, and if TCM
logic is pursued the Lung may also be implicated. Therefore, these two
Zang Fu organs may also need attention.

The most interesting thing about this TCM analysis is that it is consistent with Western thought: cellulite is trapped fat, not usually life threatening and caused mainly by poor circulation and an unsuitable diet; it
responds to physical input in the form of deep massage and exercise.

Female menopause

This is emphatically not a disease, but in Western society the menopause
has increasingly been considered as one. In both men and women, the
menopause indicates the natural passing of one phase of life into the next,
the cessation of the ability to procreate. It provides the individual with

an opportunity for self-realization of another kind – a different type of development. Free from the monthly cycles, a woman can enter a new stage of fulfilment and, perhaps, gentle preparation for the eventual end of life.

A woman who has accepted the process of menopause attains a serenity or inner peace, whereas resisted or rejected menopause can produce a chain of symptoms. This is not to say that all suffering and discomfort in this phase of a woman's life is a necessary evil, or that a positive attitude will make everything easy, but we should be careful not to regard it all as pathogenic. That said, there are some useful point combinations for both the uncomfortable and the more serious problems that arise.

Menopause has come to be associated with osteoporosis in Western medicine and this, although not described in quite these terms, has a resonance in TCM. The gradual decrease of Kidney Qi is at the root of the normal process. This leads in turn to a decrease of Qi in the Ren and Chong channels. The subsequent Blood and Jing deficiency weakening the internal organs, together with pelvic Yin deficiency allowing the Yang to rise, will cause the typical hot flushes of menopause and, if the Kidney Yin becomes exhausted as the essence decreases, the syndrome called 'Steaming Bone' may occur, and more and more of the denser Ye fraction of the Body fluids is leached from the bone marrow with resulting osteoporosis. The other organs most commonly affected are the Liver, Heart and Spleen.

Deficiency of Kidney Qi is the primary cause of the menopausal syndromes, which include:

- deficiency of Kidney and Liver Yin
- deficiency of Kidney Yang
- deficiency of Kidney Yin and Yang.

Specific treatment for these syndromes is given in Chapter 8. Preventive treatment can be undertaken utilizing the points shown in Table 11.2.

Research

There is little in the way of research evidence for acupuncture in the menopause. The best study available is that of Wyon et al (1995). The effects of two different kinds of acupuncture were studied: electroacupuncture at a current frequency of 2 Hz and a superficial needle insertion for a total of 8 weeks. Acupuncture significantly affected the hot flushes and sweating episodes by more than 50% in both groups, with effects persisting for at least 3 months after the end of treatment only in the electroacupuncture group. The researchers suggested that changes in calcitonin gene-related peptide excreted in the urine may mean that this neuropeptide, which is a very potent vasodilator, could be implicated in the mechanism of hot flushes.

Some work has been done on the false menopausal symptoms produced in women receiving the drug tamoxifen, particularly hot flushes. A small uncontrolled study by Porzio et al (2002) and a larger retrospective audit by Bolton et al (2003) indicated that acupuncture might be effective.

Table 11.2   Menopausal points

Point	Comments
Liv 14 Qimen	Overall balancing. Regulates the third phase of a woman's life
Ren 4 Guanyuan	Balances pelvic energy
Kid 4 Dazhong	Command point for the lower Jiao
Ren 7 Yinjiao	Promotes movement of Jing
UB 17 Geshu Ht 6 Yinshi Kid 7 Fuliu Du 14 Dazhui UB 43 Gaohuangshu (needle with care)	Eliminate internal Heat and restore normal Yin–Yang balance. Hot flushes

Kid 27 Shufu
UB 13 Feishu
UB 19 Danshu
  and points for
  Heat above
	'Steaming Bone' syndrome. Heat given out by the bone marrow, caused by Yin Xu with internal Heat. Symptoms include spontaneous perspiration, extreme fatigue, mild insomnia, intermittent fever, anxiety, dark urine, and heat in the palms of the hands

UB 23 Shenshu UB 52 Zhishi Kid 15 Zhongshu Kid 2 Rangu UB 11 Dashu GB 39 Xuanzhong	Early signs of osteoporosis

Myalgic encephalopathy

Myalgic encephalopathy (ME) is a modern diagnosis. It is possible that the syndrome existed in earlier times but went largely unrecognized. Victorian literature is full of people who went into a 'decline' and took to their beds. Some of these people were undoubtedly suffering from tuberculosis, but some were probably not. Viruses must have been in existence and may well have had devastating effects.

The Chinese syndromes involving collapse of Spleen energy may be something similar. Collapse of Yin and Yang would also tend to have these effects. So what is ME and how do we treat it?

The primary symptoms of ME are aching and fatigued muscles, exhaustion, a persistent low-grade 'flu-like feeling, and poor memory and lack of concentration. It is usually found as a postviral consequence, but in TCM terms it is not important exactly which virus was involved, or when. The virus as a pathogenic factor may act immediately or remain in the body as Heat or Damp Heat (Fig. 11.2).

The inclusion of immunization in this aetiology is interesting. Many TCM practitioners believe that the milder childhood fevers should be allowed to come and go, just in order to prevent this type of complication in later life. (This view depends on the general basal health of the infant

Figure 11.2 Aetiology of myalgic encephalopathy. (Redrawn with kind permission of Maciocia 1991.)

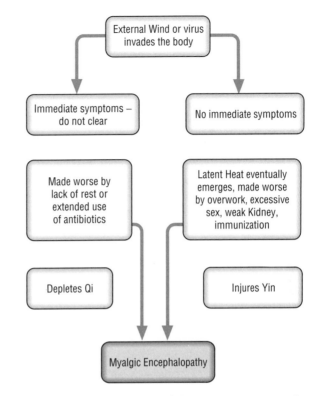

population. Where it is compromised by poor nutrition and poverty, the 'mild' childhood fevers can become killers and prevention is important.)

ME has also been linked to the Epstein–Barr virus, which causes glandular fever or mononucleosis.

Maciocia (1991) has identified three ME syndromes:

- residual pathogenic factor
- latent Heat
- Lesser Yang pattern.

Residual pathogenic factor

The invading Pathogen, usually Wind, may remain in the interior, usually as Heat or Damp Heat. It tends to weaken the body's defences, exposing it to further Pathogens and weakening Qi and Yin generally. One of the more important effects of this is a further increase in Damp produced by the functional failure of the Spleen and Stomach. The Dampness itself leads to further impedance of Stomach and Spleen. Antibiotics are associated with this type of situation and their widespread use is considered sometimes to be inappropriate. Maciocia (1994, p 632) gives a useful analogy:

> *If we hear a burglar entering the house in the middle of the night, we could react in one of two different ways, either we could get up and make a noise and scare the burglar off, or if we had a gun we could shoot the burglar dead.*

The point is made that shooting the burglar or invading Pathogen with the use of antibiotics is all very well but leaves the problem of the burglar's body. If the burglar is frightened away, as in TCM, there is no further harm to the body.

The problem lies not with the action of the antibiotics, which is obviously beneficial, but more with the fact that antibiotics also destroy 'friendly' bacteria within the body. If prolonged exposure to this type of drug is anticipated, a medical herbalist experienced in the use of Chinese herbs should be consulted in order to counteract the possible side-effects. Acupuncture treatment should concentrate on supporting the Qi deficiency and expelling the Damp (Table 11.3).

Latent Heat

This is similar to the previous concept, requiring some sort of pathology or serious emotional stress stimulus to cause a fairly sudden onset, probably appearing as an external invasion but betraying signs of latent internal Heat on examination. This is more likely to damage Yin. The Kidneys are often severely weakened, and it is not clear whether this is the cause or the effect. Wei Qi is responsible for defence but supported by Kidney Essence and Qi; in these cases there is a decreased immune response. All of this is made worse by overexertion and lack of adequate rest.

Lesser Yang pattern

The two previous syndromes may develop into a Shao Yang syndrome. Shao Yang Chiao, or Lesser Yang, is formed from the Sanjiao and Gall Bladder channels. It is regarded as a hinge or transition layer between the two other Yang Chiaos, as described in Chapter 6. Typical symptoms usually involve the two organs and may include:

- fever with shivering
- pain over the heart
- bitter taste in the mouth.

Again, this is likely to be the result of a long-term stress pattern or weakness produced by some other factor.

The points suggested in Table 11.3 will be appropriate for all three subdivisions of ME, but care must always be taken with this type of patient not to overtax them with the acupuncture; the re-establishment of natural defences should be encouraged. The aim should be expulsion of the Pathogens Heat or Damp Heat, and the tonification of Qi and/or Yin. In the case of the Lesser Yang pattern, treatment should be aimed at harmonizing the Gall Bladder and Sanjiao. This is likely to be a slow process (see Case study 11.1) and may need more than just acupuncture.

Table 11.3 Suggested points for residual pathogenic factor

Symptom	Points
Damp	Sp 9 Yinlingquan
	Sp 6 Sanyinjiao
	Sp 3 Taibai
	Ren 12 Zhongwan
	Ren 9 Shuifen
Damp Heat	LI 11 Quchi
Foggy feeling in head	St 8 Touwei
Support for Stomach and Spleen	UB 20 Pishu
	UB 21 Weishu
General muscle pain, 'Pain of the hundred joints'	SJ 5 Waiguan
Chronic 'hidden Heat'	Du 14 Dazhui

Chronic fatigue syndrome is considered by most TCM practitioners to be very similar to ME in aetiology, and for practical purposes can be treated in a similar way. A similar collection of symptoms was described by MacPherson & Blackwell (1992) under the heading 'tired out', which groups together the following syndromes: Spleen Qi Xu, Kidney Yang Xu, Liver Qi stagnation, Kidney–Heart Yin Xu, Kidney–Heart Blood Xu and general Phlegm patterns. A distinction is made between the different types of tiredness, ranging from 'I can't be bothered' in Liver Qi stagnation, 'tired but unable to sleep' in Liver–Heart Blood Xu to 'low-level chronic fatigue' in Spleen Qi Xu and really disabling fatigue in Kidney Yang Xu. The detached 'fuzzy feeling' and accompanying lethargy distinguish the Phlegm and Damp patterns. The TCM reasoning behind the differentiation into the different syndromes is complex and sophisticated, but it is the character of the 'tiredness' that initially dictates the treatment. The authors link the fatigue syndromes, ME and postviral stress in this way, suggesting logical TCM treatment strategies.

CASE HISTORY

Case study 11.1

Physiotherapist, aged 36, suspected ME sufferer.

Main problems: feels 'tired all the time', frequent need for time off, generally feeling ill, swollen glands, total lack of energy, feels 'out of control', 'weighed down', frequent dull 'foggy' headaches, shortness of breath relieved by sighing, often very cold, quietly spoken and pale, feels symptoms started after a bad dose of 'flu 2 years ago.

Tongue: pale with frilled edge.

Pulse: weak.

Predominant impressions:
Dampness distressing the Spleen
Liver Qi stagnation

Treatment
Points used were:

- Sp 6 Sanyinjiao
- Sp 9 Yinlingquan
- SJ 5 Waiguan
- St 8 Touwei
- St 40 Fenglong
- Pe 6 Neiguan, used occasionally.

These points were used for several weeks. As the condition improved, St 36 Zusanli was introduced in place of St 40 to support general metabolism, and Stomach, Spleen and Kidney back Shu points, UB 20, 21 and 23, were sometimes used.

Good outcome: headaches became rare and general energy levels were restored.

Fibromyalgia

Fibromyalgia is also a relatively modern concept but is now accepted by the medical community as a rheumatological complaint involving widespread pain and tender, focal sites in specific muscle areas. It was originally termed 'fibrositis' and has been referred to as non-articular rheumatism. Described as fibrositis, the condition has been in non-medical parlance for at least 30 years. These days it is often associated with ME, and a trawl for information on the internet can be quite confusing. There is no doubt that the painful symptoms could be contributory to the TCM syndromes described above, but fibromyalgia may not necessarily have an original viral trigger. Indeed, the so-called 'Fibro Five' are listed as shown in Table 11.4.

The difficulty with a list such as that in Table 11.4 is that almost the entire population will have suffered from symptoms of two or more of the conditions at one time or another. There is now a suggestion that fibromyalgia may be linked with types 1 and 2 diabetes (Tishler et al 2003). However, TCM would be able to link these quite amorphous conditions by symptomatology. When the main sites of fibromyalgic pain are examined, they correspond very clearly to acupuncture points and, in fact, largely to classical physiotherapy trigger points (Fig. 11.3).

The American College of Rheumatology (1990) has established a set of diagnostic criteria for fibromyalgia that include the illustrated tender points, general malaise, poor muscle condition and interrupted sleep pattern.

Depression is a common finding in these patients and antidepressant drug therapy is common. This type of patient is being referred to National Health

Table 11.4 The 'Fibro Five' diseases

Disorder	Characteristics
Fibromyalgia	Characterized by muscle pain, stiffness and easy fatiguability. Cause unknown. Symptoms adversely affected by weather conditions. Sometimes confused with polymyalgia rheumatica (PM), where the main joints affected are the shoulder and hip (erythrocyte sedimentation rate is raised in PM)
Interstitial cystitis	Chronic inflammatory condition of the bladder, more common in females. Difficulty urinating, pain on urination, increased frequency and urgency
Chronic fatigue	Unexplained fatigue, weakness, muscle pain, lymph node swelling and general malaise
Migraine headache	Vascular headache, usually temporal and unilateral in onset, commonly associated with irritability, nausea, vomiting, constipation or diarrhoea, and often photophobia. Attacks are preceded by constriction of the cranial arteries, usually with resultant prodromal sensory (especially ocular) symptoms and commence with the vasodilatation that follows
Irritable bowel	Functional bowel disorder characterized by recurrent crampy abdominal pain and diarrhoea

Figure 11.3 The 18 tender points of fibromyalgia.

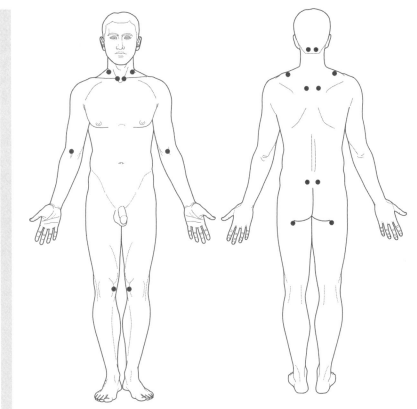

Service hospital pain clinics in increasing numbers, and they present quite a treatment problem because they are not amenable to the 'quick fix'. However, acupuncture can be fairly successful, even though quite long treatment programmes will be necessary. Acupuncture treatment is better accepted by the consulting physicians than previously, but should not be expected to be an immediate cure. It takes some time for the hyperalgesia to settle down and often acupuncture tends to exacerbate pain in initial treatments.

As overtreatment is a real issue with this condition, the points should be limited. Pearce (2000) recommends the points shown in Table 11.5 but sometimes the patient will tolerate only three or four at a time.

Research

The US National Institutes of Health (NIH 1998) made the following statement about fibromyalgia and acupuncture: 'Acupuncture may be useful as an adjunct to treatment or as an acceptable alternative, or may be included in a comprehensive management programme.'

A recent literature review concluded that there was only a limited amount of high-quality evidence but, based mostly on one high-quality study, real acupuncture was more effective than sham acupuncture for improving the symptoms of patients with fibromyalgia (Berman et al 1999). The best study suggested that acupuncture raised the pain threshold and reduced morning stiffness, but the duration of this effect has not yet been shown. Another small study of 29 patients with chronic fibromyalgia (Sprott et al 1998) demonstrated a decreased concentration of serotonin in

Table 11.5 Acupuncture points for fibromyalgia (after Pearce 2000)

Point	Comment
SI 12 Bingfeng	Local to one of the tender areas and an important reunion or Luo point. Passes close to several other tender areas
SJ 5 Waiguan	Opening point for Yang Wei Mai (See. Ch. 4). Relaxes tendons, dispels Wind. Balances Yin and Yang
Ren 4 Guanyuan	Tonifies Blood and Yuan Qi. Tonifies all Yang in body
St 36 Zusanli	Earth point. Regulates circulation of Blood and Qi throughout the body. Regulates activity of Stomach and Spleen; increases Wei Qi
Sp 6 Sanyinjiao	Meeting point for three Yin channels: Liver, Kidney and Spleen. All important for a fibromyalgia sufferer
UB 62 Shenmai	Key point for Yang Chiao Mai. Clears and cools the spirit
UB 17 Geshu	Influential point for the circulation. Reunion point for Yin and Yang
UB 18 Ganshu	Back Shu point for the liver. Eliminates Damp Heat and stagnant Qi. Nourishes Blood. Clears the head, quietens the spirit
UB 20 Pishu	Back Shu point for the Spleen. Tonifies the middle Jiao. Eliminates Damp, strengthens Blood
UB 23 Shenshu	Back Shu point for the Kidney. Supports Kidney energy. Eliminates Damp
Du 4 Mingmen	Strengthens Kidney Qi. Tonifies Yang

the platelets and increased levels of serotonin and substance P in the serum, alongside a decreased number of tender points and lower Visual Analogue Scale (VAS) pain scores. In a further study, Sprott et al (2000) also found that there was a reduction of regional blood flow above tender points in patients with fibromyalgia compared with healthy controls. A slight rise in temperature and an increase in pain threshold served to confirm the usefulness of acupuncture in fibromyalgia.

Children's diseases

Acupuncture is increasingly used for the treatment of children and is applied for conditions that, while not exactly modern diseases, are certainly more likely to be recognized than previously. Also it is only recently in the West that acupuncture has even been considered therapeutically in these situations.

Treatment of children is a specialist field. The essential thing to remember is that children respond very quickly to acupuncture needling because their Wei Qi is close to the surface and very strong. They usually require only pricking on the appropriate points, and the needles are not left in the skin. While it is a simplistic division, it does seem that children tend to polarize into two general groups, those exhibiting excess symptoms and those exhibiting deficiencies, as listed in Box 11.2.

The treatment of children is a specialized skill and Julian Scott (1986) has written extensively about it. It is relatively easy to use Eight Principle

Box 11.2 Polarities in childhood diagnosis

Excess	Deficient
Strong, sturdy	Floppy, frail
Loud	Quiet
Alert	Dull eyed
Red cheeks	Pale face
Good appetite	Poor appetite
Strong reaction to pain	Milder response to pain
Illness tends to be severe, but rare	Becomes ill easily
Needs less sleep	Needs lots of sleep
Lots of energy	Physical energy low, watches television
Difficult to ignore	Easy to be with
Excess Body fluids, snotty nose, etc.	Lack of fluids

diagnostics with children, but there are some syndromes that are more commonly seen. To paraphrase Scott: 'Treatment of children is simple, they only catch cold or have bad digestion'. Catching cold is easy to understand, school-aged children are exposed to the richness of the current germs and infections in their close society, and do indeed suffer more than adults.

Bad digestion is explained by the fact that the Spleen is relatively poorly developed because it is not needed by the fetus in the womb and is not really stressed until solid foods are started. This makes Spleen Qi Xu a common diagnosis, with symptoms such as picky eating and poor appetite associated with a failure to thrive. Acupuncture treatment has a good clinical track record in this type of case.

Acupuncture is used clinically in China for many childhood ailments, including asthma and epilepsy, but there is no Western research evidence base as yet. It is advisable to consult an acupuncture practitioner who specializes in the treatment of children for the best results at present.

Repetitive strain injury

Finally, a modern classification of disease that is purely physical, and that may well have existed previously, is the repetitive strain injury (RSI). It is certain that people required continuously to make repeated small hand and wrist movements (e.g. computer operators) probably have a lot in common with skilled workers over the ages. Fine embroidery, needlework, knitting, lace-making, etc. are all similarly damaging to the small muscles and probably produced just as much tendon damage, being dismissed as 'rheumatics' in the past.

RSI is characterized by pain occurring in a very precisely localized area, usually the wrist or forearm, as a result of a repetitive muscle activity. The diagnosis is made when the pain is no longer reduced or relieved by normal rest periods. It has only recently been recognized as a true medical condition, perhaps because of the implications for litigation. It is probably much better to prevent RSI than try to cure it. Ergonomic studies in the workplace and substitutes for the triggering movements, where possible, are more likely to have a lasting effect than any treatment.

Nevertheless, physiotherapists often find themselves asked to treat this condition. Adverse neural tension techniques will help, together with gentle acupuncture at distal points. The acupuncture points can be selected on a segmental basis once the affected muscles have been identified. Use of acupuncture can be very helpful: the local changes produced in the tissues appear to have an effect on either the stagnation (in the TCM sense) or the microcirculation (in the Western sense).

Acupuncture for the pain will not be enough; some degree of retraining or a change in activity is also essential. The flexor tendons at the wrist are commonly involved, as are those at the elbow; the tendons, tendon sheaths, muscles and nerves can all be affected. Occasionally there will be swelling, numbness, tingling and sometimes a sensation of heaviness. Overuse in sport can sometimes trigger this kind of problem in the ankle and knee.

RSI is really a form of Bi syndrome (see Ch. 2). The symptoms are quite variable and seem to be adversely affected by emotional stress. The most useful treatment is, first, a mixture of rest from the causal activity and advice on ergonomics, and, second, acupuncture for the pain. Use local points according to the tendons involved, and distal points either on the affected meridian or elsewhere in the body. GB 34 Yanglingquan and St 36 Zusanli can be added. There may also be symptoms of stagnant Liver Qi and Blood stasis, and these should be tackled to achieve long-term resolution. Quick results are rare, but over a period of time the outcome can be good as long as the patient understands the causative activity and can change it in some way (Case study 11.2).

CASE HISTORY

Case study 11.2

Hospital administrator, male, aged 44, with a stressful job. Spent a long time on a computer or laptop each day.

Right forearm: dull pain over and proximal to the wrist on palmar aspect. Pain originally worse after long sessions, producing stabbing pain, but by the time the patient was referred to physiotherapy it was made worse by any use at all. Complained of some tingling and numbness in the area.

Symptoms much worse on NHS Trust Executive meeting days. Felt very run down, but also angry; unable to sleep through the night. Occasional severe one-sided headaches.

Impression: RSI, carpal tunnel syndrome, underlying Liver Qi stagnation.

Basic points:

- Pe 6 Neiguan
- Pe 7 Daling
- GB 34 Yanglingquan
- Liv 3 Taichong.

Not able to tolerate both Pericardium points at first treatment, but relaxed on subsequent visits. Treatment given twice a week for 6 weeks.

Slow to gain a lasting response but always felt easier the day after treatment. Spent a long time looking into wrist support cushions and ways to make the keyboard more comfortable. Patient took up Shiatsu; said it helped him relax.

Good overall result, but patient aware that he still had good and bad days.

Conclusion

As time passes there will no doubt be other combinations of symptoms, adding up to further discomfort for patients. Until we are quite certain of what the mechanism of acupuncture is, sorting the symptoms into TCM patterns will remain a helpful exercise and may well provide relief for the patient. We can investigate exactly how it works later.

References

American College of Rheumatology 1990 Criteria for the classification of fibromyalgia. Report of the Multicenter Criteria Committee. Arthritis and Rheumatism 33: 160–172.

Andersson S 1997 Physiological mechanisms in acupuncture. In: Hopwood V, Lovesey M, Mokone S, eds. Acupuncture and related techniques in physiotherapy. London: Churchill Livingstone; 19–39.

Berman BM, Ezzo J, Hadhazy V, Swyers JP 1999 Is acupuncture effective in the treatment of fibromyalgia? Journal of Family Practice 48: 213–218.

Blackwell R, MacPherson H 1993 Multiple scterosis. Staging and patient management. Journal of Chinese Medicine 42: 5–12.

Bolton T, Filshie J, Browne D 2003 An overview of hot flushes and night sweats and clinical aspects of acupuncture treatment in 194 patients. BMAS Spring Scientific Meeting, Coventry, UK, April 2003.

Gardner-Abbate S 1996 Holding the tiger's tail. Santa Fe, New Mexico: Southwest Acupuncture College Press.

Lee M 1992 Insights of a senior acupuncturist. Boulder, CO: Blue Poppy Press.

Maciocia G 1991 Myalgic encephalomyelitis. Journal of Chinese Medicine 35: 5–19.

Maciocia G 1994 The practice of Chinese Medicine. Edinburgh: Churchill Livingstone.

MacPherson H, Blackwell R 1992 Tired out. Journal of Chinese Medicine 40: CD Rom.

NIH Consensus Development Panel on Acupuncture 1998 Acupuncture. Journal of the American Medical Association 280: 1518–1524.

Pearce L 2000 Fibromyalgia – a clinical overview. Journal of the Acupuncture Association of Physiotherapists October: 34–40.

Pirog JE 1996 The practical application of meridian style acupuncture. Berkeley, CA: Pacific View Press.

Porzio G, Trapasso T, Martelli S et al 2002 Acupuncture in the treatment of menopause-related symptoms in women taking tamoxifen. Tumori 88: 128–130.

Scott J 1986 The treatment of children by acupuncture. Hove: Journal of Chinese Medicine.

Sprott H, Franke S, Kluge H, Hein G 1998 Pain treatment of fibromyalgia by acupuncture. Rheumatology International 18: 35–36.

Sprott H, Jeschonneck M, Grohmann G, Hein G 2000 Microcirculatory changes over the tender points in fibromyalgia patients after acupuncture therapy (measured with laser-Doppler flowmetry). Wiener Klinische Wochenschrift 112: 580–586.

Tishler M, Smorodin T, Vazina-Amit M et al 2003 Fibromyalgia in diabetes mellitus. Rheumatology International 23: 171–173.

Wyon Y, Lindgren R, Lundeberg T, Hammar M 1995 Effects of acupuncture on climacteric vasomotor symptoms, quality of life and urinary excretion of neuropeptides among postmenopausal women. Menopause: The Journal of the North American Menopause Society 2: 3–12.

Old age problems

KEY CONCEPTS

- ☙ Work with elderly patients occupies an increasing portion of total therapy time.
- ☙ Unfortunately there are many pain problems to tackle but regular courses of acupuncture treatment would seem preferable to long-term medication.
- ☙ There are many factors complicating health problems in this age group.
- ☙ Acupuncture has something to offer in most circumstances.
- ☙ Two problems underlie most conditions: stagnation of fluid circulation and Kidney deficiency.

Introduction

Old age comes to us all – if we are lucky. The problems associated with old age can, in fact, occur at any time when they are understood from a Traditional Chinese Medicine (TCM) perspective. It is their slow and steady accumulation that can be so damaging to the general health. We have seen the rich diversity of the syndromes and how to treat them – both the ancient patterns and the newer ones. This chapter aims to relate them to a particular field of work that is constantly increasing in both the NHS and private practice. The decline due to the ageing process is known in TCM as Shuai Lao. The symptomatology may seem slightly repetitive (because Chinese Medicine is really very simple), but the message is that, although the patterns repeat endlessly, the age, condition and internal Zang Fu balance of the patient are important factors too.

Role of the Kidney

The Kidney is at the heart of the major structural changes that take place in the body as it grows to maturity and then, inevitably, older. The quality of the Kidney Essence, or Jing, and the Kidney Yin and Yang energies drive many of the physiological processes. The Kidney never shows a true excess, always tending to a deficiency. It is, however, possible to alleviate the symptoms of this deficiency even if a cure is not really possible.

The other common problem for the elderly is the slowing down of the Body fluids discussed in the Bi syndrome (see Ch. 2). This starts as a channel problem and is not actually life threatening – it just makes life more uncomfortable and, when the pain is severe, almost unbearable. However, if the other Zang Fu organs are failing, the obstructions to the flow of Qi and Blood can become much more serious over time. This idea of increasing stagnation of fluids and Qi is fundamental to some TCM approaches to geriatric medicine (Yan 2000).

The balance of Fire and Water is crucial. Fire is essential to all physiological processes, representing the flame that keeps alive and continues to feed all metabolic processes. The root of this TCM physiological fire is in the Kidneys, and is accessible with acupuncture at Du 4 Mingmen and UB 23 Shenshu.

There are more Kidney syndromes than are listed in Chapter 8, but using the classification from that chapter they can still be divided between Xu (deficiency) or Shi (excess), but it should be noted that those complicated by Shi aspects tend to be displaying false Heat (Box 12.1).

Kidney energies are more clearly divided into Yin and Yang aspects than any of the other Zang Fu organs. Recognition of these subtle differences is useful when dealing with the elderly patient. Figure 12.1 indicates the symptoms common to all Kidney problems and the specific symptoms that characterize Yin or Yang deficiencies.

The function of Yin energy is to nourish, moisten and support all aspects of growth, development and life in the body. The Yang energy is a little different, being more concerned with reproduction and general warming and the provision of energy for all physiological activities. Kidney Jing is part of Yin, but is described as the basic physical energy that

Box 12.1 Classification of Kidney syndromes

Xu

- Kidney Yin Xu
- Kidney Yang Xu
- Kidney Qi not firm
- Kidney failing to receive Qi
- Kidney Jing Xu

Xu complicated with Shi

- Kidney Xu – Water overflowing
- Kidney Yin Xu – Fire blazing

Figure 12.1
Differentiation of basic Kidney symptoms.

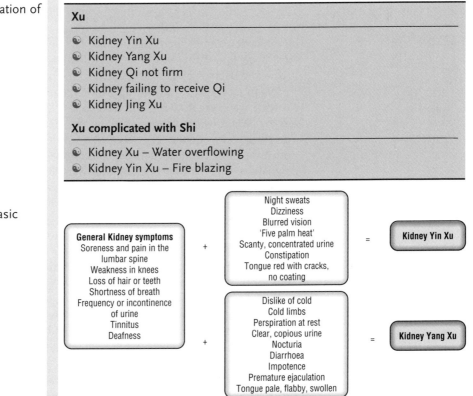

General Kidney symptoms		
Soreness and pain in the lumbar spine		Night sweats
Weakness in knees		Dizziness
Loss of hair or teeth		Blurred vision
Shortness of breath	+	'Five palm heat'
Frequency or incontinence of urine		Scanty, concentrated urine = Kidney Yin Xu
Tinnitus		Constipation
Deafness		Tongue red with cracks, no coating

		Dislike of cold
		Cold limbs
		Perspiration at rest
		Clear, copious urine
	+	Nocturia = Kidney Yang Xu
		Diarrhoea
		Impotence
		Premature ejaculation
		Tongue pale, flabby, swollen

one is born with. It is seen as a fluid substance. It is the basis of fertility; strong Jing in females leads to a relatively late menopause. It is also the basis of the energy in the Kidney itself, leading to some confusion in the syndromes. The separate descriptions will be given here, but sometimes one has to generalize and give a broad supportive treatment to the Kidney.

Kidney Yin deficiency has some characteristics that differentiate it from Kidney Yang deficiency, and they are simply identified as having too much Heat or not enough. Having too much Heat leads to signs of the consumption of the controlling Yin factors such as night sweats. These occur because the night should belong to cool, regenerating Yin; the sweating indicates that Yin is losing its normal controlling influence over the hotter Yang. Too little Heat is indicated more clearly in cold limbs, particularly cold feet, and fear or dislike of cold.

Kidney Qi not firm

This is an interesting concept, involving a collection of symptoms that all give an image of looseness or slow leaking. The symptoms manifest in the bladder as frequent urination with a weak stream, and often with dribbling after the act. There may be true incontinence, particularly at night. Certainly the frequency of urination is most troublesome for these patients at night. A major symptom is low back pain with a feeling of weakness in the lumbar spine.

There are sexual symptoms with premature ejaculation, vaginal discharge and prolapsed uterus. The tongue is pale with a white coating.

Kidney fails to receive Qi

This syndrome involves the Kidney–Lung relationship and is characterized by shortness of breath and wheezing. Breathing is rapid but weak, with difficulty on inhalation and is often diagnosed as late-onset asthma in Western medicine. There is sweating and sometimes slight swelling of the face. The tongue is pale and flabby. The limbs are cold and the patient is said to be 'spiritless'.

Two more Kidney syndromes commonly found in the elderly are Kidney Xu with Water overflowing and Kidney Yin Xu with Fire blazing. Extending the 'Water overflowing' metaphor, the Heart or Lungs can be flooded. The Lung connection is relatively easy to understand. The previously mentioned dynamic connection between Lung and Kidney is vital to keep the circulation of Jin Ye fluids through the Sanjiao. When this fails, or there is long-standing retention of Cold in the Lungs, fluid collects in the lower half of the body leading to oedematous legs, abdominal distension and a general chill in the body. There is thin, frothy sputum.

The link to the Heart is caused by long-standing retention of Dampness and the accumulation of untreated symptoms of this, which are quite likely to occur in an elderly patient with many subacute medical problems. In both cases the tongue tends to be slightly swollen, often tooth-marked, with a pale coating.

Kidney Yin Xu with Fire blazing is the result of the Kidney Water not controlling the Fire aspect. The Fire will tend to escape upwards, producing signs of what is really a false Heat in the upper body. These may include red cheeks, restlessness, low-grade fever, insomnia, scanty red urine, backache and a dry throat, especially at night. Sometimes there is excessive sexual desire; this syndrome is associated with long-standing emotional problems. It will be apparent that it is quite difficult to differentiate between chronic Kidney problems and Liver syndromes, and indeed they are often linked. The preceding symptoms would also fit a condition of Kidney and Liver Yin Xu.

Table 12.1 outlines the common combinations with suggested acupuncture points. 'Cock crow diarrhoea' is an apt description for loose motions

Table 12.1 Kidney combined syndromes

Syndrome	Symptoms	Key points
Kidney and Liver Yin Xu	Blurred vision, dizziness, tinnitus, dry throat, night sweats, sore or weak back, weak knees, and scanty menstruation or delayed cycle	UB 23 Shenshu UB 18 Ganshu UB 17 Geshu Kid 3 Taixi Kid 6 Zhaohai Liv 3 Taichong Liv 8 Ququan Ren 4 Guanyuan
Kidney and Heart Yin Xu	Insomnia, mental restlessness, palpitations, poor memory, dizziness, tinnitus, dry throat, sore back, night sweats	UB 23 Shenshu UB 15 Xinshu Ht 7 Shenmen Kid 3 Taixi Kid 9 Zhubin Ren 4 Guanyuan Pe 6 Neiguan Sp 6 Sanyinjiao
Kidney and Lung Yin Xu	Cough with a small amount of sputum, dry throat and mouth, sore or weak back and/or knees, night sweats and afternoon fever, 'five palm heat', emaciation	UB 23 Shenshu UB 13 Feishu Kid 3 Taixi Kid 6 Zhaohai Lu 7 Lieque UB 43 Gaohuangshu Ren 4 Guanyuan
Kidney and Lung Qi Xu	Asthmatic breathing, shortness of breath, worse on exertion, low voice, spontaneous sweating, cold limbs, incontinence on coughing	UB 23 Shenshu UB 13 Feishu Kid 3 Taixi Kid 6 Zhaohai Lu 7 Lieque Lu 9 Taiyuan UB 43 Gaohuangshu Ren 4 Guanyuan Sp 6 Sanyinjiao
Kidney and Spleen Yang Xu	Pale with cold limbs, sore or weak back and/or knees, facial and/or limb oedema, loose stools – 'cock crow diarrhoea'	UB 23 Shenshu UB 20 Pishu Kid 3 Taixi Kid 7 Fuliu St 25 Tianshu UB 25 Dachangshu Ren 6 Qihai

that occur only early in the morning. 'Five palm heat' is a term describing sweating on the four palms, hands and feet, and also on the upper chest.

The Back Shu points are used frequently in these conditions to deal with the perceived deficiency. Otherwise, points are used for their ability to stimulate the Yin energies and support the Zang Fu physiology.

As with any other situation in medicine, the patient is in need of information and good advice. For instance, incontinence on coughing should not be ignored; it is quite possible that strengthening of the pelvic floor muscles would be of more use than acupuncture. Correcting poor dietary habits, perhaps of a lifetime, may help with the bowel problem and eating less raw salad and sweet foods will certainly allow the Spleen to conserve a little energy.

The basis of many of these problems is suggested in Figure 12.2. Often, the circumstances of life combine to produce a decrease in the levels of Kidney Jing (see Jing Qi in Ch. 2). Modern life also makes Liver Qi stagnation much more common; this can lead into Liver deficiency syndromes, often linking back to the Kidney.

Figure 12.2 Pathologies increasing vulnerability to disease in old age.

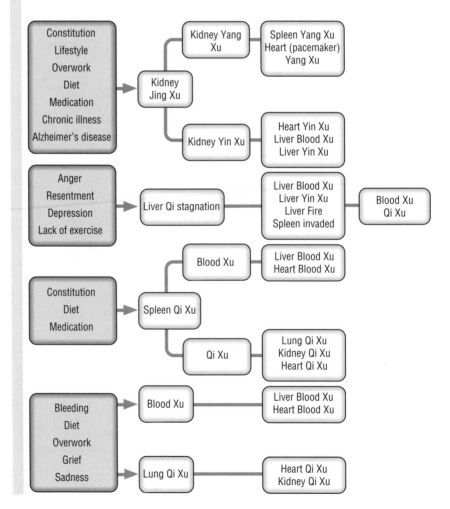

Other factors

Spleen deficiency, usually caused by damage from the Pathogen Damp working in conjunction with an unsuitable diet, or possibly the side-effects of long-term medication, can lead to further pathologies affecting all the other organs through the poor quality or lack of Blood. Simple deficiency of Blood caused by internal bleeding, menopausal disease or haemorrhoids can lead to the other syndromes. Internal bleeding may also result from long-term use of non-steroidal anti-inflammatory drugs (NSAIDs).

Lifestyle is a major factor. Habits of a lifetime are difficult to break and the effect of smoking, alcohol consumption and heavy eating all tend to be exaggerated in a system that is gradually losing the ability to cope with these toxins.

Medication is another problem. Long-term use of NSAIDs can be damaging to the gastrointestinal tract, and over-the-counter painkillers can make this much worse. Drug absorption is slower in old age, and changes in body chemistry mean that what was a normal adult dose becomes too strong.

The result may be slow bleeding or just an impaired ability to process food substances. The modern idea of a 'leaky bowel', in which some of the larger protein molecules leak from the gut into the tissues, may not be so far-fetched. NSAIDs have also been shown to slow down the healing of fractures, as the inflammatory process may be part of the healing cycle in normal tissues.

In old age there are more frequent calls on the body for healing energy (Fig. 12.3). The likelihood of surgery, regarded now as normal mainte-

Figure 12.3 Pain and stress as a secondary cause of disease.

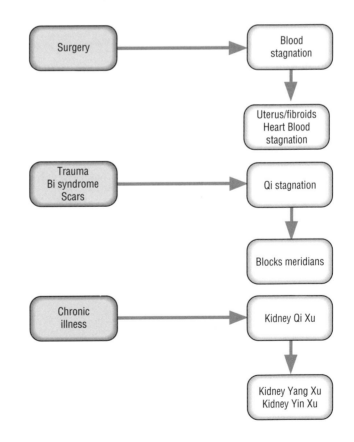

nance in Western society, can make great demands on the Qi. Common operations, replacement of hips or knees, cataract removal, insertion of pacemakers, etc. all require a period of recuperation. Often the older patient fails to 'bounce back', needing a few months to recover fully to what they themselves would regard as normal health. Co-morbidity or coexisting medical problems may complicate the picture further, slowing the healing process. Even when the recovery seems complete, the scars may remain painful with a 'locked energy' in them that needs to be released and redirected. A simple treatment with a needle at each end of the scar and a relevant distal point can often relieve a lot of discomfort.

Bearing in mind the other Kidney functions and the fact that the Kidney controls the will in a complicated relationship with the Heart, the fact that it can be damaged by fear is not surprising. The Kidney can, however, be equally damaged by bereavement. The first effects will be felt in the Lung Qi, the Lung being particularly vulnerable to the Pathogen Grief. If the Lungs are already at risk, then the secondary condition of depleted Kidneys failing to grasp Qi will be the predictable result.

Lack of exercise is a self-perpetuating cause of stagnation. Combined with the symptoms of Bi syndrome in one or more major joints, it is clear that the cycle will not be broken until the pain is relieved. Depression is quite understandable; the complaint that 'everything is an effort' may be an indication of this.

Frustration and anger at the lack of mobility will serve only to damage the Liver further – a vicious circle resulting in more general symptoms from the general slowing and stagnation of Qi and Blood.

Shen disturbances

The Shen, or inner spirit, is visible in the face, particularly with the eyes being bright and sparkling if all is well and dull and opaque if it is not. The state of the Shen will predict the motivation of the patient and thus the prognosis. This is sometimes referred to as the 'drive' of the patient. Many of the problems that beset older people – bereavement, retirement, relative poverty, failing eyesight and hearing – will all have an effect on the Shen. Stress and anxiety may accompany high blood pressure and patients may be taking beta-blockers, which themselves have a tendency to cause depression.

One of the most obvious signs of Shen disturbance (Fig. 12.4) is insomnia. This may take many forms. First, it should be noted that it is natural to sleep less as one grows older, perhaps because the physical demands of the day are not so great. However, if it is more difficult than usual to go to sleep or to remain asleep, this may indicate an imbalance in the Heart, Kidney or Liver.

Figure 12.4 Shen disturbances.

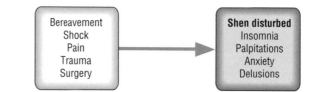

As a rough guide, if it is difficult to fall asleep, but once asleep the pattern is normal, this is probably a Blood Xu pattern. If the patient wakes often during the night, feeling hot, this is a form of Yin Xu. If palpitations or even panic attacks wake the patient, this is a sign of Heart and Kidney Xu. Recurring frightening and vivid dreams indicate the involvement of both the Heart and the Gall Bladder. If the Gall Bladder is also implicated, this may indicate a timid personality type easily disturbed by relatively trivial events, a classic 'worrier'.

Treatment with acupuncture is likely to be successful if the deficiencies are addressed (Case study 12.1). Many patients with chronic insomnia will be taking some sort of sedative and they need to be weaned slowly off these drugs. No treatment of this type should be attempted without consulting the patient's doctor. Relaxation techniques can be helpful if used in conjunction with acupuncture treatment.

CASE HISTORY

Case study 12.1

Retired teacher, aged 74 years. Suffering from insomnia. Able to go to sleep but has vivid dreams that often wake him. Worried by heart palpitations. Thinks he is losing his memory. Poor appetite and no enthusiasm for his hobbies, which include bowls.

Suffers from blocked sinuses, dull head pain. Pale tongue, thin coating, weak pulse.

Impression: a mix of Heart and Spleen Qi Xu.

Treatment 1
Points:

- Ht 7 Shenmen – calms Heart
- Ht 9 Shaochong – tonifies Heart and Blood
- LI 4 Hegu – calming, head pain
- Sp 3 Taibai – Source point for Spleen
- Sp 6 Sanyinjiao, St 36 Zusanli – boost and nourish Qi and Blood.

Treatment 2
Improved, willing to lie prone while Back Shu points are needled:

- UB 15 Xinshu
- UB 20 Pishu
- UB 21 Weishu
- UB 23 Shenshu.

No other treatment was given.

Treatments 3–8
Points as above, alternating treatments.

Patient says he feels much improved: 'head is clearer'. Now sleeping much better. Has started bowling again, twice a week. In his own words: 'It's so good to know that I don't have to feel run down and miserable because I'm old'.

Benefits of TCM

The intention in this chapter is not to paint a universally gloomy picture of old age, but to emphasize that here the TCM philosophy of the interconnectedness of all things becomes very clear. Most people survive quite well even with these complex health pictures, often experiencing only occasional discomfort or upset. Unfortunately orthodox medicine tends to collude with the patient, transmitting the message that all these problems are a natural result of old age and must just be tolerated. It seems from an evening of television viewing or reading a popular magazine that all old people are expected to be forgetful, to suffer from ill-defined aches and pains, to have difficulty getting around, to be depressed and confused by the pace of life and by new inventions such as computers.

TCM takes a different view, identifying the imbalances in detail so that some attempt can be made to rectify them. Many patients respond to acupuncture treatment with comments such as: 'I'm not sure I'm better, but I feel better about it'. Researchers have suggested that the calming, tranquillizing effect of acupuncture is a response to the regulation of metabolism of serotonin, noradrenaline, adenosine triphosphate, acetylcholine and other neurotransmitters, as well as its ability to alter brain potentials (Shi & Tan 1986). The acupuncture 'Valium' – the use of the Four Gates, Liv 3 Taichong and LI 4 Hegu – can also do wonders for the mood and tranquillity of a distressed or anxious patient. It is, however, worth bearing in mind that acupuncture is far from a miracle cure: a naturally gloomy person will stay gloomy.

Where the problems are relatively superficial, as in the initial invasions of Pathogens in the Bi syndrome, the stuck energies in the joints can be released with acupuncture and much unnecessary pain relieved. Treatments aimed at improving the digestive process will have a far-reaching effect, enabling a more efficient metabolism and helping to prevent dietary deficiencies leading to mature-onset diabetes. If nothing else, they will prevent a great deal of money being wasted on over-the-counter 'remedies'.

Finally, there may be insurmountable residential or neighbourhood problems. Distances that were previously no problem become difficult due to decreasing mobility; there may be a loss of driving ability, local transport may be unreliable and neighbours may unwilling to help or non-existent.

Acupuncture is not able to cure any of the above, unfortunately, but if the physiological problems are recognized then the quality of life may at least be improved. That said, a good combination of points for depression is given in Table 12.2.

Application to physiotherapy

It is not necessary to have a deep knowledge of TCM in order to give helpful acupuncture to elderly patients, but careful observation of the ageing process and the knowledge and humanity evident in the structure of the TCM diagnostic framework will be helpful when formulating treatments. It is in this field that the traditional ideas really begin to make sense.

Certainly, the treatment of pain, most often manifesting in a variation of Bi syndrome, will be helpful to these patients. A small addition of points, perhaps St 36 Zusanli and Sp 6 for 'indigestion' or Kid 3 or Liv 3 for more serious evidence of deficiency, could have a useful prophylactic effect.

Table 12.2 Acupuncture points for depression

Point	Comments
Pe 6 Neiguan	Apprehension, fear, fright, sadness
Ht 7 Shenmen	Fear and fright. Calms the spirit
Sp 6 Sanyinjiao	Calms the spirit. Insomnia due to Heart and Spleen Qi Xu
Liv 3 Taichong	Clears the head and eyes. Activates Qi and Blood throughout the body
St 40 Fenglong	Clears Phlegm from the Heart and calms the spirit. Manic depression
St 36 Zusanli	Calms the spirit. Insomnia due to Heart and Spleen Qi Xu
Ren 12 Zhongwan	Harmonizes the middle Jiao. Eliminates Phlegm Wind

The philosophical tradition of Chinese geriatrics contains a strong preventive element, closely tied to the concept a balanced body–mind relationship. A sound mind in a sound body is a prerequisite for longevity. Moderation in both physical and emotional activities is recommended. Tai Chi or Qi Gong combinations of gentle exercise, relaxation, breathing and meditation are believed to be helpful in promoting longevity. Certainly these two activities can be practised by anybody, no matter how physically unfit. For a good clear guide to Chi Kung (Qi Gong) with plenty of helpful photographs, McKenzie (1999) is worth reading.

Research

There have been some studies on the effect of acupuncture on ageing, but most of these have been performed on animals, chiefly senescence-accelerated mice. Neurons in the neocortex of these animals have been shown to undergo accelerated atrophy, resulting in significant age-related deterioration in learning and memory; consequently these animals are used as a model to study ageing and dementia.

A study undertaken by Shi et al (1998) looked at the relationship between brain atrophy and the possible therapeutic effects of acupuncture in this type of mouse. Apoptosis is the term describing a form of programmed or physiological cell death that is expected to occur as part of the normal ageing process. Shi et al found that mice treated with acupuncture experienced a significantly lower incidence of apoptosis or cell death in specific cerebral areas than the control group that received no treatment. The points used were Pe 6 Neiguan and Liv 3 Taichong, both used bilaterally, together with Du 26 Renzhong. They further found that mice treated at non-acupuncture points showed no observable effect when the brain tissues were examined. Regulation of apoptosis is thought to have possible practical applications in gerontology. While these results are interesting, and perhaps provide some evidence for changes occurring in the brain tissue after acupuncture, it must be accepted that this stimulus would be fairly major for something as tiny as a mouse, and the findings may not be directly generalizable to humans.

Although the research jury is still out on most of the applications of acupuncture suggested in this chapter, the problem with damage caused by the routine prescription of NSAIDs continues to grow. One conservative estimate suggests that about 2000 deaths per year in the UK are due to gastroduodenal complications after taking NSAIDs for at least 2 months (Tramer et al 2000). The side-effects of acupuncture are mostly benign; serious adverse events are very rare. Two major safety studies conducted in the UK with a total of 63 000 acupuncture treatments between them made this very clear (MacPherson et al 2001, White et al 2001).

There is considerable scope for research into the economics of acupuncture treatment costed against the rising drug bills. Physiotherapists, already employed widely by the National Health Service with this patient group, treating pain and associated problems of old age on a regular basis, should have their service evaluated in comparison to the costs of NSAIDs with regard to both economy and morbidity.

References

MacPherson H, Thomas K, Walters S, Fitter M 2001 The York acupuncture safety study: prospective survey of 34 000 treatments by traditional acupuncturists. British Medical Journal 323: 486–487.

McKenzie E 1999 Chi Kung, cultivating personal energy. London: Hamlyn/Octopus.

Shi X, Wang S, Kiu Q et al 1998 Brain atrophy and ageing: research on the effect of acupuncture on neuronal apoptosis in cortical tissue. American Journal of Acupuncture 26: 251–254.

Shi Z, Tan M 1986 An analysis of the therapeutic effect of acupuncture treatment in 500 cases of schizophrenia. Journal of Traditional Chinese Medicine 6: 99–104.

Tramer MR, Moore RA, Reynolds JM, McQuay HJ 2000 Quantitative estimation of rare adverse events which follow a biological progression: a new model applied to chronic NSAID use. Pain 85: 169–182.

White A, Hayhoe S, Hart A, Ernst E 2001 Adverse events following acupuncture: prospective survey of 32 000 consultations with doctors and physiotherapists. British Medical Journal 323: 485–486.

Yan D 2000 Ageing and blood stasis. 2nd edn. Boulder, CO: Blue Poppy Press.

Further reading

A problem with acupuncture texts, with the possible exception of this one, is that they tend to be polarized (i.e. written either from a TCM or from a 'scientific / modern' point of view). One of my aims has been to encourage further reading, but in order to direct the reader the lists need to be categorized.

The following books are recommended for their comprehensive cover of the theory of Traditional Chinese Medicine, not exclusively acupuncture but always including some suggestions for points:

- Maciocia G 1989 The foundations of Chinese Medicine. Edinburgh: Churchill Livingstone.
- Maclean W, Lyttleton J 1998 Clinical handbook of internal medicine, vol 1: Lung, Kidney, Liver, Heart. Campbeltown, New South Wales: University of Western Sydney.
- Maclean W, Lyttleton J 2002 Clinical handbook of internal medicine, vol 2: Spleen and Stomach. Penrith South DC, New South Wales: University of Western Sydney.

For a complete list and description of all the acupuncture points – probably containing more information than is strictly necessary, but utterly fascinating – see:

- Deadman P, Al-Khafaji, Baker K 1998 A manual of acupuncture. Hove: Journal of Chinese Medicine Publications.

The following books give an overview of some of the research into how acupuncture actually works:

- Ernst E, White A, eds 1999 Acupuncture, a scientific appraisal. Oxford: Butterworth Heinemann.
- Filshie J, White A 1998 Medical acupuncture. Edinburgh: Churchill Livingstone.
- Litscher G, Cho ZH, eds 2000 Computer-controlled acupuncture. Lengerich: Pabst Science.
- Stux G, Hammerschlag R, eds 2001 Clinical acupuncture: scientific basis. Berlin: Springer.

These books are interesting as background reading, giving a historical perspective and offering new ideas for extending and enriching basic treatments:

- Birch S, Felt R 1999 Understanding acupuncture. Edinburgh: Churchill Livingstone.

- Chen J, Wang N 1988 Acupuncture case histories from China. Seattle: Eastland Press.
- de Schepper L 1995 Acupuncture in practice. Santa Fe, New Mexico: Full of Life Publishing.
- Kaptchuk T 1983 Chinese Medicine: the web that has no weaver. London: Rider.
- MacPherson H, Kaptchuk T, eds 1997 Acupuncture in practice: case history insights from the West. Edinburgh: Churchill Livingstone.

The following books are particularly useful to physiotherapists, combining an appreciation of the typical caseload with useful theory:

- Baldry PE 1989 Acupuncture, trigger points and musculoskeletal pain. Edinburgh: Churchill Livingstone.
- Pirog JE 1996 The practical application of meridian style acupuncture. Berkeley, California: Pacific View Press.

Finally, some books giving an eccentric but interesting view:

- Campbell A 2003 Acupuncture in practice: beyond points and meridians. Oxford: Butterworth-Heinemann.
- Mann F 1992 Re-inventing acupuncture: a new concept of Ancient Medicine. Oxford: Butterworth-Heinemann.
- Scheid V 2002 Chinese Medicine in contemporary China: plurality and synthesis. Durham: Duke University Press.

Symptom check

The table below offers syndrome or Eight Principle suggestions for a common collection of symptoms. This is not meant to be a complete diagnosis but simply an indication of where a practitioner beginning to think in TCM terms should start. Looking up several symptoms will often produce conflicting ideas, but the final decision as to what is most important to the internal balance of the patient – and most urgently in need of treatment – lies with the practitioner.

Symptoms	TCM	Comments
Appetite		
Poor	Spleen Qi Xu	Intestinal stasis
Always hungry	Stomach Fire	
Hungry but unable to eat	Retention of Phlegm Fire	
Prefers hot food	Internal Cold	
Prefers cold food	Internal Heat	
Constipation		
Dry stools	Spleen Qi Xu or Liver stagnation	
With shortness of breath	Qi Xu	
Night sweats, dry mouth	Yin or Blood Xu	
Mild	Full Heat, Yin Xu	
Severe with other Heat signs	Collapse of Yin	
Diarrhoea		
Foul smell	Heat	
No smell	Cold	
Early morning	Kidney Yang Xu	
Chronic diarrhoea	Kidney or Spleen Yang Xu	
Undigested food	Spleen Yang Xu	
After eating	Stomach or Spleen Xu	
Mucus in stools	Damp in Intestines	
Alternating with constipation	Liver invades Spleen	
Occult Blood in stool	Blood stagnation	
Dizziness		
Slight, gradual onset	Deficiency	
Severe, sudden onset	Excess	
Hazy vision, worse when tired	Blood or Qi Xu	
Slight, foggy head	Damp	
Loses balance	Liver Yang rising, internal Wind	

Continues

Symptoms	TCM	Comments
Eyes		
Black shadow underneath	Kidney Xu	
Swelling underneath	Kidney Xu	
Twitching	Liver	
Glitter	Spirit	
False glitter	Yin Xu	
Dry eyes, failing vision	Blood, Yin, Kidney, Liver Xu	
Blurred, floaters	Liver Blood Xu	
Red, irritated	Liver Fire, Wind Heat	
Flatulence		
General	Liver Qi stagnation	
With foul smell	Damp Heat in Spleen and Stomach	
No smell	Spleen Yang Xu	
Gastrointestinal		
General discomfort	Spleen Xu or Damp	
Better after food	Deficiency	
Worse after food	Excess	
Worse with bowel movement	Deficiency	
Better after bowel movement	Excess	
Dull pain	Deficiency	
Severe pain	Excess	
Painful, distended, lumpy feeling	Retention of food	
Headaches		
Slight	Deficiency	
Severe	Excess	
Chronic	General internal imbalance	
Sudden onset, short duration	External Pathogen	
Worse with activity, better with rest	Qi Xu	
Aversion to Wind and/or Cold	External invasion	
Forehead	Stomach or Blood Xu	
Temple or side of head	Wind Cold, Wind Heat, or Liver or Gall Bladder syndrome	
Vertex	Blood Xu or Liver Yang rising	
Whole head	Wind Cold	
Heavy feeling	Damp	
Empty head	Kidney Xu	
Stabbing, boring	Blood stagnation	
Throbbing	Liver Yang rising	
Daytime	Qi or Yang Xu	
Evening	Yin or Blood Xu	
Incontinence		
Incontinence	Kidney Xu	
Dribbling urine	Kidney Xu	

Continues

Symptoms	TCM	Comments
Insomnia		
Difficulty falling asleep	Heart Blood Xu	
Waking at night	Heart or Kidney Yin Xu	
Dream disturbed	Heart or Liver Fire	
Waking then unable to get back to sleep	Gall Bladder Xu	
Itching		
General	Damp Heat in the Blood	
Jaundice		
General	Dampness depressing Spleen and Liver	
Lips		
Dry with cracks	Spleen and Stomach Heat	
Red	Heat	
Pale	Yang or Blood Xu	
Purple	Blood stasis	
Menopause		
Hot flushes	Kidney or Liver Yin Xu, Kidney Yin and Yang Xu, Liver Yang rising	
Menstruation		
Long cycle, pale scanty flow	Deficiency or Cold	
Short cycle, heavy flow	Excess or Heat	
Irregular	Liver Qi Xu, Spleen Xu, Blood stasis	
Clots, purplish blood	Blood stasis, Cold	
Thin, scanty, light in colour	Blood Xu	
Heavy loss	Heat in Blood	Spleen not controlling
Mouth		
Cold sores	Stomach Yin Xu or Damp	
Spots	Damp Heat	
Movement		
Restless, excess	Yin Xu or Heat	
Bradykinesia (lack)	Yang Xu or Cold	
Tremor, twitch	Wind	
Heavy and slow	Damp	
Heavy, forceful	Liver Shi	
Nausea		
In pregnancy	Stomach Xu	Chong Mai Xu
Nose		
Red	Lung or Stomach Heat	
White	Qi Xu	
Yellow	Damp Heat	
Flared nostrils	Heat in Lung	

Continues

Symptoms	TCM	Comments
Numbness		
Extremities	Blood Xu	
Upper limb only	Phlegm Wind, neck problems	
Pain		
Better with pressure	Deficiency	
Worse with pressure	Excess	
Intermittent, chronic	Deficiency	
Persistent, acute	Excess	
Mobile	Qi stagnation or Wind	
Hollow pain	Blood Xu in vessels	
Pricking	Blood stagnation	
Sharp and stabbing	Blood stagnation	
Heavy sensation	Damp	
Distended feeling	Qi stagnation	
Burning pain	Heat	(Also false Heat – Yin Xu)
Cold biting pain	Cold	Obstructing meridians or organs
Pain in menstruation		
Pain before period	Qi or Blood stagnation	
Pain during period	Qi or Blood stasis, Cold	
Pain after period	Blood Xu	
Perspiration		
Chronic night sweats	Yin Xu	
Daytime sweats	Qi or Yang Xu	
Oily on forehead	Collapse of Yang	
`Five palm sweat'	Yin Xu	
Profuse, listless, cold limbs	Collapse of Yang	
Hands	Lung Qi Xu	
Head only	Stomach Heat or Damp Heat	
Postnatal depression		
General	Heart Blood or Blood Xu	
Posture		
Robust	Excess	Not necessarily pathogenic
Weak	Deficiency	
Thin	Blood or Yin Xu	
Very wasted	Jing Xu	
Heavy set	Phlegm or Damp	
Overweight	Qi or Yang Xu, Damp	
Skin colour		
Pale yellow	Blood Xu	
Dull, white	Blood Xu	
Red	Heat or Empty Heat	Fire element disturbed
Yellow	Spleen Xu or Damp	Earth element disturbed
Blue-green	Liver Qi stasis or Wind	Wood element disturbed
Blue-black	Kidney Xu or Blood stasis	

Continues

Symptoms	TCM	Comments
Skin texture		
Dry	Yin or Blood Xu	
Greasy	Damp or Phlegm	
Red spots	Heat or Excess	
Oozing spots	Damp or Phlegm	
Flaky	Blood or Yin Xu, Phlegm	
Oedema	Damp	Excess Body fluids
Cellulite	Spleen Qi Xu	
Taste		
Loss of	Spleen and Stomach Xu	
Tinnitus		
Sudden onset	Liver Fire, Liver Wind, Phlegm Damp	
Gradual onset	Kidney Xu	
Worse with pressure	Excess	
Eased with pressure	Deficiency	
Sounds like running water	Kidney Xu	
High whistle	Liver Yang or Fire, Wind	
Urine		
Strong smell	Heat	
No smell	Cold	
Pain before urination	Qi stagnation in lower Jiao	
Pain during urination	Heat in Bladder	
Pain after urination	Qi Xu	
Retention	Damp Heat in Bladder	
Pale and abundant	Kidney Yang Xu, Cold	
Yellow and scanty	Kidney Yin Xu, Heat	
Cloudy, turbid	Damp	
Red	Heat	
Vaginal discharges		
White, watery, profuse	Cold or Deficiency	
Thick, yellow with odour	Heat or Excess	
Green	Damp Heat in Liver meridian	
Yellow and bloody after menopause	Toxic Damp Heat in uterus	
Vomit		
Vomiting	Rebellious Stomach Qi	
Noisy	Excess	
After eating	Heat	
Sour	Liver invades Stomach	
Bitter	Heat in Liver and Gall Bladder	Causing fluid retention in Stomach
Clear vomit	Cold	

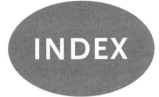

INDEX

Note: Page numbers followed by 'f' or 't' indicate figures or tables/boxed material respectively. Please also note that as the subject of this book all entries refer to acupuncture unless otherwise stated.